"Dr. Harmony Robinson-Stagg has created an excellent and integral approach of Ayurvedic treatments and protocols. This path allows for the true unfolding of the inner harmony in the form of ojas, tejas, and prana to support longevity of life. This is a masterpiece work for both the student and the healer."
—Dr Vasant Lad, BAM&S, MASc, Founder of The Ayurvedic Institute

"Dr. Harmony Robinson-Stagg brings heartfelt sincerity, dedication, and a rich blend of experience in Eastern and Western healing traditions to this book. I deeply appreciate her commitment to supporting women through the powerful transitions of life with compassion and care."
—Dr. Claudia Welch, author of *Balance Your Hormones, Balance Your Life*

"Harmony is an incredible cheerleader whose medical background and metaphysical knowledge perfectly position her in the healing space."
—Keryn Clark

"When you choose to work with Harmony, you'll get the whole package, a holistic health practitioner that goes above and beyond in order to support clients on their journey to better health and well-being."
—Jordis Wilsdorf

"I will use Harmony time and time again for the moments in my life when I need some clarity or guidance. Her ability to use her knowledge and wisdom in both Western and Eastern medicine, philosophy and psychology to help with physical and emotional situations is a skill not many people have. HIGHLY recommend, any day of the week!"
—Anna Veale

SHAKTI
Publications

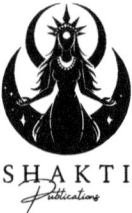

Published in Australia by
Shakti Publications
Gold Coast Australia
inspire@harmonyinspired.com.au
www.harmonyinspiredhealth.com.au

First published in Australia 2025
Copyright ©Harmony Robinson-Stagg 2025

National Library of Australia Cataloguing in Publication entry

ISBN: 978-1-7640317-0-7 (paperback)
ISBN: 978-1-7640317-2-1 (hardcover)
ISBN: 978-1-7640317-1-4 (epub)

Cover photography by Mario Colli
Cover layout and design by Neat Designs
Printed by IngramSpark

Ayurveda and the Alchemy of HER

The **Revolutionary Guide** to Women's Health, Balancing Hormones, Finding Purpose, and **Becoming Your higHERself™**

DR. HARMONY ROBINSON-STAGG

*To all the women in my life—my mother,
my mother-in-law, my grandmothers, my friends, and
my mentors—who have shaped me with their wisdom,
strength, and grace.*

*To my clients and students, the women who show up for
themselves, who ask the deep questions, who are willing
to unlearn, heal, and rise: you are the reason this work
exists. Your journeys inspire me every day, and it is my
greatest honor to walk this path with you.*

*This book is for you—the seekers, the healers,
the cycle-breakers, and the changemakers.
May you reclaim your power, honor your rhythms,
and step fully into your higHERself.*

*With love,
Dr. Harmony Robinson-Stagg*

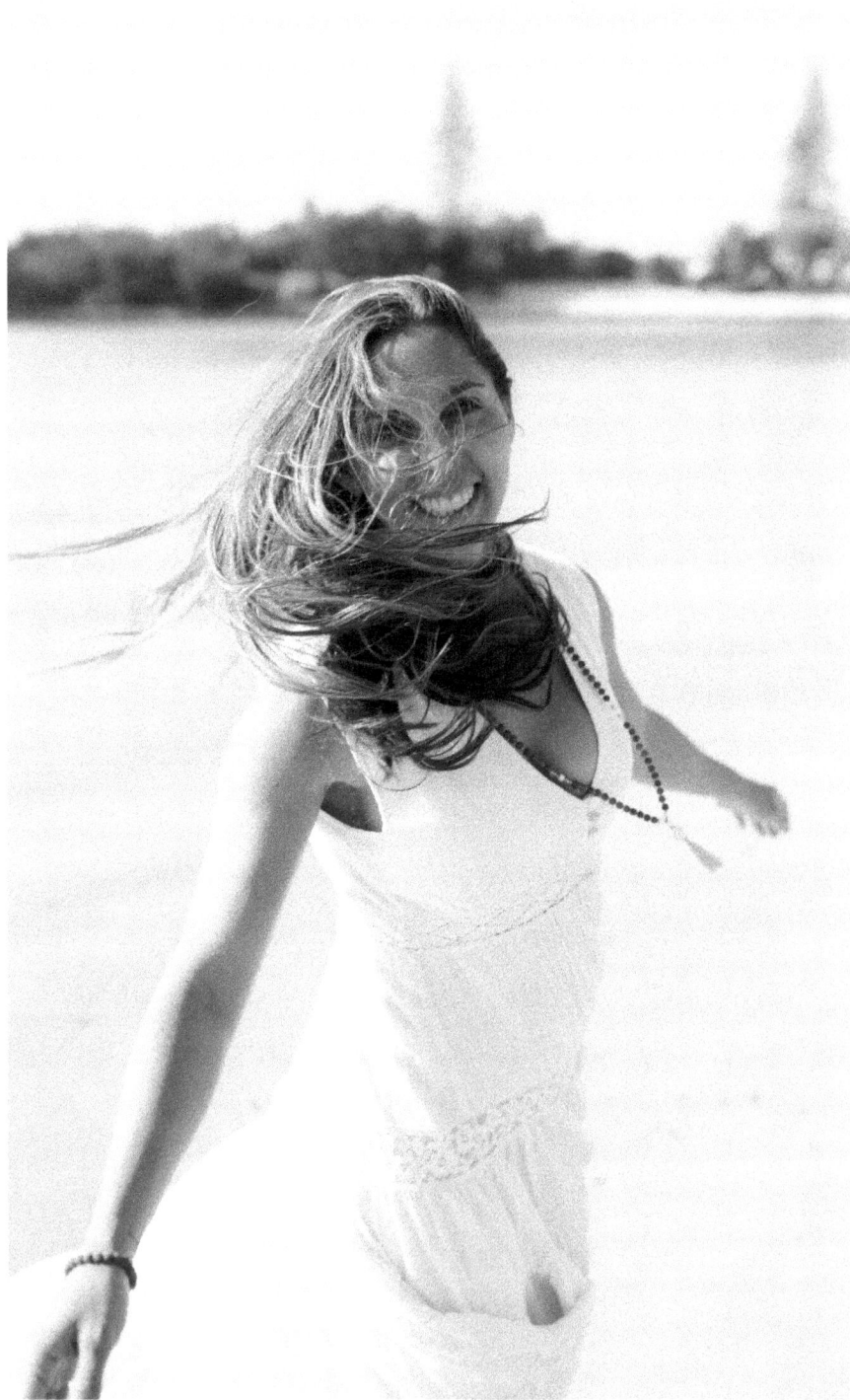

About the Author

Harmony Robinson-Stagg is a doctor of Traditional Chinese Medicine, Ayurvedic practitioner, registered nurse, and the founder and lead educator of the Ayurveda Alchemist Academy—a premier Ayurveda education school offering certifications in Ayurvedic holistic health coaching, Vedic breathwork, and Ayurvedic massage and bodywork. Dedicated to helping women reclaim their health, balance their hormones, and step into their highest expression—their higHERself™—she seamlessly integrates ancient healing wisdom with modern science.

With decades of experience in integrative health, Dr. Harmony has guided thousands of women through midlife transitions, hormonal imbalances, and deep inner transformation. Her own journey from an emergency nurse to a leader in Eastern medicine has given her firsthand insight into the physical, emotional, and spiritual challenges women face. She is passionate about bridging the gap between Ayurveda, Eastern Medicine, and modern wellness, empowering women to take control of their health and embrace their true potential.

As the visionary behind the Ayurveda Alchemist Academy, she has cultivated a community of healers and practitioners, equipping them with the knowledge and tools to create profound change in their lives and the lives of others. When not teaching, writing, or leading retreats, you'll find Dr. Harmony by the sea, hiking through nature, traveling to immerse herself in new cultures, or flowing through yoga and Pilates. She also cherishes weekends at her son's soccer games, chai in hand, and being fully present in the moments that matter most.

Her mission is clear: guide women in alchemizing their health, mind, and dharma, empowering them to rise into their higHERself™.

Contents

Introduction

There comes a point in a woman's life when the familiar paths no longer lead to the destinations they once promised. The map you've been following, drawn by society's expectations and sometimes even yourself, becomes outdated. You stand at a crossroads where the old ways no longer serve, but new terrain feels uncertain. This is not a crisis, but an awakening. A call to reclaim the essence of who you are beneath the roles, the hormones, the expectations—this is the remembrance of your higHERself™.

What once made sense now feels constraining, and the question arises: Who am I beyond my roles, beyond my past, beyond the identity I've built?

For me, this moment came after the birth of my twin boys. As a nurse and health practitioner, I had spent years studying the human body, yet nothing prepared me for the deep hormonal shifts, anxiety, and loss of identity I experienced postpartum. I felt disconnected from my body, my purpose, and even from myself. The Western medical system I had devoted nearly two decades to offered me solutions that only scratched the surface—symptom management but no true healing. It wasn't until I discovered Ayurveda that everything changed.

Ayurveda became my anchor. It helped me navigate my hormonal imbalances with clarity, understand the intricate relationship between my mind and body, and most importantly, it redefined the way I saw myself. It wasn't merely about balancing my hormones; it was about lifting the veil that had clouded my vision. Through Ayurveda, I saw myself clearly for the first time, not as a collection of symptoms or societal labels but as a woman with profound inner wisdom, an innate rhythm, and the ability to shape my own reality. It gave me a sense of connection, belonging, and understanding I had never experienced.

Once I experienced this transformation, I began to witness it in others. The women who came to see me for hormonal symptoms, stress, or digestive issues weren't just seeking physical healing; they were searching for themselves. Beneath their health struggles, there was a deeper longing for alignment, for purpose, for methods to navigate womanhood that felt empowering rather than depleting.

This book was born from that realization.

Why This Book? Why Now?

I'm Dr. Harmony Robinson-Stagg, DAC, DTCM, RN, and my life's work has been to guide women back to their bodily wisdom and clear purpose. As a doctor of Chinese medicine, an Ayurveda and women's health practitioner, and a registered nurse, I have been exploring the interplay between ancient traditions and modern health science since 2002.

Through two decades in the Western medical system, I witnessed firsthand the gaps in women's healthcare, the focus on treating symptoms rather than addressing root causes. It wasn't until I discovered Ayurveda that I truly understood the depth of healing available. Ayurveda taught me what my medical training never did: how to align with the body's natural intelligence, how to navigate hormonal transitions with grace, and how to cultivate a mindset capable of transformation.

The alchemy of a woman's health is not simply managing symptoms—it is mastery of the self. It is understanding that your mind, body, and dharma are deeply interconnected and true well-being comes from honoring all aspects of who you are.

This is not simply another wellness book. It is an invitation to explore the profound intelligence of your body, the depths of your mind, and the limitless potential of your purpose. This book is not about fixing you, because you are not broken. It is about guiding you back to yourself, equipping you with tools to navigate womanhood with clarity, vitality, and empowerment.

Ayurveda and Eastern medicine have long recognized that a woman's life is cyclical, evolving through phases that require different forms of nourishment, care, and introspection. Yet in modern society, our fifties, forties, and even our mid-thirties are often framed as a time of decline rather than a time of expansion. The truth is this is the most powerful chapter of your life. You are not fading—you are evolving. When you understand the rhythms of your body, the psychology of your mind, and the truth of your dharma, you can step into this phase with strength, wisdom, and purpose.

What You'll Gain from This Book

The higHERself™ Method is not a rigid set of rules; it is a map back to your true and authentic self. This book is structured to guide you through the four pillars of transformation:

HEALTH ALCHEMY: YOUR BODY IS YOUR FOUNDATION

We will explore how Ayurveda can help you balance hormones, optimize digestion, maintain a healthy weight and align with your body's natural intelligence. You will understand why perimenopause, menopause, and other transitions are not "medical conditions" to be feared but sacred rites of passage to be honored.

Health alchemy is not merely about your physical health; it's about alchemizing your physical, mental, emotional, spiritual, and dharmic health in alignment with your individual mind-body constitution (your Ayurvedic *dosha*).

EMPOWERED MIND PARADIGM: YOUR THOUGHTS SHAPE YOUR REALITY

We dive deep into Ayurvedic psychology, the power of neuroplasticity, and the tools to rewrite limiting beliefs. You will learn how your dosha influences your mindset and how to cultivate mental resilience for lasting transformation.

DHARMIC IMPACT: YOU ARE HERE FOR A REASON

This section guides you through discovering your unique gifts and aligning with your higher purpose. Whether you are shifting careers, stepping into a new phase of womanhood, or seeking deeper meaning in your daily life, you will gain clarity on how to live in alignment with your dharma.

ALCHEMY IN ACTION: KNOWLEDGE MEANS NOTHING WITHOUT INTEGRATION

This book is filled with actionable tools—rituals, meditations, Ayurvedic self-care practices, and real-life case studies of women who have transformed their lives through this wisdom.

This book is not only for personal health seekers, but it also acts as a guide for health and wellness professionals who want to understand their clients better so they create greater impact and meaningful transformations for their clients.

This book is for you if

✦ you feel disconnected from your body and want to reclaim your vitality

✦ you are navigating hormonal shifts and want a holistic approach to balance

✦ you struggle with self-doubt, limiting beliefs, or an anxious mind

✦ you feel a quiet longing for something more but aren't sure what

✦ you want to align with your purpose and make an impact that feels meaningful

Wherever you are on your path, know you are not alone. There is wisdom within you waiting to be unlocked, and this book will be your guide.

This is your time. Your evolution. Your reclamation.

Welcome to *Ayurveda and the Alchemy of HER*.

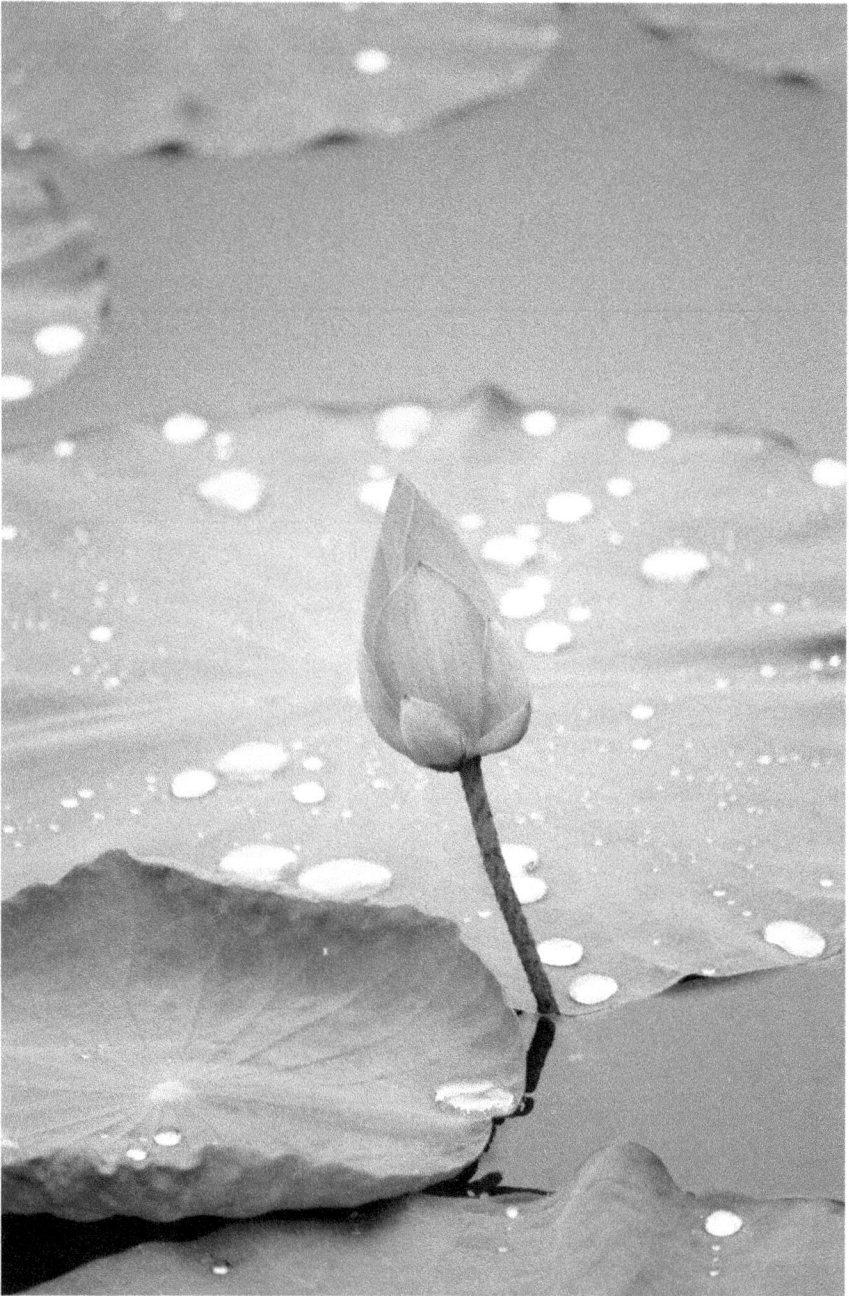

"AND THE DAY CAME WHEN THE RISK TO REMAIN TIGHT IN A
BUD WAS MORE PAINFUL THAN THE RISK IT TOOK TO BLOSSOM."
– ANAÏS NIN

PART 1

Reclaiming HER

Before transformation, there is remembrance

Reclaiming HER is about coming home to your authentic self. It is the foundation of the higHERself™ journey, rooted in ancient wisdom, lived experience, and the soul's quiet knowing that you are more than the roles you've played or the identities assigned to you.

Through the lens of Ayurveda, Vedic astrology, and personal storytelling, this section invites you to explore the original blueprint of your being—your *Prakriti*—and the cosmic energies that shape your emotional, mental, and physical nature. It's about understanding your innate strengths and reclaiming parts of yourself that may have been lost or hidden.

You'll meet the Vedic goddesses as archetypes of your feminine power, and you'll be invited to reflect on the beliefs, roles, and stories you've inherited so you can decide which to carry forward and which to release.

This is a sacred return.

A return to your inner wisdom.

A return to your wild wholeness.

A return to the woman you were always meant to be.

Let this part of the journey anchor you in self-awareness, deepen your connection to your purpose, and awaken the truth that your identity is not something to be found—it is something to be reclaimed.

CHAPTER 1

Written in the Stars

You stand at the threshold of a new chapter, finally ready to uncover the depth of what has always been within you. The alchemy of womanhood is not in resisting change but in mastering it. It is my hope that this book will not only guide you toward optimal health but also serve as a touchstone for the journey of becoming, so that you may walk through life with clarity, wisdom, and purpose.

This is not the end of who you were, it is the beginning of who you are becoming. Let us begin.

What is Ayurveda?

The word *Ayurveda* comes from Sanskrit: *Ayus* meaning "life," and *Veda* meaning "knowledge" or "science." Together, it translates to "the science of life," a system of health that extends far beyond treating illness, aiming instead to cultivate balance across the physical, mental, emotional, and spiritual layers of a human being.

Developed more than five thousand years ago in India, Ayurveda is an ancient medical system. Its foundation rests on understanding that health is not simply the absence of disease but the dynamic equilibrium of body, mind, and spirit working in rhythm with nature's laws. Every individual is seen as unique, and therefore, Ayurveda focuses on personalized approaches to diet, lifestyle, preventative medicine, and therapeutic intervention based on a

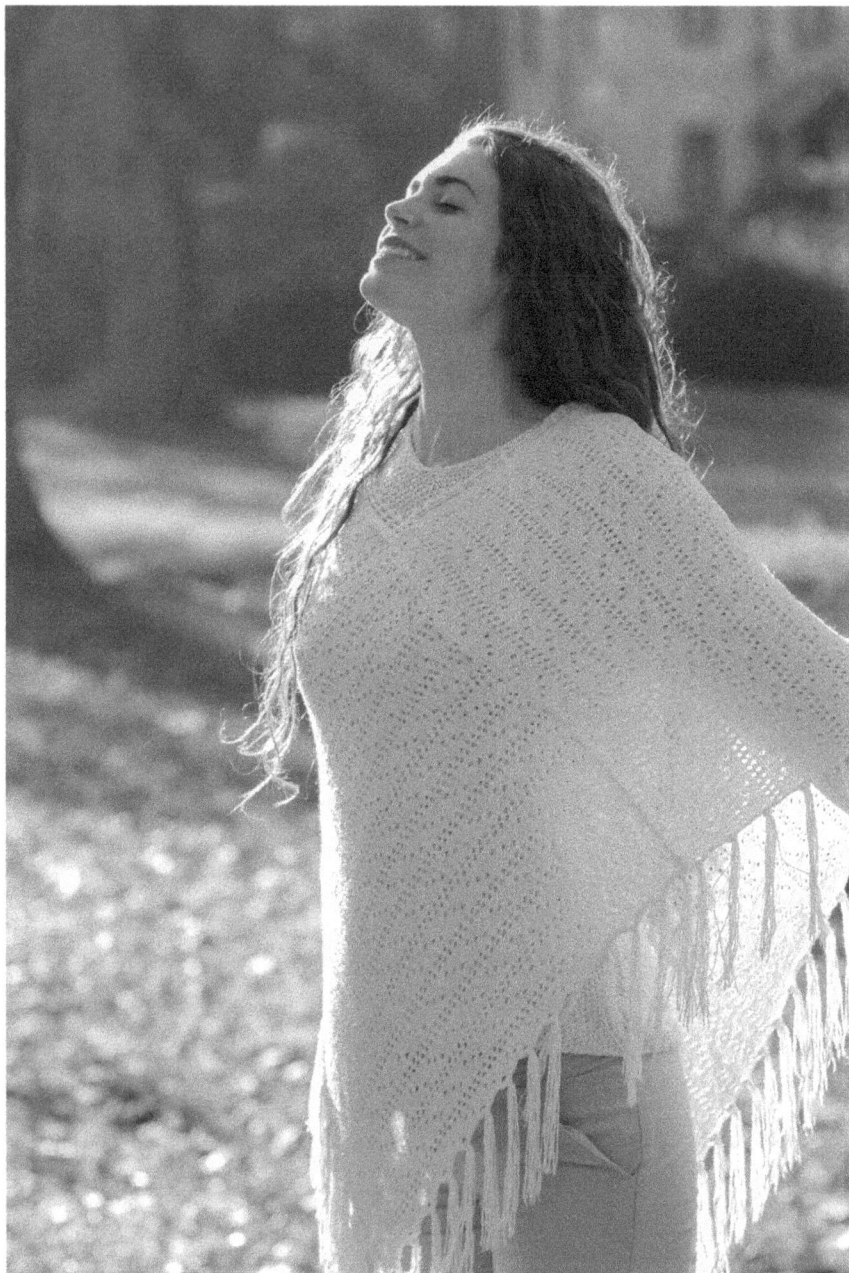

"A WOMAN IN HARMONY WITH HER SPIRIT IS LIKE A RIVER FLOWING. SHE GOES WHERE SHE WILL WITHOUT PRETENSE AND ARRIVES AT HER DESTINATION PREPARED TO BE HERSELF AND ONLY HERSELF." – MAYA ANGELOU

person's unique constitution and innate state of being (*Prakriti*), current imbalances (*Vikriti*), and environment.

In Ayurveda, health is achieved by balancing the three biological energies—*Vata*, *Pitta*, and *Kapha*—and supporting the body's natural digestive fire (*Agni*), detoxification pathways, and mental clarity. It recognises that emotional resilience, spiritual connection, and physical vitality are inseparable parts of true well-being.

Prakriti and Your Celestial Design

"Who am I, really?" This question has a way of surfacing in our lives during moments of change, growth, or challenge. For years, I sought answers in various paths of self-development, psychology, and personality typing, but it wasn't until I turned to Ayurveda and Vedic astrology that I began to understand my unique blueprint— the essence of who I am. This blueprint, known as Prakriti, is not limited to physical health. It's a cosmic map of your physical, emotional, and spiritual nature, shaped at the moment of your birth.

Understanding Prakriti: Your Unique Constitution

In Ayurveda, your Prakriti is your innate constitution, the unique combination of the three doshas Vata, Pitta, and Kapha, which is determined at the moment of your conception. It reflects your natural balance of the five elements (ether, air, fire, water, and earth), shaping everything from your physical structure to your mental and emotional tendencies. Prakriti is determined by a beautiful and complex interplay of factors: your parents' doshic balance at conception; your mother's health, emotions, and nutrition during pregnancy; the environment and season of your birth; and even deeper karmic influences. This is why even twins can have entirely different constitutions.

Unlike temporary imbalances (Vikriti), your Prakriti is unchanging and serves as a blueprint for how your body and mind are designed to function optimally.

How Ayurveda Determines Prakriti

Ayurvedic practitioners use several tools to identify your Prakriti, combining observations, palpation, detailed questionnaires, vedic astrology and pulse diagnosis.

+ **Physical characteristics**

  ✧ Body frame, skin type, hair texture, and facial features all offer clues about your dominant dosha.

  ✧ For example, a light, thin frame may suggest a Vata dominance, while a more muscular build may indicate Pitta, and a solid, sturdy frame suggests Kapha.

+ **Mental and emotional traits**

  ✧ Your natural tendencies in decision-making, creativity, and emotional expression are analyzed.

  ✧ A Vata-dominant mind may be highly creative but prone to overthinking. Pitta individuals are often focused and driven, and Kapha types tend to be calm and nurturing but can struggle with inertia.

+ **Digestion and energy levels**

  ✧ How you process food, experience hunger, and maintain energy is another key indicator.

  ✧ A Vata person may have irregular digestion, Pitta tends toward strong hunger and quick digestion, and Kapha digestion is slower but steady.

+ **Lifestyle preferences**
  - ✧ Your preferred climate, sleeping patterns, and even your reaction to stress provide insights into your dosha balance.

By analyzing these patterns, Ayurveda determines your Prakriti as a unique combination of one dominant dosha (single-dosha constitution), two primary doshas (dual-dosha constitution), or in rare cases, equal influence of all three doshas (tri-dosha constitution).

Recognising Your Own Prakriti

While working with an Ayurvedic practitioner is the most accurate way to determine your Prakriti, you can begin to recognize your natural tendencies by reflecting on your physical, mental, and emotional traits when you feel at your best—balanced, energized, and in harmony. Your Prakriti is also recognized as what is true for you most of the time and from earlier stages in life. Here's a simplified guide to help you identify which dosha(s) might dominate your Prakriti:

VATA (AIR AND ETHER)

+ **Body:** Light, thin frame, dry skin, irregular appetite and digestion
+ **Mind:** Creative, quick-thinking but prone to anxiety or restlessness
+ **Energy:** High bursts of energy followed by fatigue

PITTA (FIRE AND WATER)

+ **Body:** Medium build, warm body temperature, sharp hunger and digestion
+ **Mind:** Focused, determined but can be easily irritated or prone to perfectionism
+ **Energy:** Consistent energy but prone to burnout under stress

KAPHA (EARTH AND WATER)

✦ **Body:** Solid, sturdy build, soft skin, slower digestion

✦ **Mind:** Calm, nurturing but can struggle with motivation or emotional heaviness

✦ **Energy:** Steady but slow, with a tendency toward lethargy if unbalanced

Take time to observe yourself when you feel most aligned; this will provide insights into your true nature.

Introducing Vikriti: Your Current Imbalance

While Prakriti is your inherent nature, Vikriti reflects your current state of balance or imbalance. Vikriti shows how factors like diet, lifestyle, environment, and stress affect your doshas, often pushing them out of alignment. For example, someone with a Pitta Prakriti may develop excess Vata due to irregular routines or chronic stress, leading to anxiety, dry skin, or digestive issues.

Understanding your Vikriti is essential for bringing your body and mind back into harmony. Unlike Prakriti, Vikriti is not fixed—it can change throughout your life and even within a single season. We'll explore Vikriti in more depth in Part 2: Health Alchemy, where we'll dive into practical steps to identify and address imbalances to restore equilibrium in your body and mind.

By understanding your Prakriti and the foundational role it plays in Ayurveda, you can recognize your natural tendencies and unique strengths. This awareness is the first step in building a life that supports your authentic self, one aligned with the cosmic energies reflected in your birth chart and the wisdom of your body.

How Vedic Astrology Plays a Role in Determining Your Prikriti

I never felt a strong connection to Western astrology. While the descriptions of my Pisces sun often made sense on the surface, they never resonated deeply enough to explore the subject further. I saw astrology as intriguing but ultimately disconnected from my experiences. It wasn't until my studies in Ayurveda and other Eastern traditions that I was drawn to Vedic astrology (*Jyotish*). There was something about this ancient system, rooted in the same philosophical principles as Ayurveda, that called to me. I decided to dive in and explore.

Through this journey, I discovered something profound: Vedic astrology doesn't emphasize our sun sign (star sign) like Western astrology. Vedic astrology puts more weight on your moon sign and your rising sign. With its emphasis on the moon sign and its grounding in the sidereal zodiac, Vedic astrology offered me a deeper understanding of myself. It felt holistic, more connected to the cycles of nature and the universe.

Vedic astrology was not only about personality traits, it was about understanding the cosmic energies that shape physical, mental, and spiritual natures and how they align with our Prakriti.

WESTERN VERSUS VEDIC ASTROLOGY: WHAT'S THE DIFFERENCE?

Before we explore how Vedic astrology can reveal your Prakriti, it's important to understand the key differences between Western astrology and Vedic astrology.

✦ Western astrology is based on the tropical zodiac, which is aligned with the seasons and the equinoxes. This system, commonly used in modern times, focuses primarily on the sun sign and how the sun's position in the zodiac at your time of birth affects your personality.

✦ Vedic astrology (Jyotish) uses the sidereal zodiac, which aligns more closely with the constellations. This system accounts for the equinoxes' precession, meaning it shifts the planetary positions by approximately 23–24 degrees backward compared to Western astrology. As a result, your sun, moon, and rising signs may be entirely different in Vedic astrology than they are in Western astrology.

Additionally Vedic astrology places emphasis on the moon sign and rising sign, which are considered more reflective of your emotional and external experiences.

In Vedic astrology, the moon governs the mind and emotions, and it is seen as the most important factor in understanding your mental and emotional state. Meanwhile, the sun represents your soul's essence and life purpose, and your rising sign (Ascendant) shapes how you interact with the world and approach challenges.

When I mapped my Vedic astrology chart, I realized these differences were not merely technical—they provided a shift in how I understood myself.

WRITTEN IN THE STARS:
WHAT MY VEDIC CHART REVEALED

For years, I identified as a Pisces sun in Western astrology, which felt somewhat aligned with my love for creativity, intuition, and the spiritual world. However, when I began to explore Vedic astrology, I discovered my sun sign is in Aquarius. This shift explained why I always felt a deeper connection to humanitarian causes, innovative thinking, and independence—traits that are strongly associated with Aquarius in Vedic astrology.

Not only that, but my moon sign, which is of utmost importance in Vedic astrology, is in Cancer, placed in the eighth house. This placement gave me deep insights into why I feel so strongly about emotional depth, nurturing, and the importance of transformation and healing in my life. The eighth house represents hidden knowledge, transformation, and emotional intensity, all of which resonate deeply with the way I have always processed emotions and approached challenges.

Furthermore, my rising sign is Sagittarius, which immediately made sense. Sagittarius rising brings a thirst for knowledge, a love for travel and adventure, and a deep sense of spiritual seeking. It explained why I had always been drawn to learning, growth, and new experiences. Sagittarius is ruled by Jupiter, the planet of wisdom and expansion, which aligns with my passion for teaching and guiding others on their journeys.

Understanding Prakriti Through Vedic Astrology

Vedic astrology offers a cosmic perspective on your Prakriti by revealing how the elements and planetary energies were aligned at the moment of your birth. Each sign in Vedic astrology is connected to one of the five elements, which in turn informs which doshas dominate your constitution.

In Vedic astrology, the moon sign reflects your emotional and mental nature, which often correlates with your doshic tendencies. For example:

✦ Someone with a moon in a fiery sign, like Leo or Aries, may exhibit strong Pitta qualities, such as drive and intensity.

✦ Someone with a moon in a watery sign, like Cancer or Pisces, may lean more toward Kapha's nurturing and stabilizing traits.

Similarly, your rising sign shows how you interact with the world, often reflecting how your dominant dosha manifests externally. For example:

✦ A Vata-dominant individual with an Aquarius rising may express their creativity and quick thinking in their outward persona.

✦ A Kapha-dominant person with a Cancer rising may appear nurturing and emotionally steady to others.

Understanding these connections can help you see how your doshic constitution aligns with the cosmic energies present at your birth, deepening your understanding of yourself on every level.

My Cancer moon connects me deeply to Kapha (water and earth), bringing qualities of stability, emotional depth, and nurturing. However, this also means I struggle with emotional stagnation or heaviness if I'm not careful to balance Kapha with movement and emotional release. Aquarius, ruled by Saturn and associated with Vata (air and ether), brings creativity, independence, and a desire for innovation. The Vata influence can lead to restlessness or anxiety when unbalanced, reminding me to stay grounded.

Finally, my Sagittarius rising aligns with Pitta (fire and water), fueling my ambition, drive for knowledge, and desire for spiritual growth. When in balance, this energy is empowering, but when imbalanced, Pitta can lead to overexertion or burnout.

Understanding these elements and their interplay helps me stay balanced in my life and health. By aligning my lifestyle and choices with the wisdom of Vedic astrology and Ayurveda, I support my Prakriti and minimize the imbalances (or Vikriti) that arise from stress, environment, or lifestyle choices.

Exploring the Moon Signs and Their Qualities

As you begin to explore Vedic astrology, the moon sign is your first point of reference for understanding your emotional nature and mental tendencies. The moon governs your subconscious, your emotions, and how you process the world on an internal level. Here are the moon signs in Vedic astrology, along with their general qualities:

1. **Mesha (Aries):** Courageous and energetic but can be impulsive and headstrong

2. **Vrishabha (Taurus):** Grounded and patient, loves comfort but can be resistant to change

3. **Mithuna (Gemini):** Curious, adaptable, and communicative but can become scattered or anxious

4. **Karka (Cancer):** Nurturing, intuitive, and emotional but can hold on to the past or become moody

5. **Simha (Leo):** Confident, creative, and charismatic but can be prideful or crave attention

6. **Kanya (Virgo):** Analytical, practical, and detail-oriented but can be overly critical or worrisome

7. **Tula (Libra):** Diplomatic, balanced, and harmonious but can struggle with indecision or people-pleasing

8. **Vrischika (Scorpio):** Intense, passionate, and transformative but can be secretive or possessive

9. **Dhanu (Sagittarius):** Adventurous, optimistic, and philosophical but can be overly idealistic or reckless

10. **Makara (Capricorn):** Disciplined, ambitious, and practical but can be rigid or pessimistic

11. **Kumbha (Aquarius):** Innovative, independent, and humanitarian but can be detached or unpredictable

12. **Meena (Pisces):** Compassionate, imaginative, and spiritual but can be overly idealistic or escapist

How to Find Your Moon Sign in Vedic Astrology

To find your Vedic moon sign, you will need to know the exact time, date, and location of your birth. Your moon sign is calculated based on the moon's position in the sidereal zodiac at the moment you were born. Because the moon moves quickly through the zodiac— changing signs every two-and-a-half days—your exact birth time is crucial for an accurate reading.

You can access your Vedic moon sign and full birth chart using several free resources online. I have a webpage that will link you to a free personalised Vedic astrology chart **harmonyinspiredhealth. com.au/VedicChart**. This chart will provide your moon sign, sun sign, rising sign, and other planetary positions, offering you deep insights into your Prakriti and life path.

Why Understanding Your Vedic Chart Matters

Your Vedic birth chart isn't simply about astrology—it's a blueprint of the elemental forces and cosmic energies that shaped your physical body, emotional tendencies, and mental patterns from the beginning. In Ayurveda, we don't guess at health or personality traits, we study the influences present at birth to understand your true nature—your Prakriti. By understanding your moon sign, rising sign, and elemental composition through Vedic astrology, you gain a powerful entry point into self-discovery.

This insight becomes an important building block in unlocking your health, resilience, emotional balance, and dharma. Rather than trying to fit into someone else's path, you learn how to align with your natural constitution, creating more ease, vitality, and fulfillment. When you work with your cosmic design rather than against it, life doesn't just feel more meaningful—it becomes more sustainable, empowered, and true to who you really are.

Using Your Vedic Astrological Chart

+ What did your moon sign, sun sign, and rising sign reveal about your emotional nature, soul purpose, and the way you show up in the world?

+ In what ways do you feel aligned with your natural constitution? Where do you sense opportunities for deeper balance?

+ How can you use this cosmic insight as a tool for self-awareness, healing, and growth moving forward?

Prakriti and Vikriti Reflection

1. Based on what you've learned about Prakriti (your inherent constitution), what are some ways you can honor your natural design more fully in your daily life?

_____

_____

_____

_____

_____

2. Reflect on areas where you feel imbalanced right now. Are these imbalances temporary (Vikriti) or long-standing patterns?

_____

_____

_____

_____

_____

3. If you could offer your body and mind one commitment this month to support your unique constitution, what would it be?

_____

_____

_____

_____

CHAPTER 2

A New Paradigm of Womanhood

The Goddess Within: Reclaiming Your Sacred Wholeness

Every woman carries an innate power—whole, wise, and unshaken. It's never lost, only buried beneath expectation and noise. Reclaiming it is not becoming someone new but returning to who you've always been—the Goddess within.

To step into your highest self is to align with the truth of who you are. It is not a quest for perfection but a journey toward wholeness—a state where all parts of you, the graceful and the messy, the light and the shadow, are embraced as sacred.

When we talk about becoming our highest self, we're speaking about the process of returning to our natural state of alignment— where body, mind, and spirit are in harmony.

In Ayurveda, this alignment is reflected in the balance of your inherent constitution (Prakriti) and the imbalances that may develop over time due to lifestyle, environment, and stress (Vikriti). Much

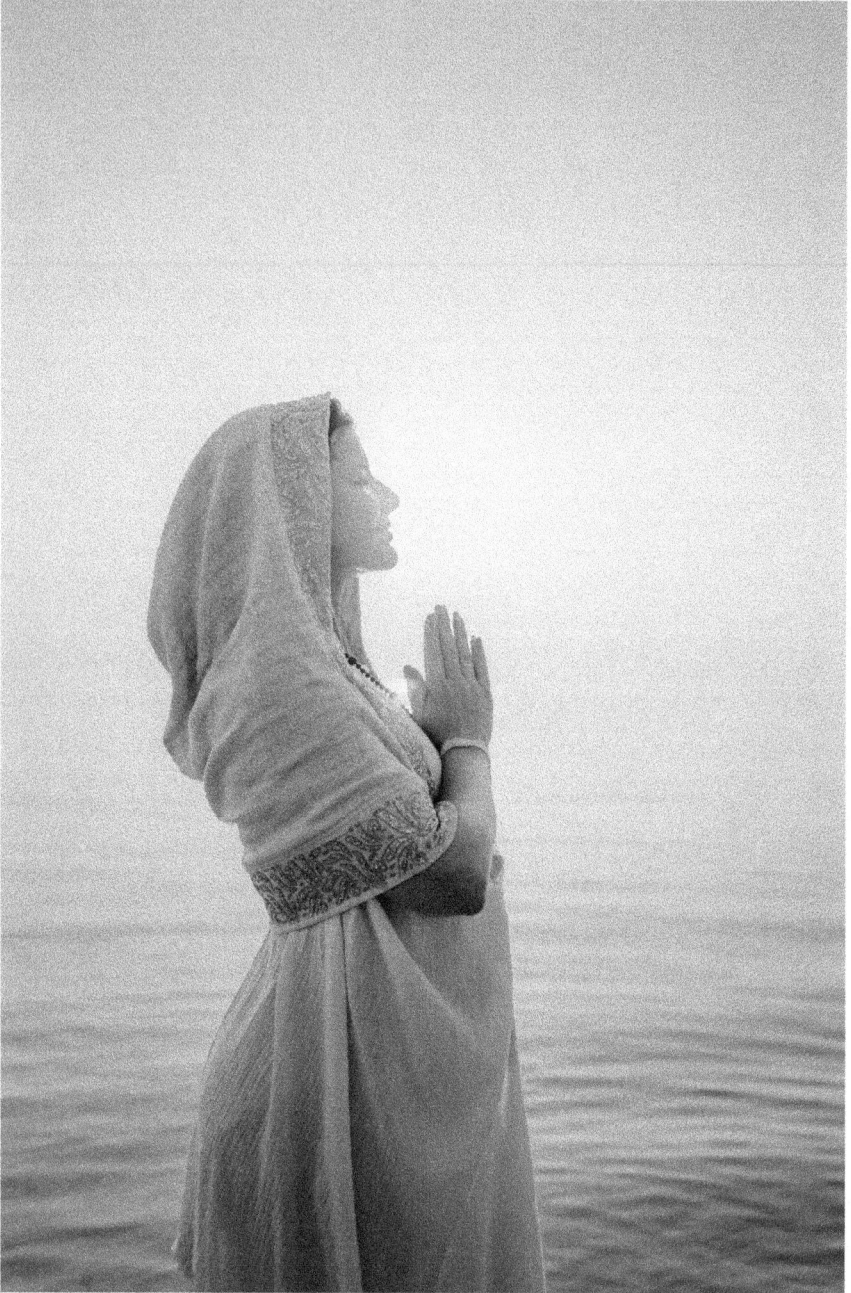

"YOU ARE NOT A DROP IN THE OCEAN. YOU ARE THE ENTIRE OCEAN IN A DROP." – RUMI

like the Goddesses of ancient traditions, each of us has a unique expression of power, beauty, and wisdom, but we also face challenges that pull us out of balance. The journey to your higHERself™ is one of acknowledging both your strengths and your struggles, and learning how to harmonize them to live in alignment with your true nature.

The Archetypes of Femininity: Lessons from the Vedic Goddesses

In the rich spiritual traditions of Vedic culture, the Goddesses represent different aspects of the divine feminine, each offering us a reflection of our own potential. They are not distant figures to be admired from afar but symbols of qualities we carry within. By understanding and embodying their teachings, we can reclaim parts of ourselves that may have been forgotten, suppressed, or undervalued.

Let us explore four key Vedic Goddesses—Saraswati, Lakshmi, Kali, and Durga—and the lessons they offer to help us embrace the fullness of our being.

SARASWATI: THE GODDESS OF WISDOM, CREATIVITY, AND LEARNING

In the pantheon of Vedic Goddesses, Saraswati embodies the qualities of intellect, artistic expression, and inner wisdom. She is often depicted seated on a lotus, holding a book, a mālā, and a vina, a stringed musical instrument. Her presence encourages us to nurture our creative potential and seek knowledge that feeds both our minds and spirits.

In your life, Saraswati's energy invites you to honor your intellect, your capacity for learning, and your creative expression. She reminds us that the path to our highest self is one of continuous growth, cultivating wisdom not only through formal education but through life's experiences, reflections, and artistic pursuits.

When we channel Saraswati's energy, we allow ourselves to speak our truth, create beauty in the world, and seek clarity in moments of confusion. She teaches us that our voice matters and that our self-expression is a sacred gift.

I've felt Saraswati's energy flowing through my life over the past few years. I've needed her gifts—the ability to absorb the wisdom I was learning during my master's degree; the intellect to break down complex subjects into simple, accessible teachings for my students at the Ayurveda Alchemist Academy; and the creativity to bring my courses to life and write this book. I keep two statues of Saraswati in my home—one in my office near my computer, and the other beside my incense bowl, where I begin my morning ritual each day.

Gazing at her figure serves as a reminder to invoke my inner wisdom and creativity.

MANTRA FOR SARASWATI

Om aim Saraswati namaha.
I honor the Goddess Saraswati,
who embodies wisdom and creativity.

LAKSHMI: THE GODDESS OF ABUNDANCE, BEAUTY, AND PROSPERITY

Lakshmi is the Goddess of abundance, both material and spiritual. She represents wealth, beauty, and the flourishing of life. Lakshmi's energy is about receiving as much as it is about giving, about being open to the universe's blessings while remaining grounded in gratitude and balance.

Too often, women are taught to shy away from their desires, particularly around prosperity or physical beauty, as though these were superficial concerns. Lakshmi teaches us that abundance is our natural state and that beauty—whether in our environment, our bodies, or our relationships—can be an expression of the divine. She invites us to take up space, to embrace our worth, and to live in a state of graceful receptivity.

Lakshmi asks us to reflect: Are we allowing ourselves to receive the blessings we seek? Are we nurturing ourselves as much as we nurture others? Her energy reminds us that when we care for our own well-being, we create a foundation from which to give generously to the world.

I must admit, in my mid-thirties, it was difficult for me to fully embrace Lakshmi's energy. I felt guilty for wanting more than others had, as if desiring abundance meant I wasn't being grateful for what I already had. But I came to realize that this way of thinking was flawed. When I am abundant, I have more to share and help other women recognize their potential. As women, we are often conditioned to believe that wanting more is ungrateful; we should simply be content with what we have. Yet abundance is not limited to material wealth—it encompasses happiness, life force energy (prana/qi), fulfilling relationships, and vibrant experiences.

Once I understood that my higHERself is fully expressed through an abundant life, I released the notion that wanting more was selfish. Now, in my forties, I embrace Lakshmi's energy with open arms. With her blessings, I have cultivated nurturing relationships, embarked on meaningful adventures, pursued an impactful career, and created a beautiful home on the Gold Coast, Australia. I have come to see abundance as a sacred force that enriches every aspect of my life. A gold Lakshmi statue resides at the top of my stairs in my home, to remind me of this abundance every day.

Lakshmi also invites us to embrace our feminine sexual energy as a sacred expression of abundance and creativity. This energy, often misunderstood or suppressed, is a powerful force that connects us to our inner radiance and capacity for joy. Embracing this aspect of ourselves might look like cultivating self-confidence, nurturing a deeper connection with our bodies, or exploring sensuality through movement, touch, or creative expression. Lakshmi reminds us that our sexual energy is not something to hide or fear but a vital source of vibrancy and empowerment, infusing our lives with pleasure, intimacy, and a profound sense of self-worth.

MANTRA FOR LAKSHMI

Om shreem mahalakshmiyei namaha.
I honor the Goddess Lakshmi,
who bestows abundance and prosperity.

DURGA: THE GODDESS OF STRENGTH, PROTECTION, AND COURAGE

If Saraswati is the Goddess of the mind and Lakshmi the Goddess of the heart, Durga represents the power of the soul. She is the fierce, protective mother, wielding weapons in each of her many arms, riding a lion into battle. Yet her face remains serene, reminding us that true strength comes from inner peace, not from aggression.

Durga is the embodiment of the warrior spirit in all women—the strength we summon when facing adversity, the courage to stand up for what we believe in, and the resilience to protect what we hold sacred. Durga's energy teaches us to claim our space in the world unapologetically, to defend our boundaries, and to act from a place of inner power.

When life becomes overwhelming or when you doubt your ability to navigate challenges, Durga is the goddess to call upon. She reminds us that we are stronger than we realize and that sometimes, our highest self requires us to wield the sword of discernment, to say *no* to what drains us and yes to what empowers us.

Reflecting on my life, I can see how I have embodied Durga's energy—the fierce, protective force that arises when we must summon courage from the deepest part of our being. Her force emerged when I was just nineteen years old. I was walking back to my apartment late one night when I noticed a man following me. The closer I got to my door, the more palpable my fear became. I felt him closing in, and as he attempted to follow me inside, something primal surged within me. I turned around, locked eyes with him, and roared like a lion. I didn't think; I just acted. My voice boomed with a force I didn't know I possessed, and in that instant, he froze, startled by the fierceness in my gaze and the power in my voice. He backed away and ran, while I stood there, heart pounding, trembling from the adrenaline. I knew, in that moment, it wasn't just me who had protected myself—Durga's energy had taken over, manifesting as a fierce warrior within me to ward off danger.

This energy also became especially palpable after the birth of my twin boys, when motherhood awakened a primal instinct within me. I found myself fiercely protective, not just of their physical safety but of their right to grow up in a world where they are empowered and nurtured. The demands of raising two babies at once taught me to draw on strength I didn't know I had. There were moments of exhaustion when I felt pulled in two directions—literally and figuratively—but Durga's energy kept me grounded. Her spirit reminded me that even in the chaos, I was capable of rising to meet every challenge head-on.

Durga's strength is not only about fighting external battles; it's also about standing up for oneself, refusing to be divided, and knowing when to draw on the protective force within. I have felt her energy in countless other moments—times when I've had to fight for my voice to be heard, defend my choices as a mother, or simply navigate the everyday challenges of life with courage and resilience. Durga is there, reminding me that I carry the spirit of a warrior within, one who is unafraid to protect what is sacred and to rise, time and time again, no matter what stands in the way.

In these moments, I don't just call upon Durga's energy—I embody her, channeling her strength, her resolve, and her fearless heart. She is an admonition that there is power in both softness and fierceness, that being protective is also a form of deep love, and that true strength emerges when we are called to protect the things we cherish most.

MANTRA FOR DURGA

Om dum Durgayei namaha.
I honor the Goddess Durga, who is fierce and protective.

KALI: THE GODDESS OF TRANSFORMATION, LIBERATION, AND FIERCE LOVE

Kali is the goddess of transformation. She does not gently nudge us toward change—she commands it. With her unyielding force, she dismantles what no longer serves us, clearing the path for freedom, authenticity, and rebirth. Her energy is raw, untamed, and deeply loving, although her lessons are often uncomfortable.

Kali's energy is a fierce, liberating force that calls us to shed layers of our identity that have grown stagnant, outdated, or false. She strips away illusions and attachments, asking us to meet the truth of who we are—unfiltered and unapologetically.

For years, I held onto my identity as a registered nurse, even after I had followed my heart and opened my practice as an Ayurveda women's health practitioner. While I knew I had found my calling in Ayurveda, part of me couldn't let go of the safety net of my career. I continued to work one shift per week at the hospital, convinced I needed to hold onto that role in case my new path didn't succeed.

Looking back, I see that it wasn't only about financial security—I was afraid to fully release that part of myself, to release the version of me I built my professional identity around for so many years.

Kali's energy called me to confront this fear and see it for what it truly was: an attachment to a self that no longer aligned with my truth. It wasn't an easy process; it felt like letting go of a tether to my old life. But in doing so, I felt a sense of liberation—a new trust in my path and my ability to thrive without needing a "backup plan."

Kali also showed up in my struggle to redefine myself after having children. I clung to my identity as a free-spirited, independent woman, finding it difficult to reconcile that version of myself with the reality of being a mother. I worried that motherhood would erase the part of me that valued freedom and the ability to pursue my passions. But Kali's energy is relentless—she asks us to step into the fullness of life, even when it means letting go of what we thought defined us. As I navigated the early years of motherhood, I began to see that I didn't have to lose myself; I simply had to evolve. Kali helped me see that true freedom comes not from clinging to the past but from embracing the person I was becoming.

As I moved further into my forties, I felt Kali's energy guiding me through the natural transitions of maturity. She helped me face the societal pressures that tell women to resist aging at all costs, to cling to youth as though it defines our worth. Kali taught me to let go of those narratives, to see the beauty and wisdom in growing older, and to step into this new phase of life with grace and confidence.

Kali's transformation isn't about destruction for its own sake—it's about creating space for something more aligned, authentic, and powerful to emerge. She forces us to confront the attachments that limit us, whether they are outdated roles, unhelpful beliefs, or fears of change. Her energy liberates us, but only when we are willing to let go of what no longer serves us.

Kali reminds us that transformation is not always easy, but it is always worth it. She pushes us to embrace the freedom that comes from letting go, showing us that the truest version of ourselves lies just beyond the illusions we've clung to.

MANTRA FOR KALI

Om krim Kalikayai namaha.
I bow to Goddess Kali, the divine force of transformation and ultimate reality, invoking her power and protection.

Goddess Reflection

SARASWATI: THE GODDESS OF WISDOM AND CREATIVITY

1. In what areas of your life are you seeking clarity or deeper understanding?

_____

_____

_____

_____

2. How can you nurture your creative energy and express your unique ideas?

_____

_____

_____

_____

3. What daily practices could help you connect with your inner wisdom?

_____

_____

_____

LAKSHMI: THE GODDESS OF ABUNDANCE AND LOVE

1. How do you define abundance in your life beyond material wealth?

_____

_____

_____

_____

2. Are there areas where you feel guilty for wanting more? How might you reframe those feelings to embrace abundance with gratitude and grace?

_____

_____

_____

_____

3. How can you invite nurturing relationships and joy into your life?

_____

_____

_____

DURGA: THE GODDESS OF STRENGTH AND PROTECTION

1. What are you fiercely protecting in your life right now, and why?

    _____

    _____

    _____

    _____

2. Where in your life do you need to set stronger boundaries to honor your energy and values?

    _____

    _____

    _____

    _____

3. When was the last time you stood up for yourself, and how did it feel?

    _____

    _____

    _____

KALI: THE GODDESS OF TRANSFORMATION AND LIBERATION

1. What beliefs, roles, or attachments no longer serve your highest self?

    _____

    _____

    _____

2. What fears are holding you back, and how might you confront them with courage?

_____

_____

_____

3. How can you create space for transformation and embrace the person you are becoming?

_____

_____

_____

CONNECTING WITH THE GODDESSES

1. Which Goddess energy do you feel most connected to at this moment, and why?

_____

_____

_____

_____

2. Is there a particular Goddess whose energy feels challenging to embody? What might this reveal about where you need to grow or heal?

_____

_____

_____

_____

3. How can you integrate the wisdom of Saraswati, Lakshmi, Durga, and Kali into your daily life to live more authentically and intentionally?

_____

_____

_____

_____

_____

_____

THE GODDESS MIRRORS YOUR OWN POTENTIAL

The Goddesses offer us mirrors of our own potential. Just as they embody creativity, abundance, and strength, so, too, do these qualities reside within you. However, in our modern world, we often compartmentalize ourselves—hiding our emotions, fearing our desires, or silencing our voices. The path to becoming your highest self is about reclaiming all aspects of yourself. It means seeing your raw, emotional, and imperfect parts as sacred. It means recognising your sensitivity, desires, and boundaries are sources of power, not weakness.

STEPPING INTO YOUR HIGHEST SELF

Stepping into your highest self is not an act of self-improvement, but an act of self-recovery. It's the recognition that you are not incomplete but rather fragmented by the demands and illusions of the world around you. Alignment is not something to be attained— it's something to be remembered. When your thoughts, actions, and desires move in unison with your true nature, you return to a state of coherence that has always existed within you.

The wisdom of Ayurveda and the Goddess archetypes offer pathways—not as ideals to aspire to but as reflections of the complex and multidimensional nature of your being.

By acknowledging your creative force, your inner strength, and your capacity to manifest abundance, you transcend the notion of healing as mere restoration.

You begin to understand it as expansion—unveiling parts of yourself that have been dormant, waiting to be awakened. This is not merely a personal transformation; it's a reclamation of the feminine presence in the world, a collective rising of women reclaiming the power to define themselves on their own terms.

The question is not whether you will step into this space, but when.

What might you discover if you chose to embrace your highest self now, without hesitation?

CHAPTER 3

Rediscovering Your Sacred Identity

The Duality of Identity

I recently attended a retreat, where I found myself sitting in a circle with women (and a few men) in their twenties and early thirties. At forty, I was among the older participants, and as I listened to their stories, I realized that identity shifts happen in every decade of life; it's not a midlife phenomenon. However, the complexities and themes evolve with age.

For younger participants, their focus was on the future: Would they make it in the world? Should they spend more years traveling, or would that lessen their chances of settling down, buying a home, or starting a family? Many had already defied societal norms— quitting high-paying corporate jobs to live out of backpacks, making the wonder of the world their only mission.

I was fascinated by their courage to break free from expectations. Some had started their journeys during COVID—a time of uncertainty for most—and were still traveling, earning through marketing, brand deals, or passion projects. They'd shed identities assigned to them in corporate offices, trading structured lives for freedom and connection. They described sitting with locals

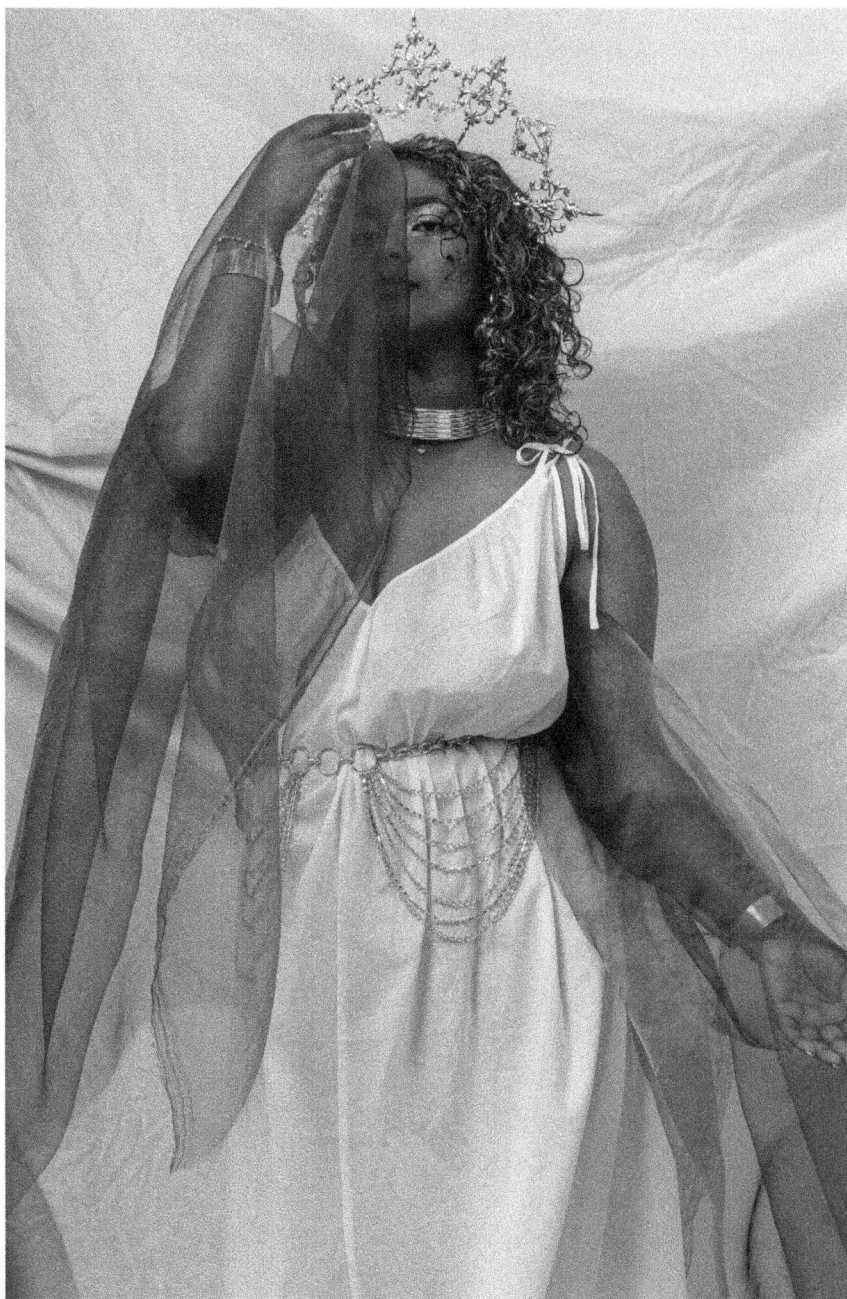

"SHE REMEMBERED WHO SHE WAS, AND THE GAME CHANGED." –
LALAH DELIA

in the mountains of Indonesia, where no English was spoken but conversations unfolded through human connection, laughter, and shared meals.

A part of me has always romanticised this kind of untethered existence—traveling the world, experiencing cultures, and feeling the profound freedom of having nowhere and everywhere to call home. I know it wouldn't be all sunshine and serenity, but I can't help imagining the possibilities.

Yet, I chose a different path—one I am deeply grateful for. We all have a dharmic journey to follow. The jungles of Costa Rica might call my name, but my journey there will look very different from the carefree, nomadic lifestyle I envisioned. My trip will be carefully planned with my family. I'll sit in the comfort of an airport lounge before boarding the flight, with a transfer waiting to whisk me to a magical resort. I'll rest in luxury before embarking on adventures— hiking through forests, diving into waterfalls, swimming in the ocean—returning each evening to a perfectly made-up room.

True freedom? That depends on perspective.

There will be interruptions—my children calling for me, emails to check, a message from the dog sitter, or a client needing something. My time won't be entirely my own, and my days will be shaped by the needs of those I love. So, have I traded raw freedom for comfort? Or have I simply redefined what freedom means? Perhaps freedom is not the absence of responsibility but the ability to choose the life that aligns with your dharma—even if it looks different from what you once imagined.

THE PULL OF TWO WORLDS

For years, I felt a pull between two identities: the barefoot bohemian gypsy who loves the rawness of mother nature, simplicity, and deep human connection, and the woman who enjoys sipping coconut water poolside in Louis Vuitton slides. I often questioned myself: Who am I? Could I truly embody both sides, or was I being inauthentic? I worried that switching between these facets of myself might make others think I was a fraud.

The more I explored this internal conflict, the clearer it became: both sides are me. They represent different facets of my higHERself, and by embracing both, I honor the complexity of who I am.

THE SHIFT OF MOTHERHOOD

I experienced a struggle with identity when I became a mother, on July 11, 2012, with the birth of my twin boys. Overnight, my old self seemed to vanish. I was a *mother* now, responsible for two tiny humans.

My new identity as a "twin mum" consumed me, but I found it difficult to connect with other mothers I met at playgroups.

Many mums seemed content to discuss baby food recipes, nap schedules, and breastfeeding. While I loved my children deeply—with a fierce, protective love I'd never felt before—I needed something more. I didn't want motherhood to be the only thing that defined me, and for those who do, I salute you for staying true to who you are and what you want in life.

For me, motherhood was a great gift, a great teacher, and everything in between, but I had another part of me yearning to be tapped into. I could confidently say it wasn't my career at the time either; nursing didn't feel like the right path anymore.

The sleepless nights and challenges of raising twins sent me into a spiral of anxiety, depression, and constant questioning of my identity. I felt alone.

My parents often drove up on Fridays to help. When my dad came, I felt a sense of relief—he gave me space to breathe. But when my mum came, it was different.

At that time, my mum was battling alcoholism, and her presence often filled me with anxiety. I never knew which version of her I'd get: the vibrant, playful grandmother who adored my boys, or the tense, unpredictable woman whose comments carried an edge that left me walking on eggshells.

Her energy was heavy, and as an empath, I absorbed it all—the disappointment, the tension, the burden. I loved her deeply, but it was a love laced with complexity, shaped by her struggles and my own.

A MOTHER'S STORY: A SEARCH FOR BELONGING

My mum has always carried the weight of an unresolved identity. She was adopted as a baby into a loving family, but beneath the surface, there was a quiet struggle—I assume it was a feeling of abandonment and unworthiness she could never quite articulate. It's a wound I imagine only someone who has been adopted can fully understand.

Her adoptive parents, my grandparents, were wonderfully supportive and always encouraged her to connect with her biological parents if she wanted. In fact, they encouraged her to search for answers and never saw it as rejecting them, only as a natural longing for missing pieces of herself.

When my mum finally reached out to her biological father, the door was firmly shut. He wanted no part of her, no acknowledgment of her existence. The first time she contacted, it was out of necessity. I was a baby, very sick, and her doctor needed a family medical history to determine possible causes. My mum reached out to his office—he was a gynecologist—only to be coldly rebuffed. There was no conversation, no curiosity about her or the grandchild he didn't even know existed.

Years later, she tried again. My brother was playing soccer at a high level, and his team had a match in her biological father's hometown. My mum thought perhaps that was a chance to connect. Surely, as a father, he might want to meet the daughter he'd never known. But the response, delivered through his secretary (who we later discovered was his wife), was as harsh as ever: He did not want to meet her.

She never tried again.

For much of my life, I didn't give this story much thought. He didn't want to know us, and frankly, he didn't seem like someone I'd want to know either. My mother's relationship with her biological mother, Maggie, was more complicated. Maggie, lived in the United States and reached out to my mum earlier in life, sending small gifts each Christmas and even visiting Australia a few times. I met her as a child, and it was clear how much my mum resembled her. Despite these interactions, their connection was fragile.

My mum flew to the US to visit Maggie when I was about eighteen, and the small bond they had formed over the years broke. Maggie, afraid of judgment from her neighbours, hid my mum from sight. She refused to give my mum her original birth certificate, denying her this piece of her identity.

My mum returned home shattered, and her pain led to a downward spiral. Her drinking worsened, and she became consumed by depression and suicidal thoughts.

Maggie's story, as I later pieced together, was one of its own heartbreak. She had fallen pregnant with my mum in her first year of medical school after a brief relationship with Mum's biological father. Though she wanted to keep the baby, her family decided otherwise, sending her away so she could give birth in secret. She was forced to give up my mum for adoption, and her dream of becoming a doctor ended shortly after. Maggie later moved to the United States, became a teacher, and married a soldier.

The pain my mum carried from the relationships with both biological parents shaped much of who she was. Being adopted, rejected, and denied her history left wounds that were never fully healed.

FINDING PURPOSE IN MOTHERHOOD

My mum's own struggles with identity mirrored those of her biological mother in some ways. Like Maggie, she became a young mother—pregnant with me at eighteen. When she told my grandma (her adoptive mother), she was given three options: "You can get rid of it, adopt it, or keep it." For my mum, there was no question. She would keep me, and our bond was formed the moment she made that decision.

I guess motherhood gave her a sense of purpose and identity that had eluded her. But it also came at a cost. My mum was incredibly intelligent—she started multiple university degrees and earned high distinctions—but juggling motherhood and work left little room to finish her education.

I remember going with her to university, sitting in lecture halls with a coloring book while she listened to her professors. At the same time, she worked tirelessly as a magazine editor and waitress to support me and my brother. My dad worked out west, often gone for long periods, so the responsibility of raising two kids fell largely on her shoulders. Something had to give, and for my mum, it was her degree.

Even so, she poured herself into being a mother with a fierce determination. Her sacrifices shaped the foundation of my life, and I carry her strength and resilience with me.

That's why it was so hard for me to reconcile my feelings when she came to help me with my boys. While I mentioned that my dad's visits felt like a relief and my mum's presence often brought a sense of anxiety, the truth is, mums carry the heavier load. She had always been my greatest support, the one who showed up for me through every challenge, and yet there I was, overwhelmed by her presence.

I felt guilty for those thoughts, for the anguish I felt when she came to help.

Deep down, I knew it wasn't about her but about the emotions her energy stirred in me. Still, I couldn't shake the shame of feeling burdened by the very person who had given me so much.

It wasn't until I went on a deep healing retreat in Bali that I came to a powerful realization: my truth was not her truth, and her truth was not mine. The way we perceive others is shaped by our own internal world and does not reflect their reality or thoughts. This understanding brought me a sense of peace and compassion—for her and for myself.

It's funny how we cling to the idea of our personal truth as if it's an absolute reality, when in fact, it is shaped entirely by our lens— our experiences, emotions, and perceptions.

Two people can live through the same event and walk away with completely different narratives.

Psychologists call this subjective reality, and it's been studied extensively in eyewitness testimony. In fact, research has shown that when multiple people witness the same accident, their recollections often vary wildly. Details like the color of a car, the speed it was moving, or even the sequence of events can be recalled differently, shaped by each person's focus, emotional state, and subconscious biases. This is why police reports often contain conflicting accounts, not because people are lying but because no two brains perceive reality exactly the same.

So while the words in this book are my deepest, most heartfelt truth, my mother may read them and see something entirely different. She may remember things I do not, interpret events through a different emotional lens, or feel that her intentions were misunderstood. Neither version is truer than the other—they are simply different reflections of the same reality, filtered through our experiences.

Understanding this through Ayurvedic psychology played a pivotal role in helping me discern this truth, guiding me to recognize the separation between my experiences and her intentions, allowing me to hold compassion for both her truth and my own.

THE REBIRTH OF IDENTITY THROUGH SOBRIETY

Through sobriety, my mum discovered a new sense of self. She shed the veil of illusion that alcohol created, uncovering the vibrant, caring person she had always been beneath the pain. As she connected more deeply to her spiritual self, she began to embrace her truth—a truth that is the essence of our ultimate identity.

Her bubbly personality and nurturing spirit resurfaced in profound ways. She started dedicating her time to rescuing and caring for koalas, working her way through ranks of volunteers to become a duty manager responsible for the care of vulnerable joeys. She now selflessly fosters orphaned wallabies as well, caring for them as if they were her own, waking every four hours to feed them exactly as a mother would.

Together with my dad, she created a sanctuary on one hundred acres of bushland, complete with a running creek and untouched natural beauty. This land has become her refuge, a space where she connects with nature daily and finds a sense of peace. It's also a place of hope for the nurtured animals. Her property was approved as a release site for koalas nursed back to health—a testament to her unwavering dedication.

Watching my mum in this new chapter of her life has taught me a valuable truth: your identity is not defined by a job title, family role, or external markers like where you live or how others perceive you. It is an evolving reflection of your experiences, values, and goals. While these may shift, they are all threads of who you are. You never lose your identity; you simply grow into new facets of it.

Legacy of Belonging: The Impact of the Mother Wound

While this is my mother's story, it is also the story of many women across generations. The details differ, but the emotional imprint—the longing to feel wanted, the ache of rejection, the search for belonging—is profoundly universal.

In Ayurveda, we understand that trauma, especially what is carried through generations, can disrupt our Prakriti (our original state of balance) and create long-standing imbalances in our Vikriti (our current state of being). When a mother carries unresolved wounds, those energetic imprints don't only live in her—they echo into the lives of her children, shaping beliefs, identities, and coping mechanisms.

Many of us inherited patterns that were never ours to carry: emotional suppression, fear of abandonment, people-pleasing, or a deep-rooted sense of not-enoughness. These patterns often begin in the womb and continue through our childhood environment, subtly influencing choices, health, and sense of self-worth.

You don't have to be adopted to understand the pain of disconnection. You may have felt unseen by your mother, unsupported in your truth, or burdened by her pain. Perhaps, like my mother, and like me, you've come to a point in life where you no longer want to pass those patterns forward.

This chapter is not simply about personal history. It is a mirror for all who have felt the ripple of unhealed lineage and seek to break the cycle—not with blame, but with compassion. You have the power to choose differently. To write a new story. To become the woman who reclaims her voice, her wholeness, and her belonging—not because she never lost it but because she finally remembered it was hers all along.

LEFT IN A BOMB SHELTER

If my mother's story reveals the ache of belonging, then my father's lineage brings forward a different wound, one etched in silence, secrecy, and survival. Where my mum's life was shaped by the search for connection, Dad's side reflects how identity can be rewritten, erased, or hidden altogether. Both threads carry the same energetic imprint: loss, fragmentation, and remarkably, resilience. As we trace ancestral paths, we see how the stories we inherit, especially the ones unspoken, shape not only our outlook but our biology, behavior, and sense of self. In Ayurveda and Vedic psychology, this is more than family history—it's karmic and energetic inheritance, influencing our Prakriti, Vikriti, and dharma. While the men in my lineage certainly carry stories of strength and survival, it is often the women—the mothers—who pass down both DNA and the emotional blueprints, beliefs, and unhealed wounds that shape us.

My nan (my father's mother) was left in a bomb shelter in England during World War II, abandoned by her mother who fled with an Irish soldier. She and her sister were the only survivors in the shelter, witnessing horrors no child should endure. Separated and fostered into different families, they were eventually reunited as adults on a reality TV show for people searching for lost relatives.

Nan's biological mother told her she was of Romani descent ("gypsy"), which explained her darker features and "gypsy blood." As a teenager, I was embarrassed by this heritage. The stereotypes of the Romani—homeless, thieving, smashing plates—clouded my perception. As I grew older, I came to embrace it. I see it now as the root of my adventurous spirit, my love for travel, and my deep connection to nature.

A FAMILY NAME AND STOLEN IDENTITY

My dad's father, my pop, also carried a story of identity shaped by tragedy. He was the youngest of seven children from a well established Irish family living in Canada. One day, his father decided to take the family on a train outing. My pop, a mischievous child, misbehaved that morning and was left behind with his mother as punishment. It saved his life.

The train exploded, killing his father and siblings. The loss was devastating, and Pop's mother spiraled into despair. Unable to cope with the grief, she gave him up for adoption to a woman who lost her son to tuberculosis.

Rather than embrace my pop for who he was, this woman gave him her deceased son's identity. From that moment, my pop carried the name and birth certificate of another child two years younger than him. It wasn't until a few years ago, when my nan had a cancer scare and Pop confided in her, that this truth came to light.

Hearing this story shook me. I had clung to my last name, Robinson, as a tether to my identity. I'd planned to keep it after marriage. To find out that this name wasn't ours but borrowed from a boy who died decades ago left me questioning everything.

A PATTERN OF IDENTITY AND LOSS

As I reflect on these stories, I see a pattern of loss and rediscovery running through generations of my family. My mum's search for her biological parents, my nan's abandonment during the war, my pop's stolen identity—all these threads have shaped who I am.

What stands out most is the resilience woven into each story.

AYURVEDA & THE ALCHEMY OF HER

My mum, despite her struggles, found purpose in raising me, my brother, and now the koalas and wallabies under her care. My nan reunited with her family after decades apart. And my pop, even after losing everything, built a life rooted in love and strength.

These stories remind me that identity isn't just something we inherit—it's something we create, layer by layer, generation after generation, through the choices we make and the connections we nurture.

Reflection on Family and Identity

1. What stories, spoken or unspoken, have shaped your understanding of who you are and where you come from?

_____

_____

_____

_____

2. Are there generational patterns in your family you feel called to break?

_____

_____

_____

3. How have your parents' or grandparents' identities influenced your own?

_____

_____

_____

4. Have you felt disconnected from your roots or unsure where you belong?

_____

_____

_____

_____

5. What does "belonging" mean to you? Do you feel "belonging" in your family of origin?

_____

_____

_____

_____

_____

_____

6. If you could speak to one of your ancestors, what would you want to ask or say?

_____

_____

_____

_____

_____

CHAPTER 4

Breaking the Cycle

Have you ever stopped to wonder if the path you're walking is truly yours, or one laid out for you by someone else's dreams, fears, or expectations? Sometimes we follow roles, careers, or life choices simply because they felt like the "right" or "safe" thing to do. What if we paused and asked: *Is this what I truly want? Is this who I really am?* In this chapter, as I reflect on the choices that shaped me and the cycles I needed to break, I invite you to do the same. Not with judgment but with curiosity and compassion. The moment we begin to question the path we're on is often the moment we begin to reclaim it.

From Nurse to Healer and Lost Along the Way

My parents always wanted me to go to university. They saw it as an opportunity to break a cycle and create a future they dreamed of for themselves. I would be the first in my family to attend and graduate. At seventeen, I left home to start my nursing degree at Griffith University on the Gold Coast. I turned eighteen during my first semester, entering adulthood as I navigated this new chapter of my life. Nursing was a mix of fascination and exhaustion. It opened my eyes to the raw realities of life and death, but it also took its toll on my spirit.

Nursing was never my dream. It wasn't that I had a burning desire to do something else—I simply didn't know what I wanted. Growing

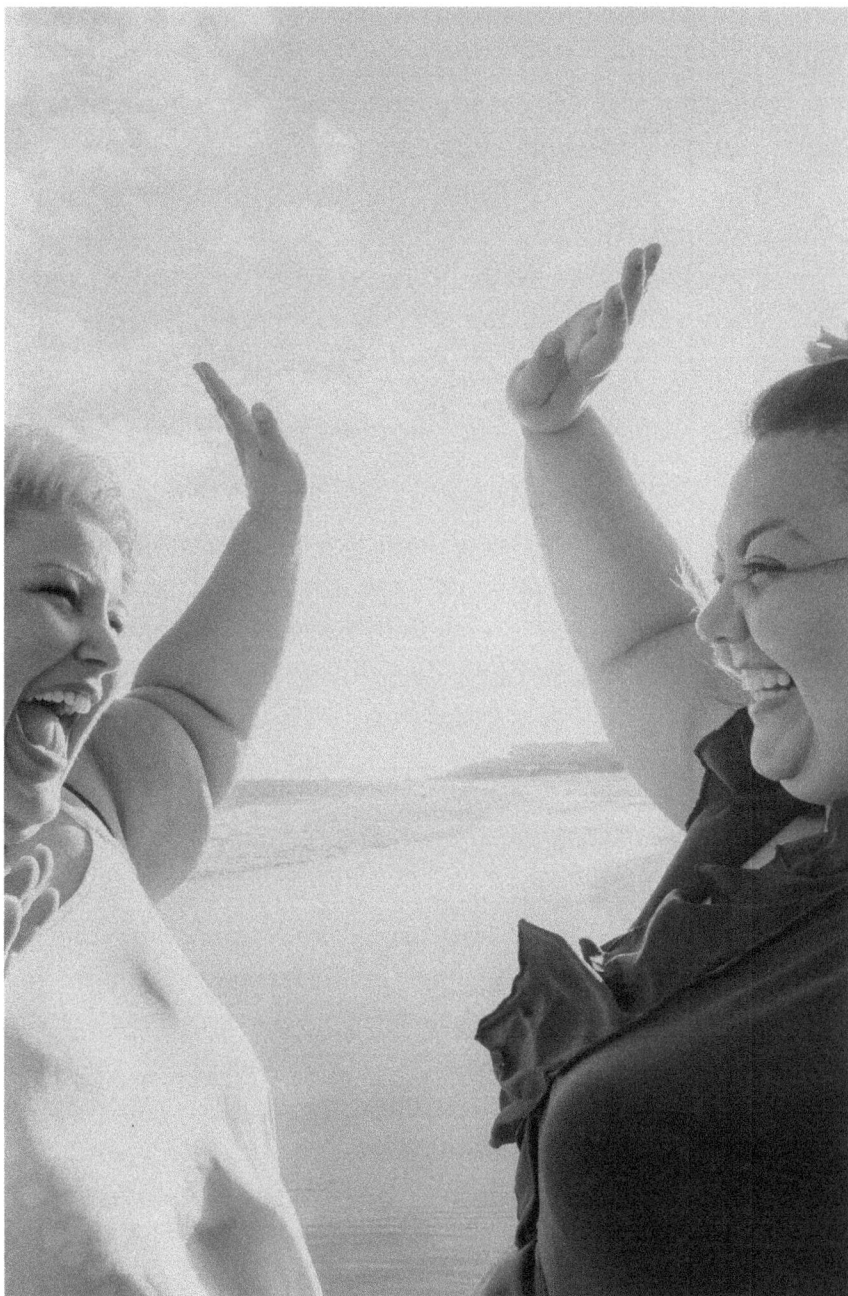

"WHAT WE DO NOT HEAL, WE HAND DOWN." - UNKNOWN

up in a small country town, the options seemed limited, and I couldn't see beyond what was directly in front of me. My mum, ever supportive, said, "You're so good with animals—you'd make an amazing nurse." She would watch me patch up imaginary wounds on our pets and insisted my nurturing nature would translate into caring for people.

She also had a bigger vision for me. As a free spirit with a longing to travel, my mum saw nursing as the passport to a life of adventure. "You can work anywhere in the world," she told me, planting seeds of possibility.

THE HARDENING OF COMPASSION

The work I encountered as a nurse was as rewarding as it was grueling. I still remember some of my earliest experiences vividly— the cries of a mother who lost her four-year-old son, a pain so raw it echoed through the emergency department. The lifeless body of a forty-year-old man in an Everlast shirt and cargo pants as I worked tirelessly to resuscitate him. The patient who grabbed my arm after being revived by CPR, her eyes wide with fear and desperation.

There were moments that cut deeply into my soul. I endured verbal abuse from a grieving mother after a miscarriage, while silently grappling with my own struggles to conceive. I cared for a heavily intoxicated mother high on drugs, giving birth to her fifth child, on a night I particularly felt the sting of my own fertility challenges. Each experience left a mark, hardening me while hollowing out the compassionate, empathetic person I once was.

Night shifts became my greatest dread. They threw my hormones and mental health into complete disarray, leaving me exhausted, irritable, and disconnected. My health deteriorated—bloating left me looking six months pregnant; my gut health was a mess; and hormonal imbalances caused anxiety, heavy cycles, and irrational mood swings.

Despite everything, I pushed forward. Nursing was all I'd known as an adult. It mattered. I mattered. But something was missing. I felt I was treating symptoms of illness rather than empowering people to heal. My patients were caught in a cycle, rebounding through the emergency room doors again and again.

THE CALL TO CHANGE

I knew something had to shift, but first, I needed to change myself. I was tired, cranky, and disconnected from my family, feeling like a failure as both a mother and a wife. My nervous system was in overdrive, and I didn't recognize the woman in the mirror.

I applied for a planning role within the emergency department, allowing me to escape the relentless toll of night shifts. Though it brought relief, the disconnect lingered. My soul felt unfulfilled, as though I was being called toward something deeper—a path I couldn't yet define.

The turning point came one evening after a long hospital shift. Sitting in my car, exhausted and disconnected, I realized I could no longer keep pouring from an empty cup. The health care system felt like it was treating symptoms, not souls, and I was a part of it. In that moment before I started the ignition, I decided to find a different path. I was listening to my higHERself with a deep openness to change. Not merely a change in career but a change in the way I lived, breathed, and understood what true healing meant.

On the drive home, I made a commitment to my yoga practice. From that day forward, I became a regular student, showing up to the mat for both my body and my spirit. I dusted off my Ayurveda textbooks that had been sitting quietly on the shelves and vowed to deepen my understanding. I immersed myself in these Vedic sciences, guided by an undeniable calling telling me this was the way to internal freedom. I finally understood that my inner environment shaped my outer world, and if I wanted a different life, I had to begin by healing from within.

Through Ayurvedic wisdom, I healed my gut and balanced my hormones. I learned to recognize the interplay of my emotional and physical health. I'll share more about that process throughout this book, but for now, know that this journey reconnected me to a deeper purpose: to inspire, empower, and help others heal—not simply treat illness.

BLENDING EASTERN AND WESTERN MEDICINE

As I transitioned into my role as a yoga teacher and Ayurvedic practitioner, I wrestled with my identity again. Was I still a nurse? Did I have to choose between Eastern and Western medicine? Could I believe in the energy and spirituality of Ayurveda while respecting the science of my clinical training?

What I came to realize was this: there is space for both. My dharma isn't about choosing one or the other—it's about bridging the gap between the two, creating a holistic, nonjudgmental approach to health and wellness. I began to see how years of nursing shaped me, not just in hardship but in resilience and insight. My experiences in emergency rooms taught me compassion, even when it was buried beneath exhaustion. My training gave me the foundation to understand the human body, but Ayurveda expanded that understanding to include the mind and soul. I discovered that true healing is not about choosing between systems—it's about integration. Western medicine excels in acute care, lifesaving interventions, and scientific advancements, while Ayurveda offers profound wisdom on prevention, longevity, and the interconnectedness of body, mind, and spirit.

As I immersed myself in Ayurvedic scriptures and psychology, I realized that my role was not to abandon one for the other but to weave them together. I saw the gaps in both—how Western medicine often overlooks the root cause of disease and how Ayurveda lacks the immediacy needed in crisis care.

By blending the precision of Western diagnostics with the intuitive, root-cause healing of Ayurveda, I found my dharma—not as just a nurse, nor just an Ayurvedic practitioner, but as a bridge between the two. I now use my knowledge of both systems, helping others reclaim their health with the best of both worlds.

This path freed me from the need to fit into a single box.

Health is not black and white;
it's nuanced, dynamic, and deeply personal.

The more I embraced this truth, the more I realized that healing is not about following a rigid set of rules—it's about aligning with what serves the individual. And in that space of integration, I found my purpose.

The Second Spring:
Awakening to Your Power Years

The Second Spring, the "power years," is a time when a woman moves into a new season of her life—of deep wisdom and untapped potential. The Second Spring is an opportunity to realign, to nurture the fire of transformation while honoring the stability we seek. Through the lens of Ayurveda, a woman's power years is a period that offers realignment with Prakriti (natural constitution), reflection on Vikriti (current imbalances), and embrace of the full spectrum of feminine power.

THE JOURNEY OF LOSS AND REDISCOVERY

In my practice, I hear it often: "I don't know who I am anymore," and "I feel like I've lost part of myself." The fear of losing who they were collides with the quiet whisper of who they are becoming.

71

Stories of Rediscovery and Feminine Power

Through Ayurveda, I've had the privilege of guiding women back to themselves, helping them rediscover their essence and reclaim their feminine power.

ALYSSA'S STORY: DANCING FOR THE SOUL

Alyssa, a forty-seven-year-old corporate executive, arrived in my practice burned out and disconnected. Despite decades of success, she felt hollow and unsure what she truly wanted from life. Her relentless drive had taken a toll on her health, manifesting as a Vata imbalance—restlessness, fatigue, and inability to focus.

We began with grounding practices to restore balance: daily *Abhyanga* (oiled self-massage), mindfulness breathing, and nourishing foods. These small steps helped Alyssa slow down and reconnect with her inner world. As she gained clarity, long-forgotten passions began to surface.

"I always loved to dance" Alyssa told me. "I competed in dance competitions until I was seventeen years old. I would love to go back to dancing, not to compete but for fun, fitness and flexibility. But I feel silly—a forty-seven-year-old corporate lady rocking up to a dance studio."

"What's sillier: a women afraid of having fun and dancing or a *woman stepping into her highest expression of creativity while having fun, getting fit, and doing something for the soul?*" I replied.

"Well, when you put it like that..."

The rest was history. To my knowledge, Alyssa still attends dance fitness classes two times per week.

As adults we customarily believe everything we do should have an important outcome or result. We forget that honoring our soul and having fun are important parts of life.

Perhaps you are reading these words, secretly acknowledging that you, too, squashed the fun out of your life. If this is you, please find the courage to schedule in more fun into your life and bear witness to the soul expansion you encounter.

NINA'S STORY: REKINDLING FEMININE POWER

For Nina, a fifty-two-year-old mother of three, her sense of identity revolved around caregiving. As her youngest child prepared to leave for university, she felt a profound void. Without the daily demands of motherhood, Nina struggled to see her purpose.

Ayurvedic wisdom guided us to nurture her Kapha energy and rekindle her inner fire. Through self-reflective journaling, energizing breathwork, and movement practices, Nina began to explore who she was beyond the role of mum. She uncovered a dream she had long suppressed: becoming a yin yoga instructor. Nina attended a yin yoga class once a week and always thought that, one day, she would love to study further; she dreamed about guiding other women through a yin yoga class. Nina looked forward to this hour of bliss every week and credited her regular attendance to the class for her peaceful demeanour. Nina, a self-confessed romantic novel enthusiast once described it as, "Yin yoga is like reading a romance novel, only your body is doing the reading and your heart is falling in love over and over again in every class."

Pursuing that dream gave Nina a renewed sense of purpose—not as a caregiver, but as a mentor for other women. She embodied a new version of her feminine power, one that was both fierce and nurturing, allowing her to step into her next chapter with confidence and grace.

Practical Exercises for Reconnecting with Your Authentic Self

Rediscovering your identity doesn't require a complete reinvention. It begins with small, intentional practices that reconnect you to your core. Here are some tools to help:

JOURNALING PROMPTS FOR SELF-REFLECTION

Who am I when I am not fulfilling a role or meeting expectations?

_____

_____

_____

_____

_____

What activities, people, or experiences make me feel most alive?

_____

_____

_____

_____

_____

What have I let go of that I would like to bring back into my life?

_____

_____

_____

_____

_____

In what ways have I silenced my true self, and how can I begin to express it?

_____

_____

_____

_____

_____

What does it mean to me to live in alignment with my highest self?

_____

_____

_____

_____

_____

_____

_____

_____

_____

_____

MINDFULNESS TECHNIQUES FOR GROUNDING

+ **Breath awareness:** Spend five minutes each day focusing on your breath, noticing the sensations of each inhalation and exhalation. Let your breath anchor you in the present moment.

+ **Body scan meditation:** Lie comfortably and scan your body from head to toe, releasing tension in each area as you exhale.

DAILY RITUALS FOR RECONNECTION

✦ Morning ritual: Start your day with Abhyanga, using warm sesame oil to ground and nurture your body.

✦ Evening reflection: Before bed, write down one moment when you felt connected to yourself and one intention for tomorrow.

Honoring the Sacred Path

This journey of honoring your sacred path to self-healing, hormonal balance, empowerment, and dharmic alignment isn't about becoming someone new; it's about remembering who you've always been. Every role you've stepped into, every challenge you've overcome, and every dream you've dared to follow has shaped the wisdom you carry today.

Allow yourself to shed the outdated stories that no longer reflect your truth and step boldly into the woman you are becoming. In this evolution lies the power to live fully as your higHERself™, anchored in authenticity, purpose, and inner strength.

Reflection on Cycle Breaking

Breaking generational or personal cycles is a courageous act of self-liberation. Take a few moments to reflect:

1. What cycles, patterns, or beliefs have you witnessed or experienced in your family, culture, or personal life that you feel called to break?

_____

_____

_____

2. When you envision your future self, or future generations, how would life be different without these cycles?

    _____

    _____

    _____

3. What resources (wisdom, strengths, support systems) do you have to help you stay committed to your path of change?

    _____

    _____

    _____

    _____

4. Where can you show yourself more compassion as you do this deep, often uncomfortable work?

    _____

    _____

    _____

    _____

5. What does true freedom look like for you?

    _____

    _____

    _____

    _____

Remember, every small decision to choose differently plants a new seed for the future. You are the one your lineage has been waiting for.

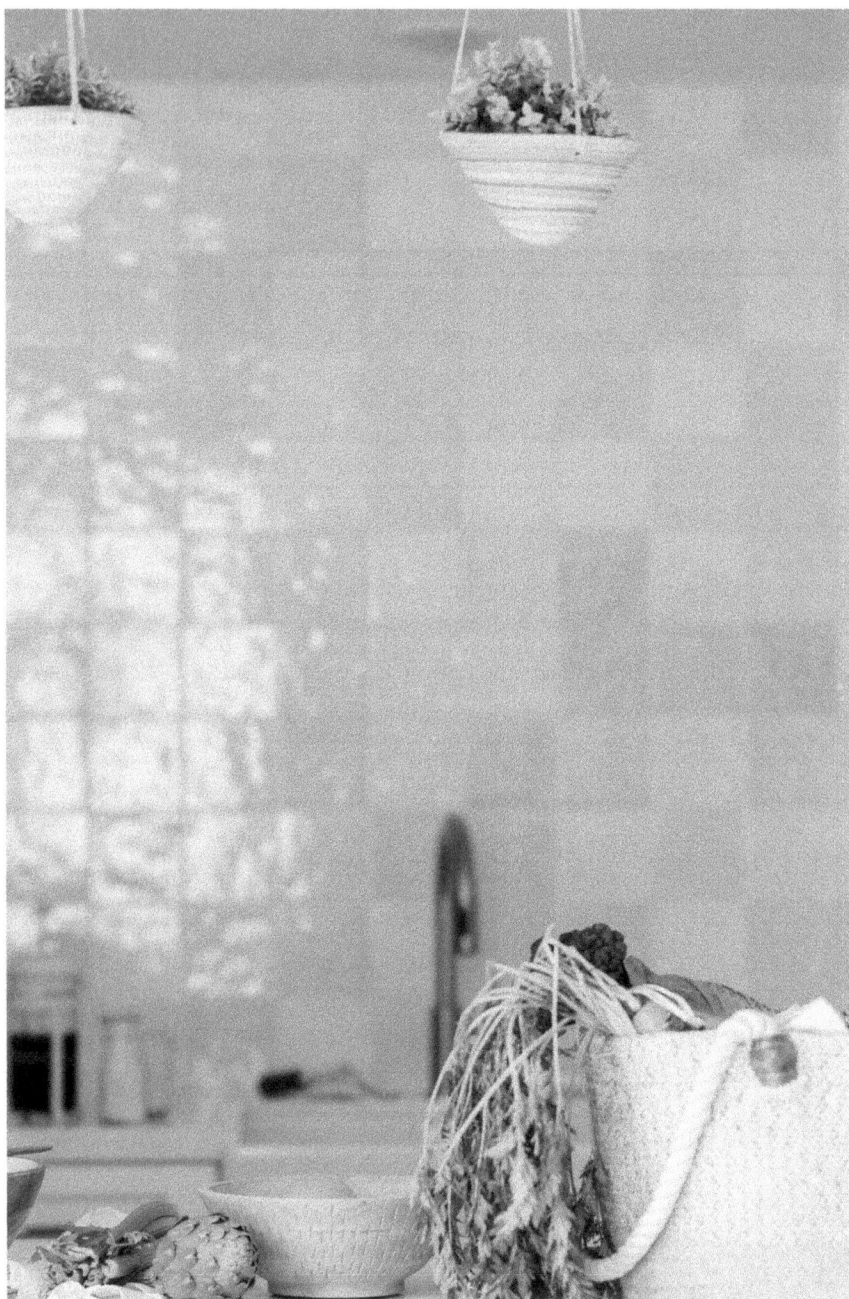

"WHEN THE DIET IS WRONG, MEDICINE IS OF NO USE. WHEN THE DIET IS RIGHT, MEDICINE IS OF NO NEED."
– AYURVEDIC PROVERB

PART 2

Health Alchemy

Integrating Ancient Wisdom and Modern Science for True Well-Being

Health is not a destination—it is a dynamic, ever-evolving relationship with your body, mind, emotions, spirit, and purpose. In this section, we step into the heart of the higHERself™ Method, the queen pillar, by exploring the multidimensional nature of well-being. Here, we bring together the best of Ayurveda, Traditional Chinese Medicine (TCM), and modern science to create a truly holistic approach to health.

This part of the journey is about integration—understanding how your biology, energy, and psychology are interconnected, and how working with natural rhythms unlocks deep healing and vitality. We explore the foundational pillars of health: physical balance, emotional regulation, mental clarity, spiritual connection, and dharmic alignment.

You will learn how your constitution, digestion, hormones, sleep, and nervous system work together, and how imbalances in one area ripple into others. We look at the concepts of *Agni*, the digestive fire, and *Ama*, the toxic residue that accumulates when we're out of sync with our true nature. You'll also discover how circadian rhythms, seasonal shifts, and ancient body clocks offer blueprints for living in flow rather than friction.

But this is more than a manual for healthy habits—it's a reclamation of health as a sacred, sovereign act. Women are taught to override their bodies, dismiss their symptoms, and ignore their intuition. Health Alchemy offers a different path—one that invites you to listen deeply, honor your inner wisdom, and become an active participant in your healing.

This is the space where ancient wisdom meets lived experience. Where clinical insight meets intuitive knowing. Where you remember that your health is not separate from your wholeness—it is a mirror of it.

Let's begin.

CHAPTER 5

Embodied Women and Layers of Physical, Emotional, and Spiritual Health

Health Alchemy is the queen pillar of the higHERself™ Method because it weaves through every aspect of our existence. It reminds us that true health is more than physical—it includes mental clarity, emotional harmony, spiritual connection, and dharmic alignment. When these elements are in balance, we thrive as whole, radiant beings.

Ayurveda teaches that health is a living, breathing state of balance, not a static condition. Over two thousand years ago, the Ayurvedic sage Sushruta beautifully articulated the definition of health in the *Sushruta Samhita*[1] that translates to balance in the doshas, optimal digestion, nourished tissues, efficient elimination, and a state of clarity and bliss in the mind and senses.

In this chapter, we'll journey through the five interconnected aspects of Health Alchemy—physical, mental, emotional, spiritual, and dharmic—offering tools to create alignment and step into your

---

1   Sushruta Samhita, Vol. 1, Sharma, P.V., 1998

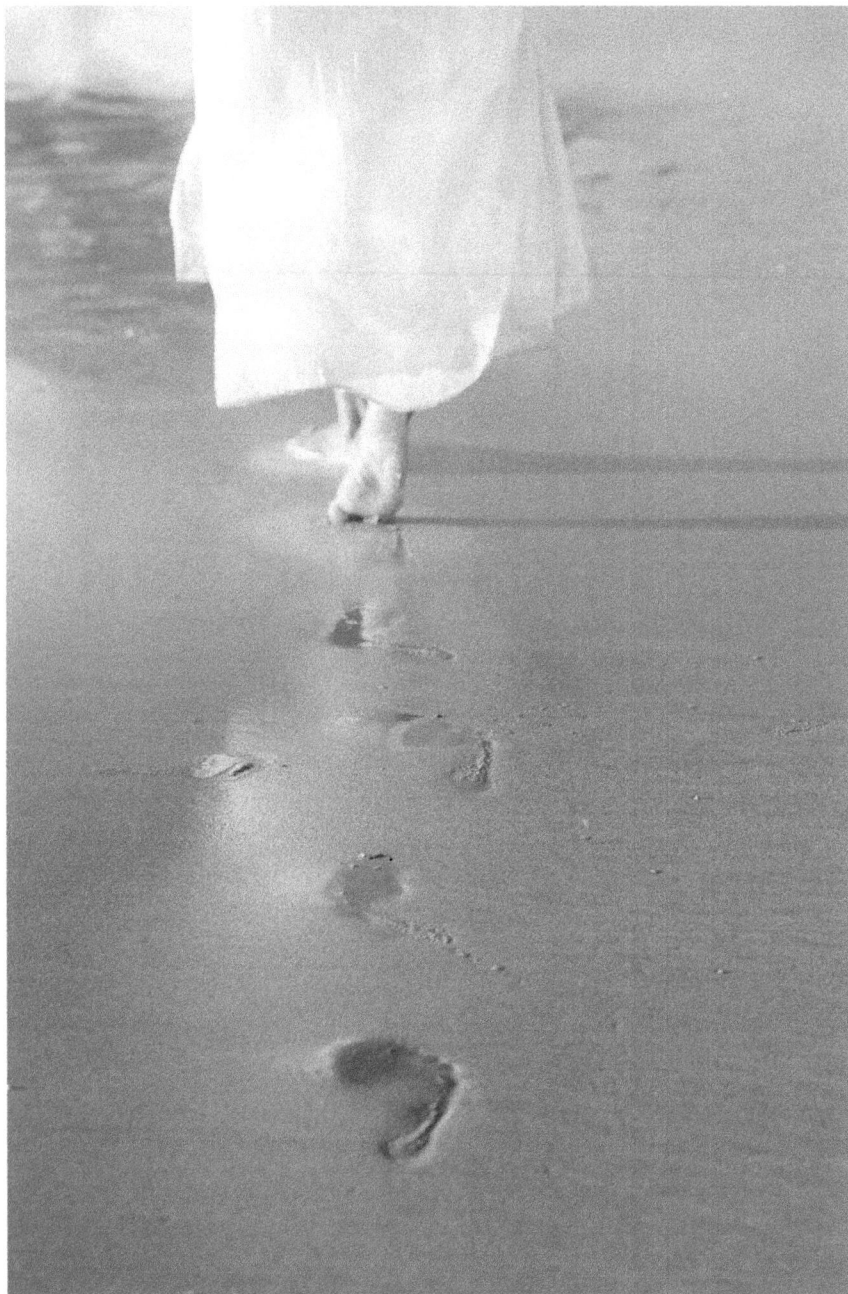

"YOUR BODY IS THE HOME OF YOUR SOUL. TREAT IT WITH
KINDNESS, NOURISH IT WITH WISDOM, AND IT WILL CARRY YOU
THROUGH LIFETIMES." – VEDIC WISDOM

highest self. Let's explore how each aspect shapes your well-being and how embracing these truths allows you to live a life of harmony, impact, and joy.

Physical Alchemy: The Foundation of Balance

Our health journey begins in the physical body; it's the vessel that carries us through life and anchors the other aspects of well-being. Ayurveda teaches that physical health is built upon the balance of the doshas and the strength of Agni, our digestive fire. A balanced Agni doesn't simply process food; it metabolises thoughts, emotions, and experiences, allowing us to thrive on every level.

Physical health is the gateway, providing energy to pursue our goals, care for loved ones, and cultivate joy. The key components of physical health include

+ hormonal balance during every stage of a woman's life

+ strategies to support strong digestion and metabolism

+ the role of movement and exercise in cultivating strength and vitality

+ the transformative power of *Dinacharya*, daily rituals that align us with nature's rhythms

This section is where you'll discover actionable tools and evidence-based insights that honor your unique needs. As we move deeper into this journey, remember that physical health doesn't exist in isolation; it's the soil from which mental clarity, emotional stability, spiritual connection, and dharmic purpose grow.

Mental Alchemy: Rewiring the Mind for Clarity and Peace

In Ayurveda, the mind, or *Manas*, is considered both a bridge and a battlefield. It is the bridge between the body and the soul, linking our physical experiences to our spiritual essence. Yet, it can also be the battlefield where imbalances play out, as conflicting emotions, desires, and doshic tendencies take center stage. Ayurvedic psychology reminds us that mental health isn't simply the absence of distress—it's the cultivation of Sattva, a state of purity and harmony, while minimizing the influences of Rajas (restlessness) and Tamas (inertia).

When the mind is out of balance, it is often dominated by doshic qualities.

+ Vata's airiness leads to anxiety, scattered thoughts, and sleeplessness.

+ Pitta's heat manifests as irritability, impatience, or perfectionism.

+ Kapha's heaviness creates lethargy, procrastination, and emotional stagnation.

True mental alchemy involves aligning the mind with Sattva, cultivating clarity, and transforming the inner narratives that no longer serve us.

TRUE STORY: MIA

One of my clients, Mia, came to me deeply affected by Vata imbalance. A mother of two in her late forties, she described herself as "a prisoner of her own mind." Chronic insomnia and a whirlwind of self-doubt left her feeling untethered, consumed by anxiety over everything from her parenting to her career. She felt caught in a cycle of restless thoughts, unable to find peace.

Ayurvedic psychology views Vata imbalance as the disruption of Prana Vayu, one of the subdoshas responsible for the movement of mental energy. This disruption causes thoughts to spiral, making the mind feel like a windstorm. To stabilize Vata, we focused on grounding her mind through small, consistent practices including the mantra meditation of "I am enough. I am whole." At first, it felt hollow, but over time, the repetition became an anchor, calming her restless mind and rewiring her self-belief. She also started taking *brahmi*, an ayurvedic herbal medicine known for soothing the nervous system and pacifying the mind.

As her Vata energy stabilized, Mia began to experience a sense of rootedness. The sleepless nights gave way to restful slumber, and her inner critic softened, replaced by a quiet confidence.

MANAS: THE MIND AS THE CHARIOTEER

In the Bhagavad Gita, the mind is compared to the charioteer steering the horses of our senses. When the charioteer is steady and focused, the journey is smooth, and we stay on the path toward our higher self. But when the charioteer is distracted or overwhelmed, the horses run wild, dragging us in directions that lead to imbalance and suffering.

Ayurvedic psychology identifies three key mind functions:

+ **Dhi (intellect):** The ability to discern truth and make wise decisions

+ **Dhriti (willpower):** The strength to follow through on decisions

+ **Smriti (memory):** The capacity to remember what is meaningful and aligned with our higher self

When the mind is dominated by Rajas or Tamas, these functions become clouded. Rajas creates restlessness and impulsivity, while Tamas leads to forgetfulness and inertia. But when Sattva is cultivated, the mind becomes clear, focused, and aligned with the truth of who we are.

The Vedic perspective on rewiring the mind is echoed by modern neuroscience. Studies show that affirmations and mindfulness practices can rewire the brain through neuroplasticity, the brain's ability to form new neural pathways. Just as Mia's mantra practice helped shift her inner narrative, consistently choosing thoughts that align with Sattva can reshape our mental landscape.

As Dr. Joe Dispenza, a leading expert on neuroscience and meditation, says, "Where you place your attention is where you place your energy. If you focus on lack, you create lack. If you focus on wholeness, you create wholeness."

REFLECTIONS FOR MENTAL ALCHEMY

Ask yourself: What stories do I tell myself about who I am? Are they rooted in fear, or do they reflect love and possibility? How can I nurture Sattva in my daily life?

The mind is like a lotus flower, as Vedic wisdom teaches: it blooms when nurtured by the waters of truth and intention. Through mental alchemy, we can rewrite the narrative, transforming the mind from a restless critic into a steady ally that guides us toward clarity, peace, and our highest self.

Emotional Alchemy: Honoring and Transforming Feelings

Our emotions are not enemies to be conquered but messengers to be honored. Ayurveda views emotions as energies tied to the doshas: fear with Vata, anger with Pitta, and sadness with Kapha. Resisting these feelings only deepens imbalance, while honoring them creates space for healing.

I was twenty-one when I first sat before a Buddhist monk in Thailand, hanging on every word he spoke. He shared a simple yet profound truth that I had never heard before: "Clouds may cover the sky, but they never change the presence of the sun." At the time, it was a completely new perspective for me, but over the years, I've heard variations of this wisdom repeated by different teachers and thought leaders. And it's true—not just for the sky, but for emotional storms too. No matter how dark or intense the moment feels, clarity and light are always there, waiting for the clouds to pass.

As I write this, I'm preparing for Cyclone Alfred, which has been dominating the news. We've been warned to expect the worst, to prepare for impact. While I've never experienced a cyclone before, and I've done all I can to be ready, I'm surprised by how calm I feel. Maybe it's because I know that, like all storms—both in the sky and within ourselves—this, too, shall pass.

But when I do find myself in darkness, when my mind feels heavy and hope seems distant, I whisper to myself, "Tomorrow, there could be a rainbow." It's a quiet reminder that no feeling lasts forever, that light and color always find their way back.

Tomorrow, there could be a rainbow.

I started saying this after a colleague of mine took her own life. In the days leading up to her funeral, the sky was gray, the rain relentless. It felt as if the world itself was mourning. The day of her funeral was heavy—dark, filled with grief.

But the next morning, the rain cleared. Two rainbows stretched across the sky. One had the deepest shade of purple, her favourite color. It was breathtaking. I remember thinking, "If only she had waited one more day, she could have seen this magic, and witnessing the beauty around her may have changed her life trajectory; it may not have ended so abruptly."

I know mental health is not that simple. I know pain can feel endless. But that moment stayed with me. Ever since, when I feel lost in the storm, I remind myself—tomorrow, there could be a rainbow. Sometimes, just that thought is enough to hold on.

When Rachel, a client reeling from a painful divorce, came to me, she felt buried in anger and sadness. I encouraged her to write letters to herself, giving voice to both her pain and her resilience. She wrote, "Even in heartbreak, I am whole." Over time, Rachel transformed her grief into strength, realizing her emotions were not obstacles but guides.

Honor your emotions. Allow them to move through you like the clouds, carrying wisdom and release. Anger sets boundaries. Sadness invites rest. Joy reminds us of life's beauty. By embracing emotional alchemy, we heal from within.

Spiritual Alchemy:
Connecting to the Divine Within

True health transcends the physical—it's about your connection to the eternal self, or *Purusha. In Ayurveda, Purusha is the divine essence within each of us, the part untouched by fear, failure, or even success.*

Connecting to this essence aligns us with something greater, offering clarity and strength.

I am reminded of a Hindu parable about a musk deer. The deer spends its life chasing a beautiful scent, not realising the fragrance comes from its own navel. Like the musk deer, we often seek fulfillment outside ourselves, forgetting that everything we long for already exists within.

In my own life, spiritual alchemy became a daily ritual through meditation and mantra. As challenges arose, I asked myself, "What am I seeking externally that I can find within?" This practice grounded me in my truth, reminding me that the sanctuary of my soul is unshaken, no matter what chaos surrounds me.

Start your day with a simple mantra:

"I am light. I am love. I am whole."

Let it anchor you in the wisdom that your spirit is infinite, divine, and always aligned.

Dharmic Alchemy: Living in Alignment with Truth

Dharma is more than a "life purpose." It's about living in alignment with universal truth—acting with integrity, compassion, and intentionality in everything you do, from grand endeavors to everyday tasks. Your dharma is the unique role you play in the cosmic order, the gifts you were born to share.

Lara, a client in her forties, had spent years climbing the corporate ladder, only to feel empty at the top. Her job was high-paying, prestigious, and demanding—everything she had once believed would bring her fulfillment.

Yet, despite her success, she felt disconnected, as if something essential was missing.

When we explored her dosha and life path, it became clear that Lara was out of alignment with her dharma. She had always been passionate about mentorship and personal growth, but in the relentless pursuit of professional achievement, she lost touch with that part of herself. Through self-inquiry and Ayurvedic practices, she began making subtle but powerful shifts—infusing meaning into her work, mentoring younger colleagues, and fostering a culture of mindfulness in her team. Rather than leaving the corporate world, she redefined her role within it. She introduced wellness initiatives at her company, led workshops on stress management, and integrated

Ayurvedic wisdom into her leadership style. What once felt like a soulless grind became a space where she could uplift others.

Lara later told me:

"I used to think my job was the problem.
But it wasn't about quitting—it was about
bringing more of myself into what I do."

Dharma isn't about abandoning your life to chase something new; it's about bringing your truth into the life you already have. When you align with your deeper purpose, fulfillment isn't something you search for—it's something you create.

The Path to Wholeness

Health Alchemy is not about perfection—it's about integration. It's about embracing all parts of yourself—the messy, the beautiful, the wounded, and the divine—and weaving them into a complex truth. Like gold refined by fire, each challenge shapes you into your most radiant self.

Ask yourself: How can I nurture my physical body, quiet my mind, honor my emotions, connect with my spirit, and align with my dharma today? Each step brings you closer to your higHERself™— the most aligned, empowered version of you.

This is your time to rise. You are not broken. You are becoming.

Reflection on Embodying
the Layers of Health

Take a moment to tune inward and reflect on how each layer of your health is currently expressing itself. Use these prompts to guide your self-inquiry:

PHYSICAL HEALTH

1. How does my body feel most days—energized, heavy, vibrant, or depleted?

_____

_____

_____

_____

_____

_____

_____

2. What daily practices nourish and support my physical body?

_____

_____

_____

_____

_____

_____

EMOTIONAL HEALTH

1. What emotions am I holding onto that may need acknowledgment or release?

_____

_____

_____

_____

_____

2. How do I allow myself to process and express emotions in a healthy way?

_____

_____

_____

_____

_____

MENTAL HEALTH

1. Are my thoughts generally supportive, clear, and focused—or scattered, critical, and draining?

_____

_____

_____

_____

_____

_____

2. What beliefs or thought patterns could I shift to cultivate a more empowered mindset?

_____

_____

_____

_____

_____

_____

SPIRITUAL HEALTH

1. In what ways do I currently nurture my connection to something greater than myself (whether through nature, prayer, meditation, or ritual)?

_____

_____

_____

_____

_____

2. How often do I pause to listen to my intuition or inner guidance?

_____

_____

_____

_____

_____

_____

DHARMIC (PURPOSE-DRIVEN) HEALTH

1. Do my daily actions feel aligned with my deepest values and purpose?

_____

_____

_____

_____

_____

_____

2. What small step can I take this week to move closer to living in greater alignment with my dharma?

_____

_____

_____

_____

_____

_____

_____

Integration: After reflecting, choose *one* small action or ritual to strengthen an area where you feel out of balance. Embodying your health is not about perfection—it's about presence, awareness, and intentional living.

CHAPTER 6

The Elements and the Doshas

A Deep Dive into the Foundations of Health

To truly understand your body, mind, and spirit through Ayurveda, it is essential to explore the foundational principles of the five elements (*Pancha Mahabhutas*) and the three doshas. These elements—ether (space), air, fire, water, and earth—form the universal building blocks of everything, including us. The doshas—Vata, Pitta, and Kapha—are dynamic combinations of these elements that govern all physiological and psychological functions.

This section will take you on an in-depth exploration of the doshas, their subdoshas, and the subtle energies that underpin them. By understanding these principles, you'll not only be able to identify your unique constitution (Prakriti) but also learn how to maintain balance and harmony throughout your life.

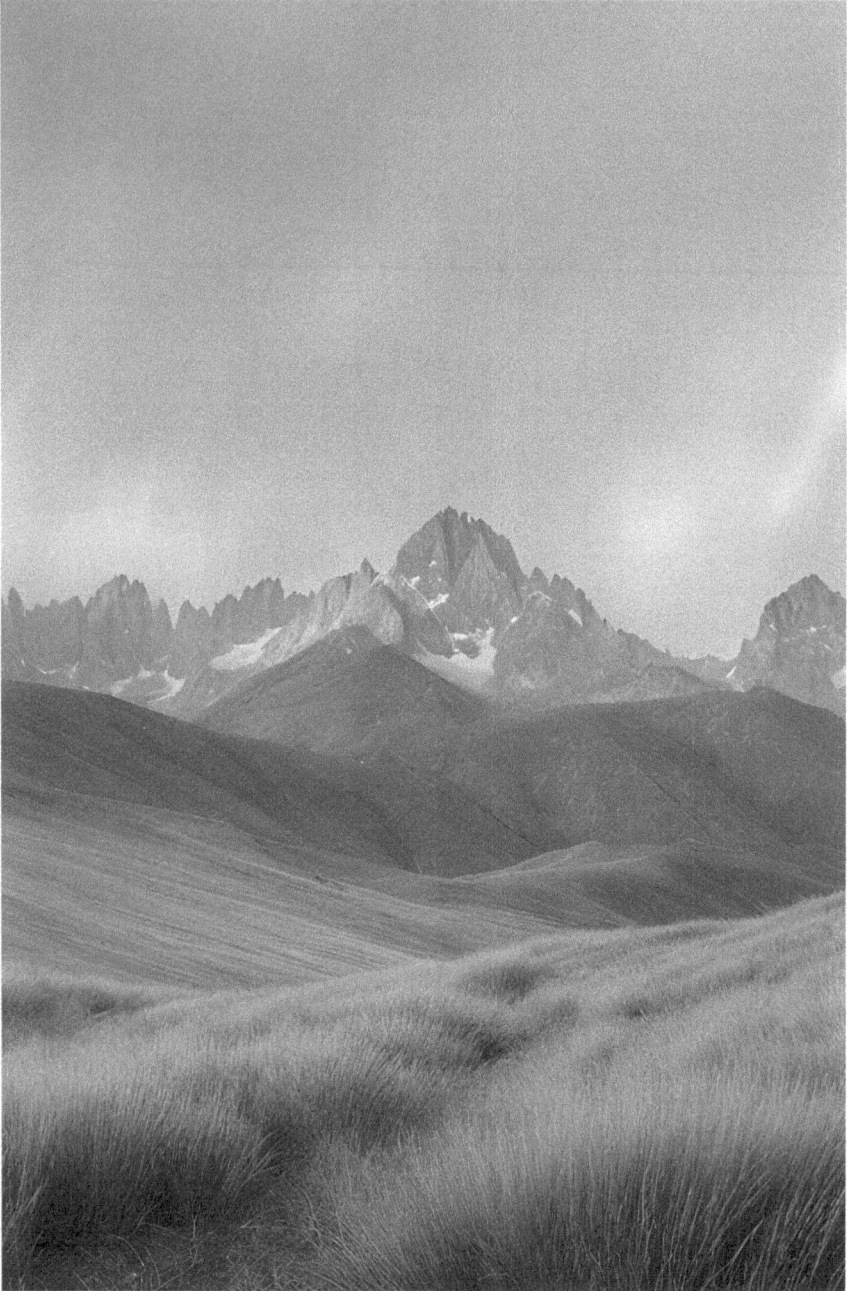

"NATURE DOES NOT HURRY, YET EVERYTHING IS
ACCOMPLISHED." – LAO TZU

The Five Elements (Pancha Mahabhutas)

In Ayurveda, everything in existence—including the human body and mind—is composed of five foundational elements known as the Pancha Mahabhutas: ether, air, fire, water, and earth. Each element not only governs physiological functions but also shapes psychological tendencies.

1. ETHER (AKASHA)

+ **Physiological role:** Ether represents space—the subtle container within which all bodily structures and processes exist. It is present in hollow spaces like the respiratory tract, digestive system, and cellular channels.

+ **Psychological influence:** A strong ether element supports intuition, expansive thinking, and creativity. When imbalanced, it may manifest as disconnection, feeling "spaced out," or difficulty focusing.

2. AIR (VAYU)

+ **Physiological role:** Air governs movement within the body, including the circulation of blood, movement of muscles, nerve impulses, and respiratory function.

+ **Psychological influence:** A healthy air element fosters flexibility, adaptability, and quick thinking. When aggravated, it can cause anxiety, restlessness, or overactive thoughts.

3. FIRE (AGNI/TEJAS)

+ **Physiological role:** Fire controls transformation and metabolism, including digestion, nutrient assimilation, and temperature regulation.

✦ **Psychological influence:** Balanced fire supports intelligence, ambition, and clarity. Excess fire can lead to irritability, impatience, and critical thinking, while deficient fire may show up as lack of motivation or dullness.

4. WATER (JALA)

✦ **Physiological role:** Water provides lubrication, cohesion, and nourishment, seen in bodily fluids like plasma, lymph, and mucus.

✦ **Psychological influence:** Water nurtures emotional depth, compassion, and connection. Imbalance may show up as emotional dependency, attachment, or lethargy.

5. EARTH (PRITHVI)

✦ **Physiological role:** Earth gives form, structure, and stability to the body, evident in the bones, muscles, skin, and tissues.

✦ **Psychological influence:** Strong earth energy brings groundedness, patience, and resilience. However, excess earth can manifest as stubbornness, resistance to change, or emotional heaviness.

The Three Doshas: Vata, Pitta, and Kapha

The doshas are dynamic energies that result from elemental interplay. Each dosha has its unique qualities, functions, and tendencies, influencing our physical, mental, and emotional health.

1. VATA DOSHA (ETHER + AIR)

✦ **Qualities:** Light, dry, cold, rough, mobile, subtle, clear

✦ **Primary functions:** Governs movement, communication, and circulation; controls the nervous system, respiration, and elimination

+ **Imbalances:** Anxiety, dryness, constipation, insomnia, restlessness
+ **Balanced state:** Creativity, flexibility, clarity, vitality
+ **Key to balance:** Grounding, warmth, stability, routine

2. PITTA DOSHA (FIRE + WATER)

+ **Qualities:** Hot, sharp, oily, light, intense, spreading, acidic
+ **Primary functions:** Governs digestion, metabolism, and transformation; oversees body temperature, vision, and hormonal balance
+ **Imbalances:** Anger, inflammation, acidity, skin rashes, irritability
+ **Balanced state:** Intelligence, courage, focus, leadership
+ **Key to balance:** Cooling, soothing, moderation

3. KAPHA DOSHA (WATER + EARTH)

+ **Qualities:** Heavy, slow, steady, cold, oily, smooth, dense
+ **Primary functions:** Provides structure, stability, lubrication; governs immunity, growth, and emotional stability
+ **Imbalances:** Lethargy, weight gain, congestion, depression
+ **Balanced state:** Compassion, patience, strength, resilience
+ **Key to balance:** Stimulation, lightness, warmth, movement

The Subdoshas: A Detailed Exploration

Each dosha is further divided into five subdoshas, which govern specific areas and functions in the body. Understanding the subdoshas adds a vital layer of nuance to your self-awareness. While the primary doshas give us a broad picture, the subdoshas explain the finer details—how your body breathes, digests, circulates, eliminates, expresses, and perceives. By recognizing which of these systems might be out of balance, you can take targeted steps to restore harmony in specific areas of your health.

As you continue reading this book, you'll notice how these subdoshas influence various aspects of your well-being—whether it's hormone health, emotional resilience, digestive function, or energy levels. Keep this framework in mind as you explore the practices, rituals, and lifestyle shifts that follow. It will help you personalize your journey, fine-tune your habits, and ultimately move toward greater alignment with your higHERself™.

VATA SUBDOSHAS

1. **Prana Vayu:** Governs inhalation, sensory perception, and mental clarity. Located in the head and chest.

2. **Udana Vayu:** Controls speech, expression, and upward movement of energy. Located in the chest and throat.

3. **Samana Vayu:** Governs digestion and absorption of nutrients. Located in the stomach and intestines.

4. **Apana Vayu:** Controls elimination, reproduction, birth, and downward energy flow. Located in the lower abdomen.

5. **Vyana Vayu:** Governs circulation and movement throughout the body. Located in the heart and circulatory system.

PITTA SUBDOSHAS

1. **Pachaka Pitta:** Responsible for digestion and metabolism in the stomach.

2. **Ranjaka Pitta:** Governs the production of red blood cells in the liver and spleen.

3. **Sadhaka Pitta:** Influences mental clarity, emotions, and memory. Located in the heart and brain.

4. **Alochaka Pitta:** Governs vision and perception in the eyes.

5. **Bhrajaka Pitta:** Responsible for skin health and complexion.

KAPHA SUBDOSHAS

1. **Kledaka Kapha:** Lubricates the stomach lining and aids digestion.

2. **Avalambaka Kapha:** Provides structural support in the chest, heart, and lungs.

3. **Bodhaka Kapha:** Governs taste and lubrication in the mouth.

4. **Tarpaka Kapha:** Nourishes the brain and cerebrospinal fluid.

5. **Shleshaka Kapha:** Lubricates the joints and maintains flexibility.

Dosha	Subdosha	Location	Function
Vata	Prana Vayu	Head, chest	*Inhalation, sensory input, mental clarity*
	Udana Vayu	Throat, chest	*Speech, self-expression, upward energy*
	Samana Vayu	Stomach, intestines	*Digestion, assimilation*
	Apana Vayu	Lower abdomen	*Elimination, reproduction, downward movement*
	Vyana Vayu	Heart, entire body	*Circulation, overall bodily movement*
Pitta	Pachaka Pitta	Stomach, small intestine	*Digestion, metabolism*
	Ranjaka Pitta	Liver, spleen	*Blood formation*
	Sadhaka Pitta	Brain, heart	*Emotions, clarity, memory*
	Alochaka Pitta	Eyes	*Vision, perception*
	Bhrajaka Pitta	Skin	*Skin metabolism, complexion*
Kapha	Kledaka Kapha	Stomach	*Lubricates stomach, aids digestion*
	Avalambaka Kapha	Chest, lungs, heart	*Supports respiration, structure, emotional holding*
	Bodhaka Kapha	Mouth, tongue	*Taste perception, oral moisture*
	Tarpaka Kapha	Head, cerebrospinal fluid	*Nourishes brain, emotional stability*
	Shleshaka Kapha	Joints	*Lubrication, joint flexibility*

The Subtle Energies of the Doshas

While the doshas govern physical and physiological functions in the body, Ayurveda also recognizes their refined, energetic expressions. These subtle energies (*Prana*, *Tejas*, and *Ojas*) are essential to our vitality, intuition, immunity, and inner strength. They serve as a bridge between the body and the mind, the mind and the spirit, helping us experience balance and wholeness on all levels of being.

Cultivating and protecting these subtle forces is as important as balancing the doshas themselves. They are the deeper essences that fuel emotional clarity, spiritual growth, and resilience in the face of life's challenges.

1. **Prana (Life Force):** Associated with Vata, it governs energy flow, inspiration, and intuition. Prana connects the physical and spiritual planes.

2. **Tejas (Inner Radiance):** Associated with Pitta, it represents intelligence, courage, and the transformative power of fire.

3. **Ojas (Vital Essence):** Associated with Kapha, it embodies vitality, immunity, and spiritual strength. Ojas is the essence of life, providing a sense of grounding and resilience.

Subtle Energy	Associated Dosha	Primary Qualities	Role & Influence
Prana	Vata	Vitality, energy flow, inspiration, Intuition	*Governs breath, life force, mental clarity, and spiritual connection*
Tejas	Pitta	Radiance, intelligence, transformation, courage	*Fuels mental acuity, digestion of experiences, and inner drive*
Ojas	Kapha	Immunity, stability, strength, contentment	*Nourishes tissues, strengthens immunity, provides emotional resilience and calm*

AYURVEDA & THE ALCHEMY OF HER

How to Identify and Balance Your Doshas

Your dosha (Prakriti) is your original constitution, while your Vikriti represents any current imbalance. Understanding both can help you live in alignment with your true nature and correct patterns that lead to dis-ease. There are several ways to begin exploring your doshic blueprint.

1. OBSERVATION

Start by reflecting on your physical, emotional, and mental tendencies. What qualities consistently show up for you; are you dry and anxious, sharp and intense, or heavy and lethargic? Dedicate five to ten minutes each morning to stillness or meditation. Observe how your body feels, where your energy is, and what your dominant emotions are. Follow this with a short journaling session to track patterns over time. This daily check-in helps you become witness to your own tendencies, rather than being ruled by them.

2. CONSULTATION

While self-awareness is powerful, working with an Ayurvedic practitioner allows for a deeper and more accurate diagnosis through tools like pulse reading, tongue analysis, and a detailed lifestyle review. A practitioner can help you uncover subtle imbalances that may not be obvious and offer personalized strategies for bringing your doshas into balance. Please remember that this book is informational; for proper herbal prescription, please see your practitioner as herbal medicine can be very powerful.

3. QUESTIONNAIRES

Online dosha quizzes, like the one I've created at **https://www. harmonyinspiredhealth.com.au/freebies**, can give you a general idea of your Vikriti. Use these as a starting point, not a final answer. Combine quiz results with observation and practitioner insight for a holistic picture.

Once you have a better understanding of your doshic profile, balancing your constitution can be done through the following foundational practices.

4. DIET

Eat with your dosha in mind. If you're Vata, favor warm, oily, grounding foods like soups and root vegetables. If you're Pitta, choose cooling, hydrating meals with bitter greens and herbs. Kapha types benefit from light, spicy foods that stimulate digestion.

5. LIFESTYLE

Match your routines to your doshic needs. Vata types do best with regularity and grounding rituals. Pitta types benefit from cooling breathwork and time in nature to unwind. Kapha types thrive on stimulation—dynamic movement, uplifting music, and a variety of experiences can keep energy flowing.

6. HERBS

Herbs can powerfully support doshic balance when used properly. For example, ashwagandha helps stabilize Vata, neem can cool excess Pitta, and Triphala gently detoxifies Kapha. Always consult a qualified practitioner before starting herbal protocols, as herbs are potent medicine.

These small but intentional shifts create powerful ripple effects. The more you understand your doshic nature, the more equipped you are to respond to your body's needs with compassion and wisdom.

Dosha	Key Qualities	Signs of Imbalance	Supportive Foods	Supportive Lifestyle	Helpful Herbs
Vata (Air + Ether)	Cold, dry, light, mobile	Anxiety, insomnia, dry skin, bloating, constipation	Warm, moist, grounding foods: root vegetables, ghee, oats, cooked grains	Consistent routine, gentle movement (yoga, walking), meditation	Ashwagandha, shatavari, licorice, triphala, hing, shankapushpi and jatamansi
Pitta (Fire + Water)	Hot, sharp, intense, oily	Irritability, acne, acid reflux, inflammation	Cooling, hydrating foods: cucumber, mint, coconut, leafy greens	Cooling activities, time in nature, regular breaks, journaling	Brahmi, neem, amalaki, shatavari, licorice, manjistha and guduchi
Kapha (Earth + Water)	Heavy, stable, slow, moist	Lethargy, weight gain, congestion, depression	Light, spicy, dry foods: lentils, ginger, bitter greens, apples	Dynamic movement, variety, upbeat music, early rising	Triphala, ginger, tulsi, guggulu, Moringa, gurmar and trikatu

Reflection on Your Doshas

Use these prompts to integrate what you've learned and begin applying it to your daily life.

1. What physical or emotional patterns show up for you most often? Are they aligned with a specific dosha?

_____

_____

_____

_____

2. Which doshic imbalance (listed earlier) resonates with how you currently feel?

_____

_____

_____

_____

_____

_____

_____

_____

_____

3. What are three lifestyle or food choices you could shift this week to better support your balance?

_____

_____

_____

_____

_____

_____

_____

_____

_____

4. Have you ever noticed how your energy changes with the seasons or time of day? How might that relate to your doshic tendencies?

_____

_____

_____

_____

_____

_____

_____

_____

_____

5. What small daily ritual could you begin (or return to) that brings your mind and body into harmony?

_____

_____

_____

_____

_____

_____

_____

_____

_____

CHAPTER 7

Kapha, My Friend; Vata, My Adventerer; Pitta, My Fearless Leader

Observing the dynamics of my friends and family through the lens of the doshas has become one of my favorite pastimes. It's fascinating to see how our individual constitutions shape not only who we are but also how we interact with one another. Even my twin boys, despite sharing the same womb and upbringing, have such distinct doshic imprints—one leans strongly toward Pitta-Kapha, grounded and determined, while the other is unmistakably Vata, brimming with creativity and restlessness.

This awareness of doshic interplay extends to my friendships. When my business bestie and I meet up for a chai, we've learned to embrace the fact that we ignite the Pitta dosha in each other. Without fail, our conversations evolve into strategic brainstorming sessions, whether we're planning events, mapping out new projects, or sharing insights for our lives. Over time, we've come to expect this synergy. Now, we always show up with a notebook and pen in hand, ready to capture the inspiration that inevitably flows when our Pitta energy blends.

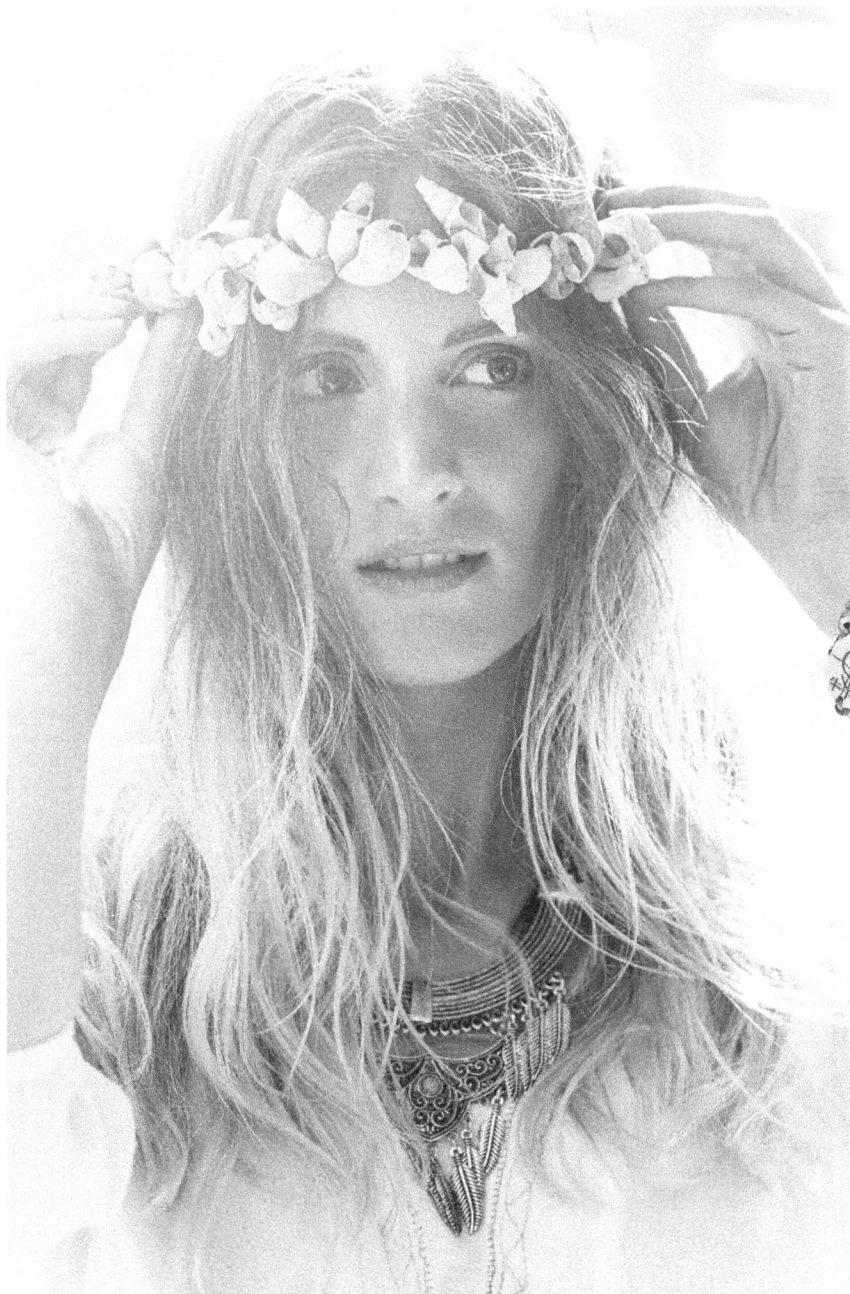

"BALANCE IS NOT SOMETHING YOU FIND, IT'S SOMETHING YOU CREATE." – JANA KINGSFORD

Doshas not only influence who we are as individuals but also how we elevate and complement each other in connection.

To truly grasp the essence of Vata, Pitta, and Kapha doshas, let's bring them to life through the lens of a relatable friendship group. Picture three women—Emma, Priya, and Lily—each embodying the qualities of one dosha.

Their personalities, work styles, relationships, and even their social habits illustrate how the doshas express themselves in the real world.

Vata: Emma, the Creative Dreamer

Emma walks into a café, her flowy boho dress trailing behind her, and immediately lights up the room with her bubbly, slightly erratic energy. She's the kind of person who talks with her hands, jumps from one topic to the next, and always has a dozen creative ideas brewing.

Work Style

Emma is a freelance writer and artist who thrives on variety. Sitting at a desk from nine to five would drain her completely, so she hops between projects, juggling a blog, her painting commissions, and a side hustle as a yoga teacher. Deadlines can be challenging because she tends to get distracted by new ideas before finishing the ones she's started.

Social Personality

As a Vata-dominant friend, Emma brings spontaneity to the group. She's the one texting, "Let's drive to the beach at sunrise!" or organizing a last-minute road trip. But if she's feeling unbalanced—too much movement or irregularity in her life—she can become forgetful, cancel plans, or feel overwhelmed by anxiety.

Desires and Relationships

Emma craves freedom and creativity in her relationships. She loves the excitement of new connections but struggles with commitment, fearing it might limit her independence. When she falls in love, it's with someone who fuels her curiosity and shares her thirst for adventure.

Balancing Vata

When Emma feels scattered or anxious, she turns to grounding practices like daily Abhyanga (self-massage with warm oil) or restorative yoga. She's learning to prioritize routine—something that doesn't come naturally to her Vata nature—by scheduling consistent mealtimes and limiting late nights.

Pitta: Priya, the Fiery Go-Getter

Priya strides into the room with purpose, her tailored blazer a reflection of her sharp, focused personality. She's the friend who's always on time, has a detailed plan for every outing, and isn't afraid to call out bad service at a restaurant.

Work Style

As a lawyer at a top firm, Priya thrives on challenges and ambition. She sets high goals and achieves them with laser focus, often climbing the corporate ladder faster than her peers. Her Pitta nature means she's an exceptional leader, but when stressed, she can become overly critical or competitive, holding others—and herself—to impossible standards.

Social Personality

Priya is the group organizer. If there's a birthday dinner or a holiday to plan, she's the one making reservations and ensuring every detail is perfect. Her fiery personality makes her loyal and protective of her friends, but it can also lead to heated debates if she feels strongly about an issue.

Desires and Relationships

In relationships, Priya is passionate and deeply committed. She values a partner who matches her drive and ambition but has learned over the years that relationships aren't projects to be managed—they require softness and balance.

Balancing Pitta

To cool her fiery nature, Priya loves moonlit walks on the beach and sips on cooling teas like peppermint or fennel. She's learning to embrace imperfection by stepping away from work at sunset and taking weekends to unwind in nature.

Kapha: Lily, the Nurturing Anchor

Lily arrives at the café fifteen minutes late, having baked cookies for everyone because she "felt like it." Her warm smile and calming presence immediately make people feel at ease. She's the friend who remembers birthdays, checks in when you're sick, and brings emotional stability to the group.

Work Style

As a teacher, Lily finds joy in nurturing others. She's patient and reliable, the type of person her students adore for her gentle guidance. Unlike Emma, she thrives in a steady routine and doesn't mind repetition—structure feels comforting to her Kapha nature.

Social Personality

Lily is the group listener, always offering thoughtful advice and a shoulder to cry on. She prefers cozy one-on-one chats to big parties but will show up to support her friends. However, if her Kapha becomes imbalanced, she might withdraw, struggling with feelings of heaviness or lethargy.

Desires and Relationships

Lily's nurturing nature makes her a deeply loyal and affectionate partner. She values emotional security and looks for a relationship that feels stable and supportive. However, she has to be careful not to over-give or lose herself in caregiving.

Balancing Kapha

When Lily feels stuck or sluggish, she incorporates energizing practices like brisk morning walks or spicy ginger tea to boost her circulation. She's learning to embrace change by trying new activities and stepping out of her comfort zone.

The Friendship Dynamic

Together, Emma, Priya, and Lily create a beautifully balanced friendship. Emma's creative spontaneity inspires Priya and Lily to step out of their routines, while Priya's drive motivates Emma and Lily to stay focused on their goals. Lily's grounding presence softens Priya's intensity and helps Emma find stability when she feels scattered.

However, when imbalances arise, their differences can create tension.

✦ If Emma cancels plans last minute, Priya's Pitta might flare, and Lily might feel unappreciated.

✦ Priya's perfectionism can overwhelm Emma, who dislikes

pressure, or Lily, who prefers a slower pace.

✦ Lily's tendency to withdraw during heavy emotions might leave Priya frustrated or Emma feeling unsupported.

By understanding their doshas, they've learned to navigate these differences with compassion. Emma knows to follow through on commitments, Priya has softened her need for control, and Lily has embraced speaking up about her needs.

The Subtle Energies: Prana, Tejas, and Ojas

Beyond their physical traits, the three friends embody the subtle dosha energies.

✦ Emma's Prana (life force) fuels her creativity and excitement for new ideas, but when unbalanced, it leads to anxiety or exhaustion.

✦ Priya's Tejas (inner radiance) drives her ambition and intelligence, but excess Tejas can manifest as burnout or anger.

✦ Lily's Ojas (vital essence) gives her a nurturing, grounded energy, but depleted Ojas can make her feel heavy, unwell, or stagnant.

By embracing practices to balance their doshas and subtle energies, Emma, Priya, and Lily are able to live in alignment with their true selves while maintaining harmony within their friendship.

Reflection on Kapha, Vata, and Pitta in Relationships

Each dosha not only shapes your physical and emotional tendencies but also deeply influences how you relate to others. Use the prompts below to reflect on your dominant dosha(s) and how they show up in your relationships—with partners, children, friends, and colleagues.

KAPHA REFLECTION

1. In what ways do I show up as nurturing, loyal, or dependable in my relationships?

    _____

    _____

    _____

2. Do I tend to hold on to relationships or emotions longer than necessary?

    _____

    _____

    _____

    _____

3. Am I resistant to change or avoid difficult conversations to "keep the peace"?

    _____

    _____

    _____

    _____

4. Where might I be over-giving or neglecting my own needs?

    _____

    _____

    _____

    _____

    _____

VATA REFLECTION

1. Do I communicate with spontaneity and creativity, or do I become inconsistent or distracted?

_____

_____

_____

_____

2. How does anxiety or overstimulation affect the way I listen or respond to others?

_____

_____

_____

_____

3. Do I find it hard to stay grounded in long-term relationships or commitments?

_____

_____

_____

_____

4. Where might I need to create more stability in how I show up for others?

_____

_____

_____

_____

PITTA REFLECTION

1. Do I bring clarity, leadership, and focus into my relationships?

_____

_____

_____

_____

2. When under stress, do I become impatient, critical, or controlling in communication?

_____

_____

_____

_____

3. How do I handle emotional vulnerability in others—do I try to "fix" instead of empathize?

_____

_____

_____

_____

4. Where might I soften my intensity and invite more compassion into my connections?

_____

_____

_____

_____

FINAL INTEGRATION

1. Which dosha do I most notice in my interactions, and which do I see in the people closest to me?

_____

_____

_____

_____

_____

_____

_____

_____

2. How can I use this awareness to create more balanced, supportive, and conscious relationships?

_____

_____

_____

_____

_____

_____

_____

_____

CHAPTER 8

Expanding the Alchemy: Integrating Ayurveda and Traditional Chinese Medicine

As a doctor of Traditional Chinese Medicine (TCM) and an Ayurvedic practitioner, I've had the privilege of witnessing the profound healing these ancient systems can bring—individually and together. While Ayurveda equips us with an insightful preventative health care system of full mind-body treatments and self-empowering tools, TCM's sophisticated understanding of the body's energetic systems, particularly the meridians and Zang-Fu organs, offers unique insights into the interconnected nature of physical, emotional, and spiritual health. Together, these systems provide a deeper lens through which we can understand the complexities of women's health.

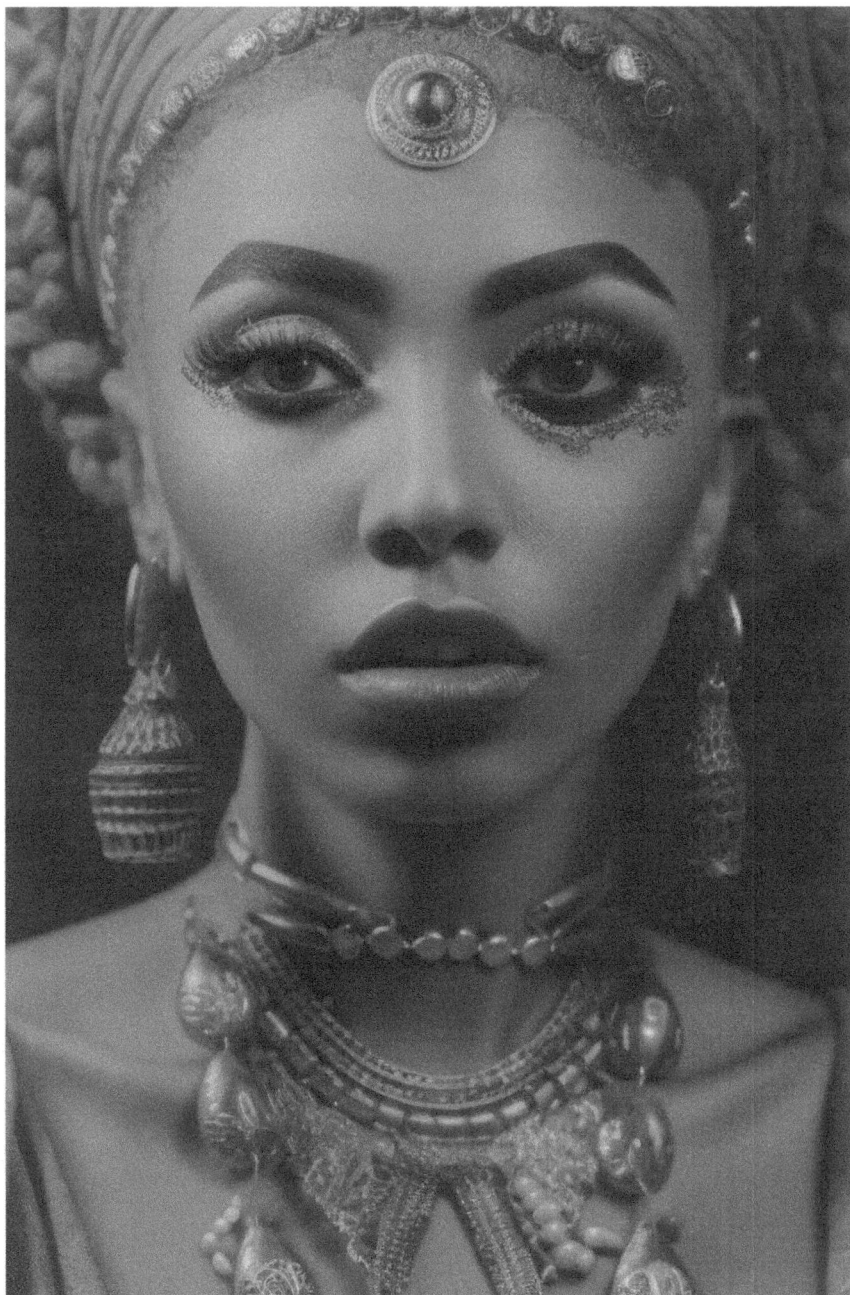

"TRUE WISDOM LIES IN EMBRACING THE KNOWLEDGE OF BOTH THE ANCIENT AND THE NEW." – UNKNOWN

The Zang-Fu Organs: Guardians of Balance

At the heart of TCM lies the concept of the Zang-Fu organs. These are not just physical structures but energetic systems that regulate and influence health on physical, emotional, and spiritual levels. The Zang organs (yin) are responsible for storing vital substances like qi, blood, and essence, while the Fu organs (yang) are more dynamic, focusing on digestion, transformation, and elimination.

Understanding Zang-Fu organs is essential for supporting women's health, as they govern key processes such as hormonal balance, emotional well-being, and reproductive vitality. Let's explore the Zang organs most relevant to women's health and draw parallels to their Ayurvedic counterparts.

THE LIVER (GAN)

✦ **Function in TCM:** The liver governs the smooth flow of qi and blood, as well as the storage of blood. It plays a critical role in regulating emotions, menstrual health, and detoxification.

✦ **Common imbalances:** Stagnant liver qi can manifest as PMS, irritability, or menstrual irregularities. Over time, it may lead to heat in the liver, causing symptoms like headaches, anger, or skin flare-ups.

✦ **Ayurvedic parallel:** The liver corresponds closely to Ranjaka Pitta, a subdosha of Pitta that governs the quality and production of blood. When Ranjaka Pitta is imbalanced, issues like hormonal swings or acne can arise.

Practical tip: Incorporate gentle twisting yoga poses to stimulate the liver, or try a warm infusion of dandelion root tea, which supports both TCM and Ayurvedic liver health.

THE SPLEEN (PI)

+ **Function in TCM:** The spleen governs digestion, transformation, and the production of qi and blood. It also helps "hold things in place," making it essential for preventing issues like prolapse or excessive menstrual bleeding.

+ **Common imbalances:** A weak spleen can lead to fatigue, bloating, poor appetite, and a "heavy" feeling, both physically and emotionally.

+ **Ayurvedic parallel:** The spleen's function aligns with Samana Vayu and Rasa Dhatu, which govern digestion, nutrient absorption, and the formation of plasma cells. Weak digestion (Agni) in Ayurveda mirrors spleen qi deficiency in TCM.

Practical tip: Strengthen your digestion by eating warm, easily digestible foods like kitchari and practicing mindful eating to support both spleen qi and Agni.

THE KIDNEYS (SHEN)

+ **Function in TCM:** The kidneys are considered the foundation of life, storing essence (*Jing*) and governing reproduction, growth, and aging. They are deeply tied to hormonal balance, fertility, and vitality.

+ **Common imbalances:** Deficient kidney Jing can manifest as lower back pain, premature aging, infertility, or exhaustion.

+ **Ayurvedic parallel:** The kidneys can be compared to Ojas, the subtle essence of vitality and immunity, as well as Shukra Dhatu, which governs reproductive health and longevity.

Practical tip: To nourish kidney energy, incorporate black sesame seeds, soak your feet in warm water before bed, and prioritize rest during your menstrual cycle.

THE HEART (XIN)

+ **Function in TCM:** The heart houses the *Shen* (spirit) and governs circulation, emotional well-being, and mental clarity. It is the seat of joy and connection.

+ **Common imbalances:** An overactive heart can lead to anxiety, insomnia, and palpitations, while a deficient heart may manifest as depression or lack of motivation.

+ **Ayurvedic parallel:** The heart corresponds to Sadhaka Pitta, which governs emotions and clarity of thought, as well as the Anahata chakra, the energetic center of love and compassion.

Practical tip: Calm the heart by meditating with rose quartz, sipping on rose tea, or practicing pranayama techniques like Nadi Shodhana (alternate nostril breathing).

THE LUNGS (FEI)

+ **Function in TCM:** The lungs govern qi and respiration, acting as a bridge between the external and internal world. They play a key role in immunity and emotional release.

+ **Common imbalances:** Lung qi deficiency can result in fatigue, shallow breathing, or frequent colds. Emotionally, grief and sadness are stored in the lungs.

+ **Ayurvedic parallel:** The lungs relate to Udana Vayu, which governs breath and upward-moving energy, as well as Prana, the life force.

Practical tip: Practice diaphragmatic breathing and incorporate warming spices like ginger and cinnamon into your meals to strengthen lung qi and support Prana.

Integrating the Wisdom of TCM and Ayurveda

The Zang-Fu framework and Ayurvedic doshas are two sides of the same coin, offering complementary approaches to understanding the body's inner workings. By combining these perspectives, we can create a more nuanced picture of health. For instance:

+ Liver qi stagnation in TCM mirrors imbalanced Ranjaka Pitta in Ayurveda. Both systems emphasize the importance of movement—whether through exercise, yoga, or breathwork—to release blockages.

+ Kidney Jing deficiency aligns with depleted Ojas in Ayurveda, reminding us of the need for rest, nourishing foods, and rejuvenating practices.

+ Spleen qi deficiency, which affects digestion and energy, finds its Ayurvedic counterpart in weak Agni and low Samana Vayu. Warm, grounding foods are universally recommended to restore balance.

Your Self-Healing Toolkit:
Marma and Acupressure Points

To empower you further, here are some self-care techniques combining Marma therapy and TCM acupressure:

1. LIVER QI RELEASE

✦ **Point**: Shankha Marma / Taiyang point (temples)

✦ **How to Locate**: Place your fingers at the outer corner of your eyes, then move them about a finger's width toward your hairline. You'll find a small soft hollow at the temples—this is the point.

✦ **Action**: Gently use your index or middle finger to massage this area in small circles. This relieves tension headaches, releases emotional buildup, and calms the mind.

2. DIGESTIVE HARMONY

✦ **Point**: Nabhi Marma / Ren 8 (navel)

✦ **How to Locate**: Simply find your belly button—this is your Nabhi Marma.

✦ **Action**: Warm some sesame oil in your palms and massage around the navel in clockwise circular motions, staying within 3–5 cm from the center. This enhances digestive fire, soothes bloating, and calms nervous digestion.

3. KIDNEY REJUVENATION

✦ **Point**: Kurcha Marma (ankle) / Kidney 3 (medial ankle)

✦ **How to Locate**: Sit comfortably and find the bony bump on the inside of your ankle (the medial malleolus). From there, slide your finger back toward the Achilles tendon—just between the bone and tendon. You'll feel a slight indentation; that's the point.

✦ **Action:** Apply gentle but steady pressure with your thumb or index finger for 30–60 seconds. This point supports reproductive health, strengthens the lower back, and boosts energy reserves.

4. HEART CONNECTION

✦ **Point:** Hridaya Marma / Ren 17 (heart center)

✦ **How to Locate:** Place your hand flat over the center of your chest, midway between the nipples, on the breastbone (sternum). This is the emotional heart center.

✦ **Action:** Rest your palm here, close your eyes, and take 5–10 deep, intentional breaths. This calms the nervous system, opens emotional pathways, and fosters self-love and inner safety.

The Relationship Between Meridians and Nadis: A Pathway of Energy

The meridians in Traditional Chinese Medicine (TCM) and the *Nadis* in Ayurveda represent intricate energy pathways that flow within the body, connecting the physical with the subtle energetic realms. While their systems differ in terminology and perspective, both recognize the importance of energy flow for maintaining health and harmony.

In TCM, meridians are channels through which qi (life force energy) flows. These pathways connect the Zang-Fu organs, enabling communication and balance between internal bodily systems. There are twelve primary meridians, each associated with specific organs, emotions, and elements, as well as extraordinary meridians that provide a deeper reservoir of energy. Blockages or imbalances in the meridians can lead to stagnation or deficiency, manifesting as physical, emotional, or mental disturbances.

In Ayurveda, Nadis are channels that carry Prana (vital life energy) throughout the body. There are said to be seventy-two thousand Nadis, with three primary ones: Ida, the lunar energy channel; Pingala, the solar energy channel; and Sushumna, the central channel associated with spiritual awakening and balance. The Nadis are closely connected to the chakras, the body's energy centers, and are essential for maintaining vitality and spiritual growth.

While the meridians emphasize organ and elemental relationships, the Nadis focus on the flow of Prana and its connection to mental clarity, spiritual awakening, and overall vitality. Despite these differences, both systems recognize that energy must move freely and harmoniously for optimal health.

The synergy between meridians and Nadis lies in their shared understanding of the body's energetics. Practices like acupuncture, acupressure, Abhyanga massage, pranayama, and marma therapy work to remove blockages in these pathways, allowing life energy to flow unimpeded. For example, where acupuncture stimulates specific meridian points to restore qi, marma therapy activates energy points to balance Prana and restore harmony in the Nadis. Together, these systems remind us of the profound interconnection between physical, emotional, and spiritual health, offering complementary approaches to align the body's energies.

A Client's Journey: Healing Heart Palpitations Through Ayurveda and TCM

One of my clients, Sophie, was a thirty-eight-year-old childcare worker who came to me experiencing heart palpitations, insomnia, and chronic fatigue. Her symptoms worsened after a difficult marriage breakdown, leaving her feeling emotionally depleted and physically unwell. She described her palpitations as "a constant fluttering in my chest, like my heart can't keep still," which made her anxious and fearful. She had Western medical tests, but her doctors assured her there were no structural heart issues—her symptoms were stress-induced.

Her work in childcare demanded constant energy and patience, yet she felt like her reserves were running dry. "I feel like I'm just going through the motions," she told me. "I love my job, but lately, I've been snapping at the kids, and then I feel even worse. It's like I'm failing everywhere—in my work, my relationships, and my health."

THE AYURVEDIC PERSPECTIVE: REBUILDING RESILIENCE AND NOURISHING THE HEART

From an Ayurvedic lens, Sophie's symptoms indicated an imbalance in Vata dosha, with its erratic, ungrounded qualities manifesting as anxiety, restlessness, and insomnia. The heart palpitations and emotional fragility also pointed to an imbalance in Sadhaka Pitta, the subdosha governing emotional processing and clarity of the heart.

Ayurvedic Plan

1. Lifestyle Adjustments

Sophie's day-to-day life needed more grounding and routine. I encouraged her to adopt a Dinacharya (daily routine), starting with waking up at the same time each day, practicing morning oil pulling, and completing a gentle Abhyanga (self-massage) with warm sesame oil.

We introduced evening rituals, including drinking a cup of warm almond milk with nutmeg and practicing Yoga Nidra to calm her nervous system before bed.

2. Dietary Changes

Sophie's diet was irregular and full of cold, processed foods, which aggravated Vata. I recommended warm, nourishing meals like kitchari, root vegetable soups, and spiced teas made with ginger, cardamom, and fennel. She incorporated foods rich in natural oils, such as ghee and soaked almonds, to support emotional and physical stability.

3. Herbal Support

I created a personalized herbal tonic that included ashwagandha to reduce her stress and nourish her adrenal glands. Ashwaganda helps improve sleep, builds strength and resilience, and replenishes Ojas (vital essence).

Arjuna was added to specifically support her heart and calm palpitations. It is a powerful herb known to strengthen the physical and emotional heart, and to support circulation, blood pressure, and grief-related depletion. Traditionally arjuna is used to balance Sadhaka Pitta (emotional processing in the heart).

Brahmi was included to enhance mental clarity and ease anxiety. It is very helpful for overthinking, emotional sensitivity, and nervous tension. From an Ayurvedic perspective, it strengthens *Majja Dhatu* (nervous tissue).

4. Ayurvedic Therapies

Sophie began a series of *Nasya* and *Shirodhara* treatments, where warm herbal oil was poured over her forehead to calm the mind and balance Vata. After each session, she described feeling deeply relaxed, often saying, "It's like my chest feels light for the first time in months." These treatments were done in conjunction with the acupuncture described next.

THE TCM PERSPECTIVE: MOVING STAGNATION AND STRENGTHENING THE HEART

In TCM, Sophie's symptoms pointed to heart yin deficiency and liver qi stagnation. The emotional stress of her marriage breakdown had depleted her heart yin, leaving her with palpitations, restlessness, and insomnia. The liver qi stagnation contributed to her feelings of frustration, irritability, and an inability to process her emotions.

TCM Treatment Plan

Acupuncture

I selected points such as Ren 17 (*Shanzhong*) to calm the chest and regulate the heart, HT 7 (*Shenmen*) to nourish heart yin and reduce palpitations, and LIV 3 (*Taichong*) to move stagnant liver qi. After each acupuncture session, Sophie reported feeling lighter and more at ease, and over time, her palpitations lessened significantly. Sophie was encouraged to incorporate gentle movement like qigong or yoga to help move stagnant qi and deepen her connection with her body.

The Synergy of Ayurveda and TCM

What was most profound in Sophie's case was how Ayurveda and TCM worked together seamlessly. Ayurveda provided her with daily self-care rituals, a nourishing diet, herbal medecine support, and deeply grounding therapies like Shirodhara. These practices helped her feel more in control of her healing process. Meanwhile, TCM's acupuncture addressed the energetic imbalances in her body with precision, releasing blockages and replenishing her reserves.

For example, while Ayurvedic herbs like ashwagandha and arjuna strengthened her resilience and soothed her heart, the acupuncture treatments targeted her physical symptoms, such as the palpitations and emotional tension. The two systems complemented each other beautifully, offering Sophie a truly holistic approach to healing.

The Unique Role of Ayurveda in Holistic Healing

What makes Ayurveda so powerful is its ability to integrate with other modalities like TCM, kinesiology, massage, naturopathy, osteo, chiropractic, and the list goes on. Ayurveda ties everything together by addressing the root causes of imbalance while giving each individual tools to participate in their healing. Whether it's through Marma therapy, herbal remedies, dosha-specific diet regimes, or lifestyle changes, Ayurveda empowers people to create lasting transformations in their lives.

In Sophie's case, she noticed profound changes within a few weeks. The palpitations subsided, her sleep improved, and she found herself smiling more often at work. She reconnected with her love for childcare.

As Sophie put it, "I feel like I'm finally coming back to myself—not just the version of me from before the marriage, but a stronger, more whole version."

Reflection on Ayurvedic and TCM in Your Life

1. What physical or emotional symptoms do you experience most often, and how might they be linked to energetic imbalances in your body (such as Vata, Pitta, Kapha or qi stagnation, yin deficiency, etc.)?

_____

_____

_____

_____

_____

2. In what ways do you already support your body's energy systems—through food, movement, breath, or self-care rituals? Where is there room for deeper alignment?

_____

_____

_____

_____

_____

3. Reflect on the organ systems discussed (liver, spleen, kidneys, heart, lungs). Which one resonates most with your current challenges or healing focus? Why?

_____

_____

_____

_____

_____

_____

4. How do you process emotions like grief, frustration, or anxiety? Do you notice these emotions manifest in your body in specific ways?

_____

_____

_____

_____

_____

5. What daily or weekly rituals could you introduce from either Ayurveda or TCM to support your vitality, balance your energy, or ground your nervous system?

_____

_____

_____

_____

_____

_____

_____

6. How do you feel about blending ancient healing systems like Ayurveda and TCM with modern life? What insights or curiosities has this chapter sparked for you?

_____

_____

_____

_____

_____

_____

_____

_____

CHAPTER 9

Hormones Unhinged: The Wild Ride of Womanhood

Hormones are chemical messengers that regulate nearly every function in the body. They are intricately interconnected, and even small imbalances ripple outward, impacting mood, energy, sleep, metabolism, and more. Here's a closer look at the primary hormones that shift during perimenopause and menopause.

Estrogen: The "Queen Hormone"

Estrogen is often referred to as the "queen hormone" because of its far-reaching influence on women's bodies. Its primary role is in reproductive health, regulating menstrual cycles and maintaining uterine health. However, its impact extends much further.

+ **Bone health:** Estrogen supports bone density by slowing the breakdown of bone tissue. When levels decline, particularly after menopause, women become susceptible to osteoporosis.

+ **Cardiovascular protection:** It helps maintain healthy cholesterol levels and supports the elasticity of blood vessels, reducing the risk of heart disease.

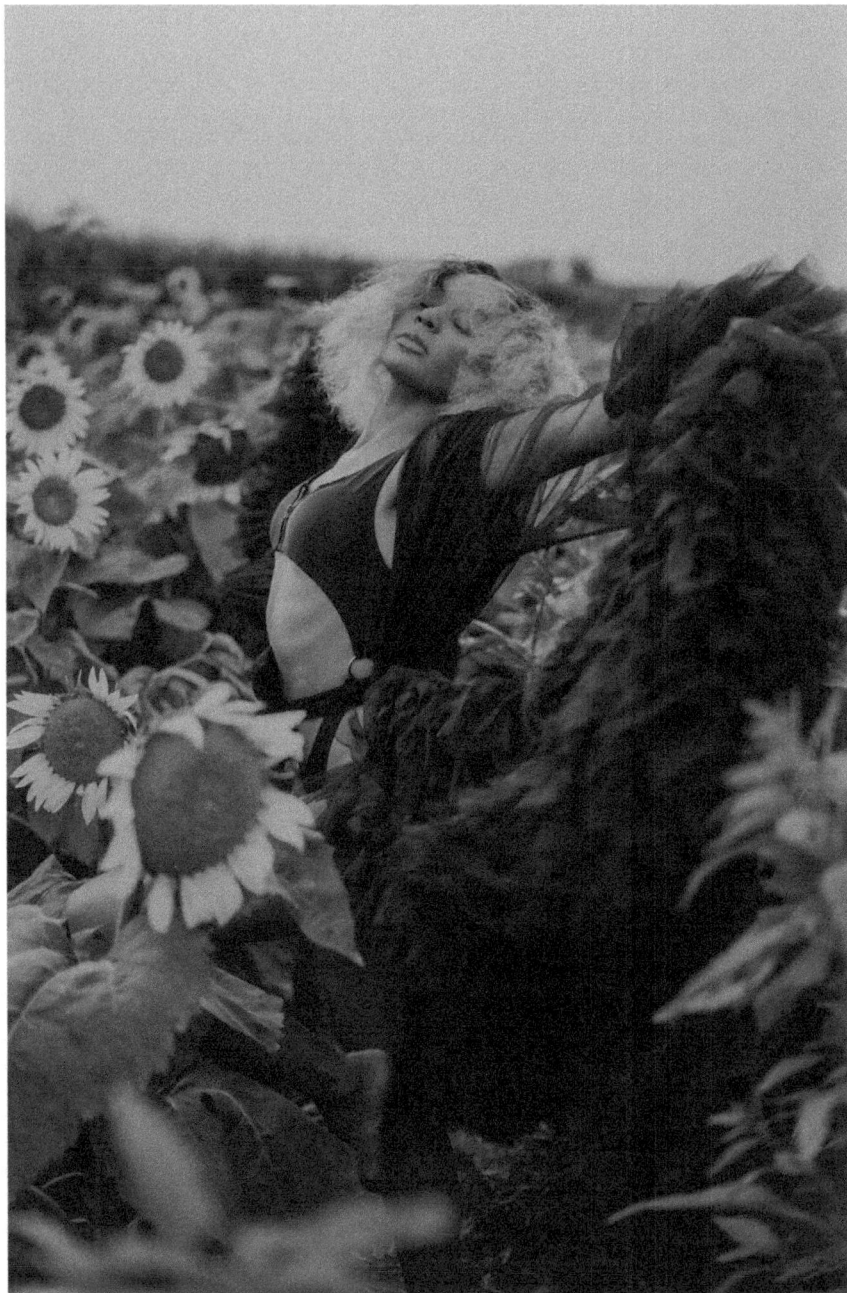

"THERE IS NO FORCE MORE POWERFUL THAN A WOMAN WHO HAS LEARNED TO RIDE THE WAVES OF HER OWN RHYTHM." – UNKNOWN

✦ **Skin elasticity**: Estrogen stimulates collagen production, contributing to firm, hydrated skin.

✦ **Mood and gut regulation**: Estrogen plays a critical role in mood regulation by influencing key neurotransmitters like serotonin and dopamine—chemicals that affect emotional stability, mental clarity, and resilience. However, what many don't realize is that over 90 percent of serotonin is produced in the gut. This means estrogen's impact on mood is deeply intertwined with gut health. When the gut microbiome is disrupted—through stress, poor diet, or inflammation—both neurotransmitter production and estrogen metabolism can be compromised. A healthy gut supports better hormonal signalling, which helps stabilize mood, energy, and even cognitive function. In this way, estrogen and gut health work in a symbiotic relationship: balance one, and you often support the other.

✦ **Hormonal interactions**: In early adulthood, estrogen supports menstrual regularity and resilience, optimizes insulin sensitivity, and helps maintain healthy metabolism and body composition. At this stage, balanced estrogen contributes to stable energy, mood, and fertility. However, imbalances—whether from stress, poor gut health, contraceptives, or environmental toxins—can disrupt this harmony, leading to symptoms like irregular periods, PMS, or weight fluctuations. In perimenopause, estrogen fluctuates more dramatically. This transition can bring a host of symptoms—hot flashes, mood swings, irregular periods—due to estrogen's wide-reaching effects on the brain, metabolism, and nervous system. By menopause, estrogen levels significantly decline, which can contribute to vaginal dryness, urinary tract issues, a slower metabolism, and a marked loss in bone density. Estrogen doesn't operate in isolation, it works closely with progesterone to balance and regulate the menstrual cycle. It also interacts with insulin, which influences how the body metabolizes carbohydrates and stores fat.

Progesterone: The Calming Hormone

Often referred to as the "balancer," progesterone has a calming effect on the body and mind. Its primary roles include:

+ **Regulating menstrual cycles:** Progesterone prepares the uterus for pregnancy and supports its early stages.

+ **Sleep support:** It promotes restful sleep by influencing the production of GABA, a neurotransmitter that calms the nervous system.

+ **Anti-inflammatory effects:** Progesterone helps regulate the immune response and reduces inflammation.

+ **Hormonal interactions:** Progesterone complements estrogen, ensuring that estrogen's effects on tissues like the uterine lining and breasts remain balanced. A drop in progesterone often precedes a decline in estrogen during perimenopause, leading to anxiety, sleep disturbances, and irregular cycles.

Testosterone: The Vitality Hormone

Though typically associated with men, testosterone is equally essential for women. It is a driver of:

+ **Libido and sexual desire:** Testosterone enhances sexual arousal and sensitivity.

+ **Muscle strength:** It supports muscle mass and strength, which are vital for overall health and mobility as we age.

+ **Energy and motivation:** Testosterone contributes to overall vitality and a sense of drive.

+ **Hormonal interactions:** Testosterone interacts with estrogen, and a decline in testosterone exacerbates the effects of low estrogen, contributing to reduced energy, diminished libido, and loss of muscle mass.

Cortisol: The Stress Hormone

Cortisol is produced by the adrenal glands and is critical for managing stress and maintaining homeostasis. Its functions include:

✦ **Energy regulation:** Cortisol helps maintain blood sugar levels by prompting the liver to release glucose.

✦ **Inflammation control:** It plays a role in reducing inflammation during times of short-term stress or injury.

✦ **Fight-or-flight response:** Cortisol is essential for short-term survival, helping the body respond to acute stress.

✦ **Hormonal interactions:** Chronic stress activates the hypothalamic-pituitary-adrenal (HPA) axis, triggering the release of both cortisol and adrenaline (epinephrine). While cortisol helps regulate long-term stress by influencing blood sugar, metabolism, and inflammation, adrenaline is responsible for the immediate "fight or flight" response—increasing heart rate, blood pressure, and alertness. When stress becomes chronic, constant release can dysregulate hormonal balance. Elevated cortisol and adrenaline suppress reproductive hormones like estrogen and progesterone, impair thyroid function, and lead to symptoms such as anxiety, weight gain (especially abdominal), irritability, and fatigue. Over time, this depletes the adrenal glands, resulting in what is sometimes referred to as "adrenal fatigue" or "hypocortisolism." Low cortisol symptoms include profound morning and afternoon fatigue, salt cravings, low blood pressure, poor stress tolerance, and difficulty concentrating. These symptoms are accompanied by sleep disturbances—difficulty waking in the morning, energy crashes mid-afternoon, and a second wind late at night. From an Ayurvedic perspective, this state reflects a Vata imbalance and diminished Ojas (vital life essence), which compromises immunity, emotional resilience, and hormonal harmony.

Thyroid Hormones: The Metabolic Regulators

Produced by the thyroid gland, these hormones are responsible for regulating the body's metabolism and energy levels.

+ **Metabolism and weight:** Thyroid hormones control how the body uses energy, impacting weight, body temperature, and energy levels.

+ **Mood and cognition:** They influence mental clarity and emotional balance, with low levels often contributing to brain fog and depressive symptoms.

+ **Hair and skin health:** Healthy thyroid function supports strong hair and radiant skin.

+ **Hormonal interactions:** Thyroid hormones interact with cortisol and insulin, creating a complex web of metabolic regulation. Thyroid dysfunction is common in women in their thirties to fifties and mimics or exacerbates menopausal symptoms, such as weight gain, fatigue, and mood changes.

DHEA: The Anti-Aging Hormone

Dehydroepiandrosterone (DHEA) is a steroid hormone primarily produced by the adrenal glands and serves as a precursor to both estrogen and testosterone. Often referred to as the "anti-aging hormone," DHEA is crucial for vitality, particularly in midlife when levels begin to decline.

+ **Energy and vitality:** DHEA helps combat fatigue and supports stamina, particularly during times of stress or hormonal transition. Many women report improved energy and mood with optimal DHEA levels.

+ **Stress adaptation:** It buffers the effects of cortisol, supporting resilience and recovery from chronic stress. When cortisol is high, DHEA often becomes depleted—contributing to burnout and hormonal imbalance.

+ **Immune function:** DHEA plays a protective role in immune health and inflammation regulation, particularly as the body ages.

+ **Hormonal interactions:** As DHEA declines with age, so does the body's ability to maintain balanced estrogen and testosterone levels. This magnifies symptoms related to perimenopause, menopause, and low libido or muscle mass.

While not always discussed as often as estrogen or progesterone, DHEA is an important piece of the hormonal puzzle, especially in relation to stress, aging, and vitality.

Insulin: The Metabolic Hormone

Insulin, produced by the pancreas, is responsible for regulating blood sugar levels by facilitating glucose uptake into cells.

+ **Energy regulation:** Insulin ensures that the body's cells have a steady supply of glucose for energy.

+ **Fat storage:** When insulin levels are consistently elevated (due to stress, poor diet, or lack of exercise), it can lead to increased fat storage and insulin resistance.

+ **Hormonal interplay:** Insulin interacts with estrogen and cortisol, influencing weight, energy levels, and inflammation.

+ **Hormonal interactions:** Imbalanced insulin levels can exacerbate symptoms of perimenopause and menopause and contribute to weight gain, fatigue, and mood disturbances. Stabilizing blood sugar through diet and lifestyle is key to managing overall hormonal health.

The Synergy of Hormonal Health

Hormones don't work in isolation; they function as a finely tuned symphony, with each one playing a vital role in maintaining balance. When one hormone is out of balance, it disrupts others, creating a cascade of symptoms. For example:

✦ Chronic stress and elevated cortisol levels suppress thyroid function and increase insulin resistance.

✦ Declining estrogen affects serotonin levels, leading to mood swings and sleep disturbances.

✦ Low progesterone amplifies the effects of high cortisol, creating a cycle of anxiety and poor sleep.

By understanding these hormones' unique roles and how they interact with each other, we begin to see our bodies not as broken, but as beautifully complex and dynamic. Hormonal imbalances are not random; they are signals. They reflect the ways we live, eat, move, think, and rest. This awareness gives us power—because once we understand our patterns, we can begin to shift them. I encourage you to get your hormone levels tested with your healthcare provider, particularly if you're experiencing persistent symptoms like fatigue, mood swings, irregular periods, or weight changes. There are also apps and journals available to help you track your cycles, moods, and energy, offering insight into your hormonal rhythms. But most importantly, listen to your body. Begin noticing how you feel at different times throughout the month. Journal your emotional and physical changes. Reflect on your stress levels, sleep, and energy. These small acts of self-awareness lay the foundation for deeper hormonal harmony—and bring you one step closer to your higHERself™.

Balancing the Scale:
How Hormones Influence Weight

Across the stages of womanhood—from puberty and the reproductive years to menopause and beyond—shifts in hormonal balance can profoundly affect how our bodies store fat, process nutrients, and respond to exercise.

HORMONES AND WEIGHT IN PUBERTY
AND THE REPRODUCTIVE YEARS

During puberty, rising levels of estrogen and progesterone initiate the menstrual cycle and shape the female body. These hormonal changes promote fat distribution in the hips, thighs, and breasts—essential not just for fertility but also for hormonal balance and reproductive vitality. Contrary to popular belief, balanced estrogen actually supports healthy weight regulation, not just weight gain. It helps maintain insulin sensitivity, supports serotonin production, and promotes metabolic function—all critical for maintaining energy and mood throughout the cycle.

Throughout the reproductive years, hormonal fluctuations continue to influence weight in more subtle ways. For example, in the luteal phase (post-ovulation), progesterone becomes the dominant hormone. This shift can naturally increase appetite and cravings for carbohydrates and sweets—a mechanism designed to fuel a potential pregnancy. While this is biologically normal, without conscious eating or proper metabolic support, it can lead to weight gain or energy crashes.

Research also highlights the critical connection between insulin and reproductive hormones. Insulin resistance, especially paired with hormonal imbalances, can contribute to unwanted weight gain and fatigue. This is particularly evident in women with polycystic ovary syndrome (PCOS), a condition marked by elevated testosterone, irregular cycles, and disrupted insulin metabolism. In these cases, higher testosterone levels promote visceral fat storage and disrupt the body's ability to regulate weight and blood sugar efficiently.

But it's not simply about hormones working against us—when hormones are in balance, they are powerful allies. They stabilize appetite, boost mood, enhance digestion, and support efficient fat metabolism. The key lies in nurturing this delicate hormonal harmony through lifestyle, nutrition, and stress management.

HORMONES AND WEIGHT DURING PREGNANCY AND POSTPARTUM

Pregnancy brings a profound hormonal surge. Estrogen and progesterone levels rise dramatically to support the growing baby, while other hormones like prolactin and human chorionic gonadotropin (hCG) shift the body's metabolism toward nourishment and preservation. Fat is stored intentionally—not as a flaw, but as a biological necessity to support breastfeeding and postpartum recovery.

However, excess weight gain during pregnancy can stem from poor dietary habits, unresolved stress, or an imbalance in Kapha dosha, which governs structure, lubrication, and stability in the body. Ayurveda teaches us that this phase is not the time for restriction but for mindful nourishment—choosing foods that support Agni, hormonal balance, and stable energy.

Postpartum, the body undergoes a steep hormonal drop. Estrogen and progesterone decline rapidly, while cortisol may increase due to sleep deprivation and the emotional intensity of new motherhood. These shifts result in slower metabolism, poor digestion, and stubborn weight retention if not addressed holistically.

Ayurvedic wisdom offers a nurturing roadmap: warm, grounding meals like kitchari; digestive herbs such as fennel, cumin, and ginger;

and Abhyanga (self-massage) to support the lymphatic system and hormone recalibration. Emotional support, rest, and connection are just as vital to help mothers rebuild their strength and reclaim their vitality.

KEY SUMMARY OF HORMONES AND WEIGHT: THE BALANCING ACT

Hormonal imbalance can contribute to weight gain by

+ increasing appetite and cravings (especially during the luteal phase)

+ disrupting insulin sensitivity and blood sugar regulation

+ raising cortisol from chronic stress or sleep deprivation, which promotes fat storage

+ elevating testosterone (as in PCOS), leading to increased abdominal fat

+ slowing thyroid function, which reduces metabolic rate

But when your hormones are in balance, they support:

+ a stable metabolism

+ balanced appetite and cravings

+ efficient fat burning

+ enhanced insulin sensitivity

+ emotional well-being and motivation

HORMONE-SUPPORTIVE STRATEGIES

Try these Ayurvedic- and science-backed approaches to support your hormones and metabolism:

+ **Support Agni (digestion):** Use spices like cumin, fennel, ginger, and coriander to enhance digestion and reduce bloating.

+ **Build muscle mass:** Incorporate resistance training at least twice a week to support metabolism and insulin sensitivity.

+ **Balance stress:** Daily meditation, Vedic breathwork, or yoga nidra can help regulate cortisol, which in turn supports hormonal balance.

+ **Prioritize blood sugar stability:** Focus on protein, healthy fats, and fiber at every meal to prevent insulin spikes and crashes.

+ **Respect your circadian rhythm:** Go to bed before 10:00 p.m. and aim for consistent wake times—even on weekends—to support hormone production.

+ **Herbs and adaptogens:** Ashwagandha, shatavari, saffron, and licorice root may help balance hormones and support adrenal function (consult your practitioner).[2]

---

2   Lovejoy J. C., Champagne C. M., de Jonge L., Xie H., Smith S. R., 2008, "Increased Visceral Fat and Decreased Energy Expenditure During the Menopausal Transition," *International Journal of Obesity, London* 32 (6): 949–958, doi:10.1038/ijo.2008.25; Santini F., Galli G., Maffei M., et al., 2021, "Thyroid Function and Body Weight: A Complex Relationship," *Front Endocrinol (Lausanne)* 12 (706619), doi:10.3389/fendo.2021.706619; Santollo J., Eckel L. A., 2008, "Estradiol Decreases the Orexigenic Effect of Ghrelin in Female Rats," *Endocrinology* 149 (11): 5353–5360, doi:10.1210/en.2008-0444.

Reflections on Hormonal Wisdom

Take a few quiet moments to explore your own hormonal landscape.
Use the following questions to guide your self-inquiry.

1. What recurring symptoms (physical, emotional, or mental) have
    I noticed that might be linked to hormonal changes?

    _____

    _____

    _____

2. How do my energy levels and mood fluctuate across my monthly
    cycle (or, if postmenopausal, across the seasons or stress levels)?

    _____

    _____

    _____

3. When do I feel most grounded and balanced? What habits or
    environments support that?

    _____

    _____

    _____

4. Have I experienced times in my life when stress clearly affected
    my hormonal health or menstrual cycle? How did I respond?

    _____

    _____

    _____

    _____

5. What role does self-care currently play in my hormonal health? Where could I offer myself more support or compassion?

_____

_____

_____

6. Do I track my cycle, energy, or moods in any form? If not, what simple tool (app, journal, etc.) could I begin using?

_____

_____

_____

7. What does hormonal balance feel like to me—not just physically but emotionally and spiritually?

_____

_____

_____

_____

8. What next step feels most aligned—consulting a practitioner, changing a habit, or simply tuning in more deeply?

_____

_____

_____

_____

Let your answers reveal patterns and possibilities. Your hormones carry wisdom. Are you listening?

CHAPTER 10

Flow State: The Phases of Your Menstrual Cycle and Doshas

The menstrual cycle is a sacred reflection of a woman's inner world—a living, breathing connection to the rhythms of nature and the moon's cycles.

Ayurveda teaches us that this cycle isn't just a physiological event but a window into our physical, emotional, and spiritual health. It's not about fitting into a one-size-fits-all definition of what a "normal" cycle should look like but about honoring the unique rhythm of your own body.

The "average" menstrual cycle is often described as twenty-eight days, divided into distinct phases, but let's be honest—rarely does life fit neatly into averages. A healthy cycle might be slightly shorter or longer, depending on your constitution (dosha), lifestyle, and even the season of life you're in. For some, it's twenty-six days; for others, thirty-two. And that's okay. Ayurveda reminds us that our cycles are as individual as we are, each one carrying its own story.

What's important is learning to attune yourself to your body's

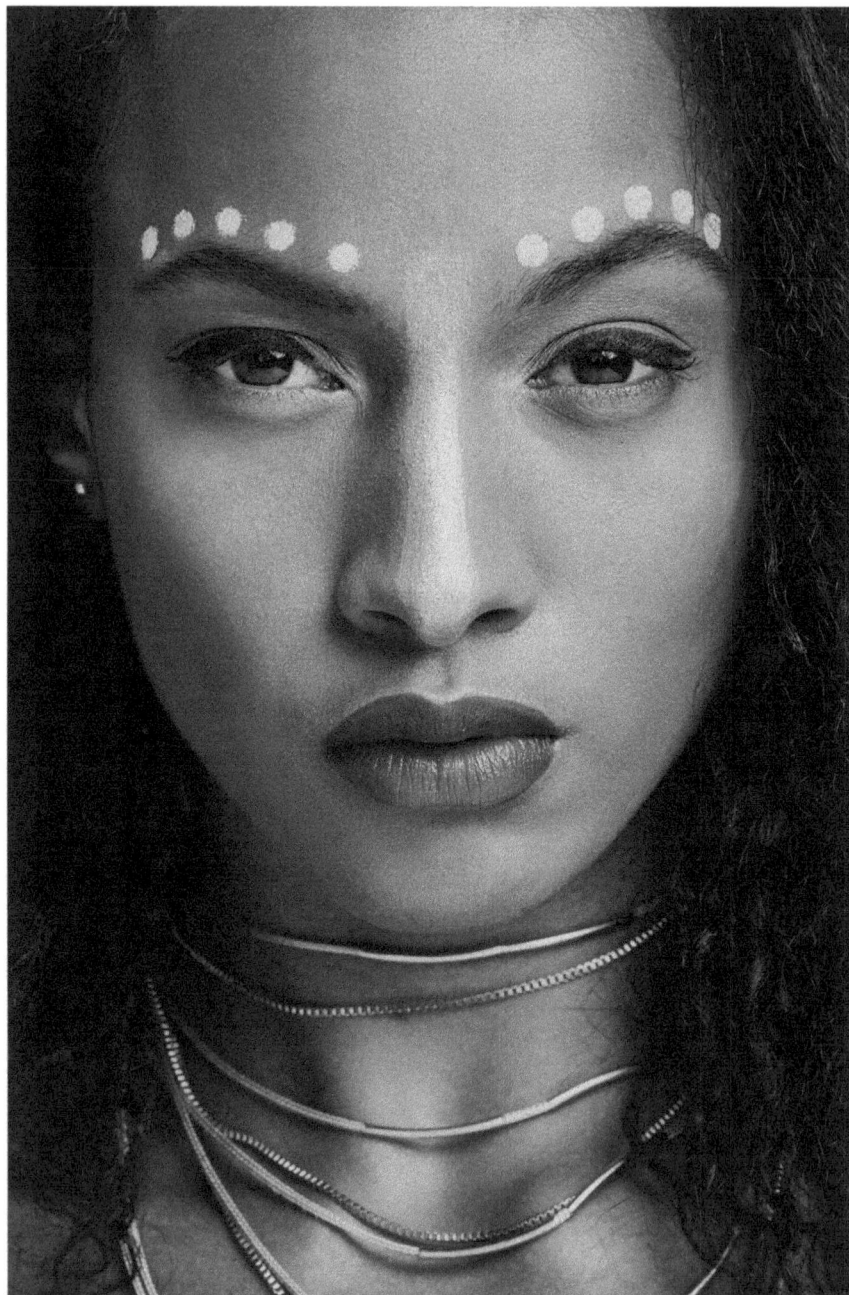

"TO UNDERSTAND THE RHYTHM OF YOUR CYCLE IS TO UNDERSTAND THE RHYTHM OF YOUR POWER." – UNKNOWN

natural flow and recognizing when it's happy—or when it's calling for support. Each cycle phase brings its own hormonal symphony and doshic interplay, influencing not just how your body feels but how you move through the world emotionally, mentally, and energetically.

This is about more than tracking dates on a calendar; it's about tuning into the subtle shifts within you, celebrating your unique rhythm, and giving your body the care it needs in each phase. Whether your cycle matches the textbook description or dances to its own beat, it is your guide—a compass pointing you toward balance and self-connection.

Let's take a deeper look at the journey of hormones and doshas through the phases of your cycle and how you can align with this sacred rhythm.

1. The Menstrual Phase (Days 1–5)

Hormonal Activity

During menstruation, estrogen and progesterone levels are at their lowest, signaling the release of the uterine lining. This is the body's natural monthly detox—a time of shedding not just physically but energetically.

Doshas at Play

Vata dominates this phase, particularly through Apana Vayu, the subdosha responsible for downward and outward flow. When Vata is balanced, menstruation can feel like a gentle release. But excess Vata can bring cramping, bloating, constipation, lower back pain, anxiety, or a feeling of being ungrounded.

How a Woman May Feel

This is often a time of low energy and heightened emotional sensitivity. Many women naturally want to withdraw and reflect, which is an intuitive response to the energetic shift. Sleep may be lighter, or you may crave more of it. It's also common to experience cravings for carbohydrates, sweets, or salty comfort foods. From a physiological perspective, the body loses iron during this time, and an increase in iron-rich or warming antioxidant foods (such as beets, dates, leafy greens, or a small portion of red meat if aligned with your diet) can be supportive.

AYURVEDIC PRACTICES FOR THE MENSTRUAL PHASE

+ **Rest and retreat:** Honor the body's need to slow down. Avoid intense workouts and overstimulation. Instead, embrace stillness, journaling, restorative yoga, or simply doing less.

+ **Warmth:** Keep your abdomen warm. Sip ginger, cinnamon, or tulsi tea. Use a heat pack on the lower back to ease tension.

+ **Nourishment:** Eat grounding, easy-to-digest meals like kitchari, soups, or stewed apples. Avoid cold, raw, or overly spicy foods, which can aggravate Vata and disrupt digestion.

+ **Supplement if needed:** If you're prone to fatigue or dizziness during your cycle, consider having your iron and ferritin levels checked and consult your practitioner for support.

SELF-CARE RITUAL:
WARM HERBAL COMPRESS OR BELLY PACK

Create a warm compress using a soft cloth soaked in a soothing herbal infusion, such as chamomile, lavender, or ginger. Alternatively, you can use a hot water bottle wrapped in a towel. Place the compress on your lower abdomen to ease menstrual cramps, calm Vata, and provide grounding warmth.

To enhance the ritual, you can apply a few drops of castor oil or a warming Ayurvedic oil like ashwagandha bala oil on your lower belly before applying the compress. This helps support detoxification and relieves muscle tension.

Pair this practice with deep, diaphragmatic breathing to further relax the nervous system and connect with your body's natural rhythm during this sacred time of rest and reflection.

---

2. The Follicular Phase (Days 6–14)

Hormonal Activity

After menstruation, estrogen levels steadily rise, stimulating growth of ovarian follicles and thickening the uterine lining. This marks a time of physiological renewal and expansion. The body prepares itself for potential conception with increased vitality and cellular rebuilding.

Doshas at Play

Kapha takes center stage during this phase, aligning with the qualities of nourishment, growth, and cohesion. Its grounding and stabilizing influence supports rebuilding the reproductive system.

How a Woman May Feel

Energy levels begin to rise, and many women notice an uplift in mood, clarity, and motivation. Emotionally, this is often a phase of creativity, vision, and sociability. Libido also naturally increases as estrogen rises, and women may feel more open, flirty, or receptive to connection. If in balance, this is a beautiful time for romantic and sexual expression. If Kapha is elevated, however, it may manifest as sluggishness, emotional clinginess, or resistance to change.

AYURVEDIC PRACTICES FOR THE FOLLICULAR PHASE

+ **Energizing foods:** Support Kapha's building nature with fresh fruits, lightly steamed vegetables, lean proteins, and whole grains. Minimize heavy or overly oily foods to avoid dampness or stagnation.

+ **Movement:** Engage in energising practices like Vinyasa yoga, brisk walks, or dance to stimulate circulation and balance Kapha.

+ **Hydration and herbs:** Stay well-hydrated to support cervical fluid production and overall vitality. Sip on teas infused with lemon zest, tulsi (holy basil), or fennel.

+ **Sacred sexuality tip:** This phase is ideal for cultivating sensual confidence and conscious intimacy. Explore physical connection with playfulness and creativity. Practices like yoni steaming or self-massage (Abhyanga) can also help enhance receptivity and body awareness.

SELF-CARE RITUAL

Dry brushing or Garshana (silk glove massage) can stimulate lymphatic flow and prevent Kapha stagnation.

---

3. The Ovulatory Phase (Days 15–17)

Hormonal Activity

Mid-cycle marks a powerful time of transformation and action. A surge in luteinizing hormone (LH) triggers the release of a mature egg from the dominant follicle. After ovulation, the follicle becomes the corpus luteum, which begins producing progesterone to prepare the uterus for potential implantation. Estrogen reaches its peak during ovulation, increasing vitality, mood, and mental clarity, while a rise in testosterone enhances assertiveness, self-confidence, and sexual desire.

Doshas at Play

This is when Pitta steps into full expression, bringing heat, intensity, and direction. Pitta governs the precision of ovulation and ignites the drive for connection—whether that's through intimacy, creativity, or purposeful action.

How a Woman May Feel

Many women report feeling radiant, magnetic, and socially open during this phase. There's often a noticeable boost in libido, sexual receptivity, and a desire for intimacy and bonding. This is a powerful time for authentic communication, boundary setting, and embodiment. When Pitta is in excess, however, it may present as irritability, impatience, or perfectionism.

AYURVEDIC PRACTICES FOR THE OVULATORY PHASE

✦ **Cooling foods:** Balance Pitta's heat by focusing on foods like cucumber, coconut, leafy greens, berries, and aloe vera juice. Minimize caffeine, alcohol, and spicy foods, which can amplify inner heat and reactivity.

✦ **Conscious movement:** Engage in strength-building but mindful practices like Pilates, weight training, moderate-intensity training, or yoga that encourages flow without burnout.

✦ **Embrace connection:** This is an ideal time for nourishing emotional and physical intimacy. You may feel more sensually alive—lean into that with awareness. Try heart-opening rituals, shared Abhyanga (oil massage), or sensual movement to connect with your body and your partner.

✦ **Sexual energy tip:** Whether partnered or solo, explore what pleasure feels like when you are fully present in your body. This is a peak time for ovary–heart coherence. Use that energy not only for physical connection but to birth creative ideas and embody your inner radiance.

SELF-CARE RITUAL

Instead of fiery stimulation, focus on cooling and calming the body and mind. Apply a cooling face mask made of aloe vera and rose water to refresh your skin and soothe Pitta's heat. Alternatively, enjoy a cooling herbal tea with mint, coriander, or fennel to balance internal warmth.

---

4. The Luteal Phase (Days 18–28)

Hormonal Activity

Following ovulation, progesterone rises, secreted by the corpus luteum to stabilize the uterus in preparation for implantation. If conception doesn't occur, both progesterone and estrogen levels fall, leading to menstruation. This hormonal drop can also impact mood, energy, and sleep patterns. For those who conceive, the corpus luteum remains, allowing continued progesterone production until the placenta takes over.

Doshas at Play

Kapha predominates in the early luteal phase, offering a sense of calm, stability, and introspection. As the cycle nears completion, Vata begins to rise, especially if there's stress, fatigue, or overwhelm, which can intensify PMS symptoms like anxiety, restlessness, bloating, and insomnia.

How a Woman May Feel

Many women notice a dip in energy, a need for solitude, and heightened emotional sensitivity. This is a time when irritability, cravings, self-doubt, or emotional reactivity may surface—especially if Vata or Pitta are out of balance. Libido may fluctuate: for some, progesterone's calming effect can heighten sensuality and a desire for comfort and connection, while for others, lower energy and irritability may reduce sexual interest. This is not a phase to push through—but rather one to honor with gentleness and attunement.

AYURVEDIC PRACTICES FOR THE LUTEAL PHASE

✦ **Grounding nutrition:** Prioritize warm, nourishing meals like root vegetables, oily foods, stews, and well-spiced grains. Increase magnesium-rich foods (like pumpkin seeds and leafy greens) to ease tension and reduce bloating. If you're craving sweets, opt for warm spiced dates or a golden milk latte instead of sugar-laden snacks.

✦ **Mood-supporting herbs:** Herbs like ashwagandha, shatavari, or brahmi help ease nervous system tension, support mood, and regulate hormones. Always consult a practitioner before use.

✦ **Womb-focused self-care:** Abhyanga (oiled self-massage) with warm sesame oil soothes Vata, supports digestion, and reconnects you to your body. Use circular motions around the lower abdomen.

✦ **Cycle-sensitive libido:** If you feel drawn to intimacy, favor slow, nurturing connection. Honor your need for emotional safety. If your libido dips, communicate your needs clearly and soften into rest.

✦ **Gentle movement:** Choose restorative yoga, slow walking, or breath-led Pilates. This is a time to prioritize ease over achievement.

SELF-CARE RITUAL

Soak in a warm bath with a few drops of lavender oil to calm the nervous system and balance Vata.

The Connection to the Moon Cycle

The menstrual cycle is often compared to the moon's phases. Many women naturally menstruate around the new moon and ovulate around the full moon, reflecting the moon's waxing and waning energies. However, if the moon cycle is not in sync with your natural menstrual cycle that is perfectly normal too, or if you are no longer menstruating—whether due to menopause, hormonal birth control, or other factors—you can still align with the moon's rhythms to connect with your cyclical nature.

✦ **New moon (menstrual phase):** A time for introspection, rest, and planting seeds of intention.

✦ **Waxing moon (follicular phase):** A phase of growth, renewal, and creativity.

✦ **Full moon (ovulatory phase):** A peak of energy, magnetism, and manifestation.

✦ **Waning moon (luteal phase):** A time for releasing what no longer serves you and turning inward.

FOR WOMEN WITHOUT A MENSTRUAL CYCLE

If you're on hormonal birth control, postmenopausal, or have irregular cycles, you can still harness the power of cyclical living by syncing your lifestyle with the moon phases.

1. **Set intentions with the new moon:** Reflect on what you want to release or call into your life.

2. **Take action during the waxing moon:** Begin new projects or cultivate positive habits.

3. **Celebrate the full moon:** Acknowledge your achievements and express gratitude.

4. **Reflect during the waning moon:** Let go of what isn't serving you and prepare for rest.

Ayurvedic rituals like journaling, meditation, or self-massage can help you deepen this connection.

Rituals and Ayurvedic Wisdom for the Menstrual Cycle

Ayurveda views menstruation as a sacred time for detoxification and renewal. In ancient texts, women were encouraged to rest and honor their bodies during this phase. Here are a few rituals to integrate into your life:

✦ **Honor rest:** Create a cozy space with warm blankets, herbal teas, and soothing music.

✦ **Use herbs for balance:** Triphala can aid detoxification, while shatavari supports reproductive health.

✦ **Practice Pranayama:** Nadi Shodhana (alternate nostril breathing) can balance the mind and calm emotions.

✦ **Create a sacred space:** Light a candle or burn sage to honor this time of renewal.

HONORING THE FEMININE CYCLE, TOGETHER

Understanding the menstrual cycle is more than a personal health tool—it's a profound act of self-awareness and empowerment. We spend decades moving through these rhythms, and even when our own cycles change or cease, the women around us—our daughters, mothers, friends, and colleagues—continue to live them. By learning to honor our own cycle and becoming attuned to the cyclical nature of others, we foster a sisterhood rooted in empathy and connection.

Whether you are menstruating or no longer bleeding, this wisdom still applies. We all hold the blueprint of cyclical living within us. Tuning into these patterns—whether through the menstrual cycle's lens or the moon's phases—allows us to live with more intention, compassion, and vitality.

By acknowledging the unique energetic landscape of each phase, we better support ourselves and others emotionally, physically, and spiritually. Imagine a world where women feel held, honored, and understood—not only by themselves but by each other. This is where collective healing begins.

Reflection on Your Own
Menstrual Cycle/Wisdom

1. How do you currently feel about your menstrual cycle (or the absence of it)? Has that perspective changed over time?

    _____

    _____

    _____

    _____

2. Which phase of the cycle do you feel most connected to? Which phase feels the most challenging for you, and why?

_____

_____

_____

_____

_____

3. What physical or emotional patterns have you noticed in your cycle that repeat each month?

_____

_____

_____

_____

_____

4. How does your energy shift across the different phases of your cycle? How might you begin to honor those shifts more intentionally in daily life?

_____

_____

_____

_____

_____

_____

_____

AYURVEDA & THE ALCHEMY OF HER

5. What messages about menstruation, positive or negative, did you receive growing up? How have those beliefs shaped your experience of being in a female body?

_____

_____

_____

_____

6. If you are no longer menstruating, how might you use the moon cycle as a guide for tuning into your inner rhythm?

_____

_____

_____

7. What rituals or practices help you feel most connected to your body during each phase of your cycle? How can you expand or deepen those?

_____

_____

_____

_____

8. How might your relationships improve if you honored both your own cycle and those of the women around you?

_____

_____

_____

_____

162

CHAPTER 11

Riding the Hormone Storm: Peri- to Postmenopause Survival

Hormonal transitions are a natural rhythm of a woman's life, yet perimenopause and menopause can often feel like being caught in an unpredictable tide—one moment calm, the next, swept away by waves of change. These phases are frequently misunderstood, reduced to a checklist of symptoms to control rather than honored as a profound transformation.

What Is Perimenopause and Menopause?

Perimenopause is the transitional phase leading up to menopause, typically beginning in a woman's late thirties to mid-forties and lasting anywhere from four to ten years. During this time, estrogen and progesterone levels fluctuate, causing irregular cycles, mood shifts, sleep disturbances, and other changes that feel destabilizing. This is the body's way of slowly adapting to the next phase of life.

Menopause is defined as the complete cessation of menstruation

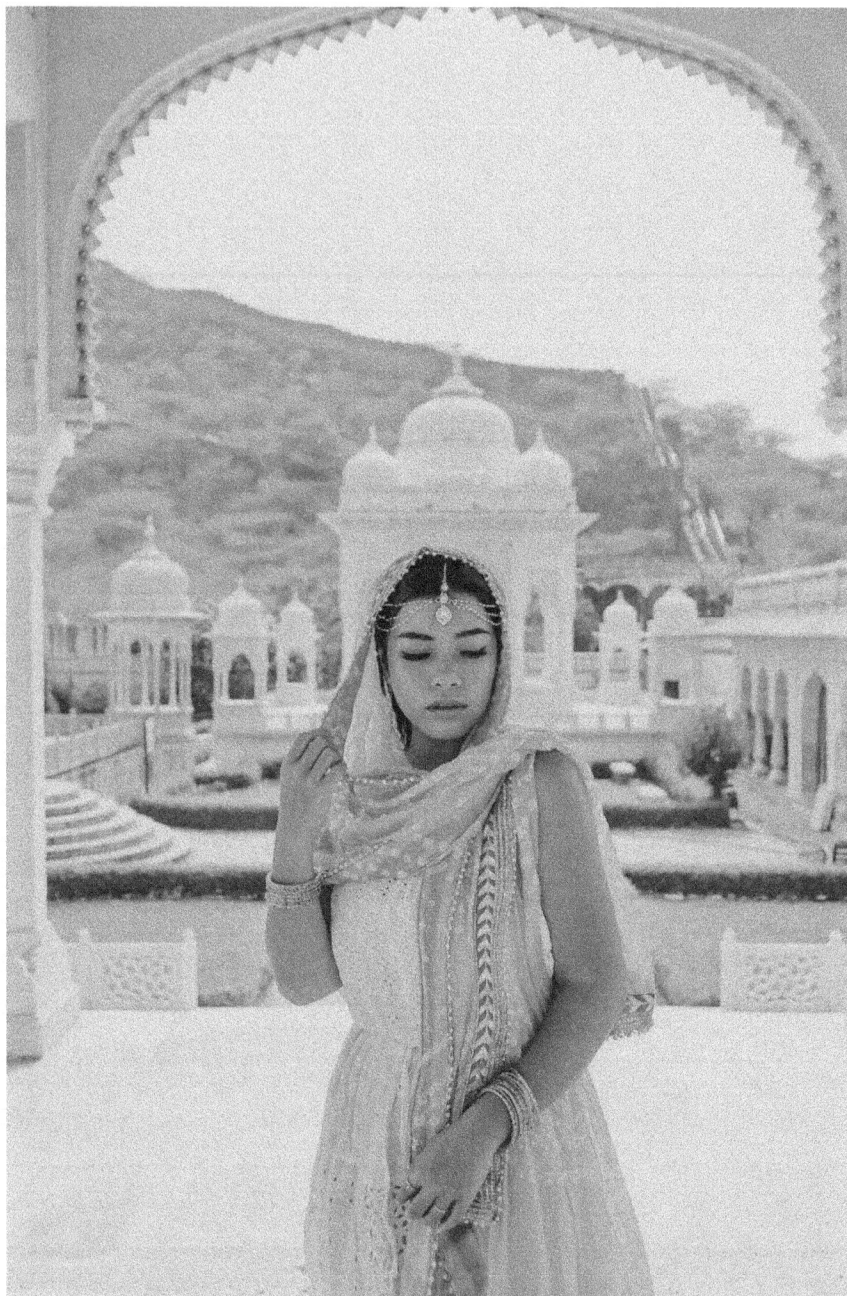

"WHAT IF THE CHANGE YOU FEAR IS THE ONE THAT WILL SET
YOU FREE?" – HARMONY

for twelve consecutive months, signaling the end of a woman's reproductive years. Most women reach menopause around age fifty to fifty-five, though this varies.

Postmenopause follows, a phase where estrogen remains low, and the body fully adapts to its new hormonal state. While Western medicine often treats menopause as a hormonal deficiency, Ayurveda and TCM see it as a natural and necessary transition—not an end, but a rebirth.

The Ayurvedic Perspective: A Time of Transformation

In Hindu philosophy, life is divided into four key stages— Brahmacharya (student life), Grihastha (householder life), Vanaprastha (retirement and spiritual reflection), and Sannyasa (renunciation and pursuit of liberation). Each phase offers a unique opportunity for growth, aligned with one's physical, emotional, and spiritual evolution.

From this lens, the perimenopausal to menopausal transition aligns with the shift from Grihastha to Vanaprastha—a turning inward from the outward focus of family, career, and societal roles to a deeper engagement with wisdom, introspection, and spiritual awakening.

In Ayurveda, this transition is honored as a sacred passage—not a decline, but a profound initiation. It marks a time when a woman steps more fully into her power, no longer defined by her reproductive function but by the depth of her presence and inner knowing.

In Ayurveda, the perimenopause to menopause transition is honored as a sacred passage—a gateway from the outward phase of reproduction to an inward phase of spiritual awakening. Rather than seeing it as a loss, it is embraced as a time when a woman steps more fully into her power.

Perimenopause is largely governed by a dynamic interplay of Pitta and Vata. Pitta's fire may manifest as hot flashes, irritability, and inflammation, while rising Vata can bring anxiety, insomnia, dryness, and scattered thinking. This duality can feel intense, but it also offers a powerful opportunity for transformation. In this phase, the energy of Goddess Kali is a potent ally—she invites you to dismantle old patterns, face truths, and burn away what no longer serves you with fierce compassion.

As we transition into menopause, the fluctuation between Pitta and Vata continues. The body may feel more sensitive, reactive, or depleted. This is the time to embrace Goddess Durga, who rides between worlds, both protector and nurturer. Durga's strength supports the need for boundaries, nourishment, and resilience.

As women enter the postmenopausal years, the body naturally shifts into what Ayurveda refers to as the Vata stage of life—contributing to the natural decline of bone density, tissue strength, and internal moisture. These changes are not inherently pathological; they are a reflection of elemental energies at play. However, when Vata becomes aggravated—due to lifestyle, diet, or unresolved stress—it can lead to imbalances such as insomnia, joint discomfort, anxiety, or accelerated aging.

While Vata dominates this phase, Kapha qualities such as stagnation, weight gain, and emotional heaviness may linger or increase, especially if they have been unaddressed in earlier years.

The wisdom and beauty of Goddess Lakshmi can be invoked here—she offers a reminder of inner abundance, harmony, and self-worth.

Throughout all stages, Goddess Saraswati, the embodiment of creative intelligence and spiritual expression, gently calls you into deeper connection with your inner truth. As your cycle ceases, your creative and intuitive energies are no longer divided—they are unified, focused, and available for deeper purpose and dharma.

By aligning your practices with these shifting doshic patterns and invoking the archetypes of these Goddesses, menopause becomes not a time of decline, but a profound reclamation of your power and presence. This is the alchemy of transformation.

The TCM Perspective: The Second Spring

Traditional Chinese Medicine (TCM) offers a reverent and empowering lens through which to view perimenopause to menopause. TCM describes this time as a woman's "Second Spring"—a return to the self, and an opportunity to reclaim inner harmony, vitality, and spirit. This new season marks the end of outward reproductive activity, but the beginning of profound inward cultivation.

In TCM, the foundation of a woman's vitality during this transition lies in the kidneys, which store Jing (essence). Jing is inherited at birth and gradually depleted through life; menopause signals a natural decline in this essence. If not replenished or preserved, symptoms like fatigue, dizziness, tinnitus, low back pain, weak bones, vaginal dryness, and forgetfulness arise.

Liver qi and blood also play central roles. The liver stores blood and regulates the smooth flow of qi throughout the body. If liver qi becomes stagnant—often due to emotional suppression, overwork, or long-term stress—it can lead to mood swings, frustration, menstrual irregularities, or digestive changes. Furthermore, a deficiency in liver blood may cause insomnia, dry eyes, or feelings of ungroundedness.

Yin deficiency becomes particularly common during perimenopause and menopause. Yin represents cooling, nourishing, moistening qualities, and as it wanes, women may experience symptoms like hot flashes, night sweats, dry skin, anxiety, and sleep disturbances. TCM interprets these symptoms not as problems to be eradicated, but as signals that the body is craving rest, reflection, and nourishment.

HOW TO SUPPORT THE BODY DURING THIS TRANSITION

To thrive through this Second Spring, we turn to time-honored practices and remedies rooted in Chinese medicine.

Nourish Kidney Jing

+ Foods such as black sesame seeds, walnuts, bone broth, goji berries, and seaweed help fortify the kidneys.

+ Rest is essential; allow ample sleep and periods of stillness.

+ Gentle breathwork and qi gong practices strengthen kidney energy without overexertion.

Pacify Liver Qi

+ Practices like journaling, walking in nature, and emotional expression can help qi move freely.

+ Chrysanthemum tea or rosebud tea support liver qi movement and emotional calm.

+ Acupressure on liver 3 (Tai Chong)—located between the big toe and second toe—can help release stagnation.

Anchor the Shen (Spirit)

+ The Shen resides in the heart and reflects our emotional and spiritual well-being. During this time, it is common for Shen to feel unsettled.

+ Calm the Shen with stillness, meditation, creative expression, and Shen-calming herbs such as reishi, Schisandra, and Zizyphus (Suan Zao Ren).

+ Acupressure on Yin Tang (the point between the eyebrows) can promote calm and mental clarity.

Cool the Fire of Yin Deficiency

✦ Incorporate cooling yin-nourishing herbs like rehmannia root (Shu Di Huang), Chinese yam, and lily bulb.

✦ Favor foods like cucumber, tofu, pears, mung beans, and barley.

✦ Avoid stimulants, excessive heat (both food and emotional), and late nights, which can further deplete Yin.

Create Rituals

✦ In Chinese culture, menopause is sometimes marked with ceremony—a symbolic acknowledgment of transition. You might light a candle, write yourself a letter of release, or create space for stillness at the new moon.

MENOPAUSAL TRANSITION AS A PORTAL TO POWER

In both TCM and Ayurveda, menopause is not an illness to cure but an awakening. It is a sacred passage into a new archetype—the wise woman, the sage, the teacher.

When we soften the fight against aging and tune into our body's messages, we gain more than energy—we gain sovereignty. Wisdom is distilled through experience, and this is your invitation to live from your inner knowing rather than societal noise.

From ages thirty-five to sixty-five, women are often at the height of their insight and creative potential. With the right support—nutritional, emotional, and spiritual—this season can feel not like a decline, but like the most deeply rooted and empowered time of your life, moving you into your highest form of self-leadership.

More and more women are turning to Eastern medicine because they're no longer satisfied with being told their symptoms are "just part of aging" or handed a prescription without a deeper conversation. They're craving a system that sees them as whole, honors their bodily complexity, and offers tools rooted in both prevention and personal empowerment. Ayurveda and Eastern medicine are not relics of the past—they are blueprints for our future. These traditions offer a compassionate, cyclical, and embodied approach to health that modern medicine is beginning to understand. By sharing this wisdom now, we not only support ourselves—we become cycle-breakers and wisdom-keepers for our daughters, granddaughters, and every woman who walks this path after us.

Perimenopause and Menopause: Understanding Hormonal Shifts and Weight

Perimenopause can begin as early as your mid-thirties, although most women notice stronger shifts in their forties. It marks a natural transition, but one that often comes with confusion around weight, mood, and metabolism. Knowing what's really happening in your body can help you navigate this phase with more confidence and less frustration.

During this time, estrogen and progesterone levels fluctuate significantly. Progesterone often declines first, which may lead to symptoms like water retention and bloating. Meanwhile, estrogen levels rise and fall unpredictably before gradually decreasing. This can contribute to changes in fat distribution, particularly an increase in abdominal fat, which many women find difficult to manage.

There's a common belief that metabolism "slows down" in midlife. While basal metabolic rate doesn't dramatically drop all at once, research shows that hormonal shifts—combined with changes in muscle mass, physical activity, and thyroid function—can make weight maintenance more difficult. One study found that the metabolic rate in midlife women declines by about 2 percent per decade, and this effect may be more pronounced if thyroid function is impaired.

Estrogen also affects appetite-regulating hormones like leptin and ghrelin. With lower estrogen, leptin sensitivity decreases (making it harder to feel full), while ghrelin increases (stimulating hunger), which can contribute to overeating. Add in poor sleep, high cortisol from chronic stress, and the demands of this life stage, and it becomes clear why weight gain feels inevitable for many women.

But it isn't a losing battle. It's simply a new phase that requires new strategies.

Reflection on Midlife and Menopausal Goals, Fears, Dreams, Anxieties, Excitements, an Identities

1. What are the most significant internal or external shifts you have experienced during midlife, and how have they influenced your sense of identity?

    _____

    _____

    _____

    _____

2. Which fears or anxieties about aging or menopause have surfaced for you, and how might they be pointing you toward areas that need healing or attention?

    _____

    _____

    _____

    _____

    _____

3. What dreams or goals have emerged in this stage of life that feel more aligned with your true self than ever before?

_____

_____

_____

_____

4. In what ways has menopause challenged your perception of femininity, power, or worth—and how has it also expanded your understanding of those concepts?

_____

_____

_____

_____

5. What aspects of your younger identity are you ready to release, and which new facets of yourself are you beginning to embrace?

_____

_____

_____

_____

6. How can you consciously redefine this phase of life as a time of initiation and transformation rather than decline or loss?

_____

_____

_____

_____

CHAPTER 12

Womb Wisdom: The Subtle Energies of Womanhood

There is a sacred intelligence held within the womb—a wisdom that transcends biology and speaks directly to a woman's creative essence, intuition, and emotional truth. In both Ayurveda and TCM, the female reproductive system is not merely a set of organs—it is viewed as a powerful energetic center, a temple of vitality, and a mirror for the soul. Yet in modern medicine and culture, the womb is often reduced to its function: fertility, menstruation, reproduction. When challenges arise—painful periods, fibroids, hormonal imbalances—we look at the symptoms in isolation rather than asking deeper questions: *What is my body trying to tell me? What emotions or stories are stored here? What part of me is asking to be heard, healed, or expressed?*

This chapter invites you to explore the womb not only through the lens of anatomy and hormones but as an energetic and emotional landscape that holds our lived experiences. Here, we begin to understand how unprocessed grief, suppressed creativity, ancestral patterns, and the cultural wounds of womanhood take root in the body. The womb becomes not only a center for creation but

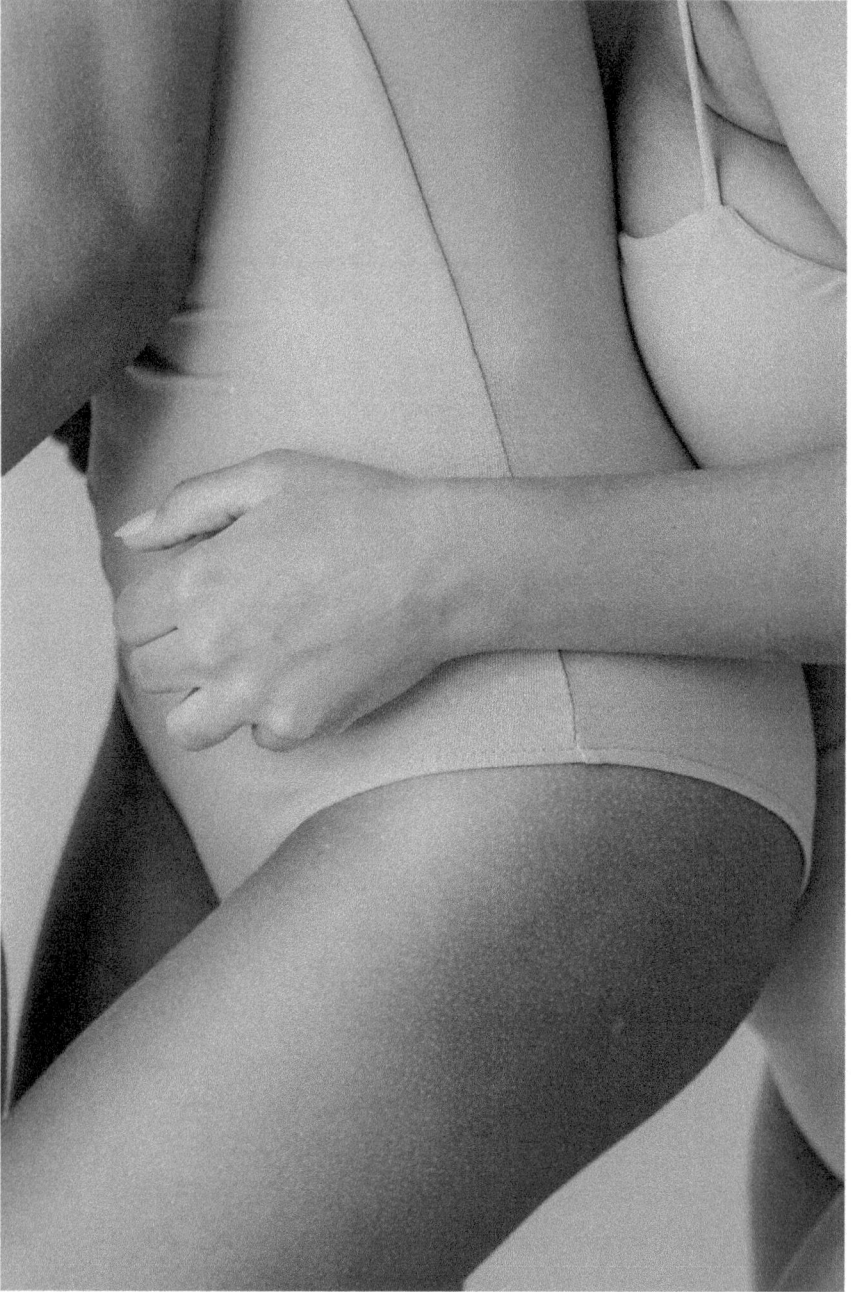

"A WOMAN'S WOMB IS NOT JUST A PLACE WHERE LIFE IS CREATED. IT IS WHERE SHE CREATES HERSELF OVER AND OVER AGAIN." – UNKNOWN

a container for what has been silenced or unmetabolized. When this space is acknowledged, nurtured, and brought into balance, it becomes a powerful catalyst for transformation.

In this chapter, we explore subtle energies of the female reproductive system from both Ayurvedic and TCM perspectives, and how disruptions in this sacred center may reflect more than physical dysfunction. We'll examine the links between reproductive health and emotional well-being and begin to unravel how conditions like adrenal fatigue, PCOS, amenorrhea, and others are not only medical syndromes but energetic messages calling us home to ourselves.

By returning to the womb as a source of inner knowing rather than pathology, we open the door to a deeper form of healing—one that honors our cycles, our power, and our wholeness. This is womb wisdom: ancient, embodied, and uniquely yours.

Ayurvedic Perspective

+ **The womb** (*Garbhashaya*): Seen as the seat of creation, the womb represents not only the ability to give life but also the creative potential of a woman's essence. Imbalances here often mirror unexpressed emotions or suppressed desires.

+ **Subtle energies**: Ayurveda speaks of Apana Vayu, the downward-moving energy responsible for menstruation, childbirth, and elimination. When Apana Vayu is disturbed, it can lead to irregular cycles, prolapse, or emotional instability.

TCM Perspective

✦ **The uterus** (*Zi Gong*): Known as the "palace of the child," the uterus is nourished by the kidney essence (Jing) and regulated by liver qi. Emotional stress or trauma can disrupt the flow of qi, leading to menstrual irregularities or infertility.

✦ **Subtle energies:** The concept of *Ren Mai* (conception vessel) and *Chong Mai* (penetrating vessel) in TCM highlights how the body's energy channels regulate reproductive health and connect to overall vitality.

The Reproductive System as a Mirror for the Soul

The metaphysical lens of Ayurveda and TCM invites us to see the reproductive system as more than a physical organ—it is a sacred space that reflects the state of our emotional, mental, and spiritual health. When we suppress our emotions, ignore our creativity, or carry unprocessed trauma, this energy can manifest in physical conditions.

For instance:

✦ Heavy periods may symbolize an emotional "overload."

✦ Painful cramps may reflect a subconscious resistance to change or a struggle to express anger.

✦ Irregular cycles can indicate a lack of rhythm or flow in daily life.

Let's take a closer look at some common women's health syndromes from the scientific and energetic aspects.

The Metaphysics of Disease: Emotions and the Feminine Body

In both Ayurveda and TCM, the body is understood as a physical and energetic vessel where unresolved emotions take form and manifest as physical symptoms. The reproductive system, as a center of creation, transformation, and emotional memory, is particularly sensitive to these energetic imbalances. This view parallels what Western medicine might categorize under the term psychosomatic symptoms—physical conditions that are influenced or triggered by mental or emotional factors. However, while Western approaches may often regard these manifestations as byproducts of psychological stress, the Eastern lens sees them as integral signals from the body's intelligence, urging us to acknowledge what has been suppressed or left unprocessed. This perspective offers a holistic understanding of women's health—one that invites us to look beyond surface-level symptoms and instead ask: What part of me is asking to be seen, heard, and healed?

Let's take a closer look at some common women's health conditions that can arise throughout the lifespan. The following conditions are listed alphabetically, so feel free to skip ahead and explore the ones that resonate most with your personal journey or professional focus.

ADRENAL FATIGUE: THE CURSE OF OVERACHIEVEMENT AND PEOPLE-PLEASING

Western Medical Understanding

Adrenal fatigue, though not officially recognised in Western medicine, describes a state of chronic stress where the adrenal glands first over-produce cortisol in response to stress then are unable to produce sufficient cortisol to meet the body's demands. Symptoms include fatigue, brain fog, low energy, and difficulty managing stress. This condition is often linked to HPA (hypothalamic-pituitary-adrenal) axis dysfunction, rather than adrenal gland dysfunction itself.

Emerging Science

Research into the effects of chronic stress on the HPA axis highlights the importance of stress-reducing practices in restoring cortisol balance. Adaptogenic herbs like ashwagandha, licorice, and rhodiola have shown promise in clinical studies for reducing stress and improving adrenal function. Lifestyle interventions, such as improving sleep quality and reducing blue light exposure, are also emphasised in adrenal recovery.

Ayurvedic Energietics

Adrenal fatigue aligns with a Vata-Pitta imbalance, reflecting overexertion (Vata) and burnout (Pitta). Depleted Ojas (vital energy) is a hallmark of this condition, leaving the body susceptible to fatigue and stress. Adrenal fatigue often reflects an imbalance between "doing" and "being." It symbolizes being caught in a cycle of overachievement or people-pleasing, leading to a depletion of personal reserves.

To heal from adrenal fatigue, favor grounding and rejuvenating foods like warm milk with ashwagandha, almonds, and saffron. Avoid stimulants like caffeine and refined sugar. Ingest supportive herbs such as ashwagandha (adaptogen and stress-reliever), Brahmi (calms the mind), and guduchi (restores Ojas). Prioritize restorative practices like yoga nidra, self-massage with ashwagandha oil, and daily meditation.

AMENORRHEA (ABSENCE OF PERIODS): DISCONNECTION FROM FEMININE ENERGY

Western Medical Understanding

Amenorrhea refers to the absence of menstruation—either when a young woman hasn't begun her cycle by age fifteen (primary amenorrhea), or when menstruation stops for three or more months after previously being regular (secondary amenorrhea). From a conventional perspective, this condition is often linked to factors such as low body weight, intense physical training, emotional stress, hormonal imbalances (such as PCOS or thyroid dysfunction), or a disruption in communication between the brain and ovaries (the hypothalamic-pituitary-ovarian axis).

Emerging Science

New research focuses on the role of energy balance and leptin (a hormone involved in regulating appetite and metabolism) in hypothalamic amenorrhea.[3] For women with PCOS-related amenorrhea, myo-inositol supplementation has been shown to improve ovulation. Mindfulness-based stress reduction programs are also being studied for their effectiveness in regulating cycles by reducing cortisol levels.

Ayurvedic Perspective

Many, but not all, women I have seen in my clinic who suffered from amenorrhea were eating a calorie-deficient diet that was not suited to their individual constitution, were overexercising, and led a high-stress lifestyle. When these aspects were corrected through Ayurvedic lifestyle medicine, the results were wonderful.

---

3   Sharon Chou et al., October 26, 2010, "Leptin Is an Effective Treatment for Hypothalamic Amenorrhea," Proceedings of the National Academy of Sciences of the United States of America, https://pages.ucsd.edu/~mboyle/COGS163/pdf-files/Leptin%20is%20an%20effective%20 treatment%20for%20amenorrhea-2011-Chou-6585-90.pdf.

Amenorrhea is often linked to a severe Vata imbalance, leading to dryness, depletion, and lack of flow in the body. It may also be connected to Kapha stagnation if weight gain or hormonal suppression is involved.

Amenorrhea can symbolise disconnection from feminine energy, creative suppression, or a fear of stepping into one's power. It may reflect a sense of being "frozen" emotionally or spiritually.

Ayurvedic support includes incorporating warm, nourishing foods like soups, stews, and ghee to pacify Vata and avoiding cold, raw, or overly processed foods. Take herbs such as Dashamoola (strengthens reproductive tissues), shatavari, bala (for nourishing and grounding), and Vitex (support healthy ovulation). Rituals like Abhyanga (self-massage) with sesame oil and yoga poses like child's pose and forward fold promote grounding and relaxation.

LIGHT PERIODS (HYPOMENORRHEA): FEAR OF "TAKING UP SPACE"

Western Medical Understanding

Light periods or hypomenorrhea are characterised by unusually low menstrual flow, which may be caused by hormonal imbalances, thyroid disorders, excessive exercise, or the use of hormonal contraception. Scar tissue in the uterus (Asherman's syndrome) or endometrial thinning due to long-term birth control use may also contribute.

Emerging Science

Emerging studies emphasise the importance of endometrial health in supporting menstruation. Hormonal therapies that focus on estrogen balance and improving uterine blood flow are gaining traction. Nutritional factors, including adequate intake of iron, zinc, and B vitamins, are increasingly recognized as crucial for maintaining a healthy endometrium.[4]

Ayurvedic Energetics

Light periods are often a result of Vata or Kapha imbalances. Vata may cause dryness and insufficient flow, while Kapha contributes to stagnation and weak endometrial lining. Light periods may symbolize a reluctance to fully express emotions or creativity. It may reflect a fear of "taking up space" in one's personal or professional life.

To nourish the body, include iron-rich foods like beets, dates, and leafy greens. Use spices like cumin and turmeric to stimulate Agni. Take shatavari, ashwagandha, and Vidarikand to build Ojas and strengthen reproductive tissues. Rituals of warm oil massages and grounding yoga practices promote blood flow and relaxation.

DYSMENORRHEA (PAINFUL PERIODS): RESISTANCE TO LETTING GO

Western Medical Understanding

Dysmenorrhea refers to pain during menstruation, often described as cramping in the lower abdomen. In conventional medicine, this pain is linked to elevated levels of prostaglandins—hormone-like compounds that trigger stronger uterine contractions. Primary dysmenorrhea occurs without an identifiable medical cause, while secondary dysmenorrhea is associated with underlying conditions such as endometriosis or fibroids.

Emerging Science

Anti-inflammatory diets rich in omega-3 fatty acids have been shown to reduce prostaglandin production and alleviate menstrual pain. Acupressure and acupuncture are gaining scientific support

---

4   Rhiana-Lily Smith, "How Do Minerals Affect the Menstrual Cycle?," Technology Networks: Proteomics & Metabolomics, April 18, 2024, https://www.technologynetworks.com/proteomics/news/how-do-minerals-affect-the-menstrual-cycle-385891.

for their ability to relieve dysmenorrhea by promoting endorphin release and improving pelvic blood flow.

In my practice, I have observed that combining 600 mg of magnesium with 1,000 mg of ginger daily has provided significant relief for clients experiencing menstrual discomfort. This combination leverages the muscle-relaxing effects of magnesium and the anti-inflammatory properties of ginger to address menstrual pain effectively.

Magnesium is believed to help by relaxing the uterine muscle and reducing the inflammation that causes period pain. Ginger, known for its anti-inflammatory properties, has been shown to reduce the severity of menstrual cramps.[5]

It's important to consult with a health care provider before starting any new supplement regimen to ensure safety and appropriateness for individual health needs.[6]

Ayurvedic Energetics

Painful periods often reflect the body's resistance to releasing physical and emotional stagnation. Dysmenorrhea is linked to Vata imbalances, as Vata governs all movement in the body, including the downward flow of Apana Vayu (elimination). Pitta imbalances may also contribute through inflammation and heat. Emotionally, dysmenorrhea can signal a struggle with releasing old patterns, grudges, or beliefs.

---

5 Lara Briden, "Magnesium and the Menstrual Cycle," Clue, March 7, 2018, https://helloclue.com/articles/cycle-a-z/magnesium-and-the-menstrual-cycle.

6 Bajalan, Z., Alimoradi, Z., & Moafi, F., 2019, "Nutrition as a Potential Factor of Primary Dysmenorrhea: A Systematic Review of Observational Studies," *Gynecologic and Obstetric Investigation* 84 (3): 209–224; Armour, M., Dahlen, H. G., Zhu, X., Farquhar, C., & Smith, C. A., 2018, "The Role of Treatment Timing and Acupuncture Type in the Management of Primary Dysmenorrhea: An Exploratory Randomised Controlled Trial," *PLOS ONE* 13 (3): e0193037.

Healing Practices

Warm castor oil packs on the lower abdomen can ease pain and promote flow. Cooling herbs like shatavari can calm inflammation, while mindfulness practices help identify emotional blocks.

MENORRHAGIA (HEAVY PERIODS): OVERWHELEMED BY LIFE'S RESPONSIBILITES

Western Medical Understanding

Menorrhagia refers to abnormally heavy or prolonged menstrual bleeding that can disrupt daily life. Common causes include hormonal imbalances (excess estrogen or insufficient progesterone), uterine fibroids, adenomyosis, polyps, or underlying conditions like thyroid disorders or bleeding disorders. Iron deficiency anemia is a frequent consequence of chronic menorrhagia, which can worsen fatigue and other symptoms.

Emerging Science

Advances in hormonal therapies, including low-dose progestin IUDs, are providing more targeted treatment options for heavy periods. Research also suggests a link between chronic inflammation and heavy bleeding, with anti-inflammatory diets and supplements like omega-3s showing promise in alleviating symptoms.[7]

Ayurvedic Energetics

Heavy periods result from a Pitta imbalance. Excess Pitta creates heat and inflammation, or excessive flow. Poor liver health (seat of Ranjaka Pitta) may also exacerbate heavy bleeding.

---

7   Rahbar N, Asgharzadeh N, Ghorbani R., January 17, 2012, "Effect of Omega-3 Fatty Acids on Intensity of Primary Dysmenorrhea," *International Journal Gynaecology and Obstetrics*.

Metaphysical Meaning

Heavy periods may reflect an inability to release emotional burdens or unprocessed grief. It may also signify unresolved feelings of loss or being overwhelmed by life's responsibilities.

Ayurvedic Support

Customized dosha-specific diets will help. Favour cooling and anti-inflammatory foods like cucumbers, coconut water, and leafy greens. Avoid spicy, sour, and salty foods. Herbal support like ashoka (balances Pitta and supports uterine health) and Guduchi (anti-inflammatory) are common. Rituals are important: rest during menstruation and avoid overexertion. Perform cooling pranayama, such as Sheetali breath.

ENDOMETRIOSIS: THE WEIGHT OF FRUSTRATION AND GRIEF

Western Medical Understanding

Endometriosis is a condition where tissue similar to the endometrial lining grows outside the uterus, often on the ovaries, fallopian tubes, and pelvic lining. This tissue responds to hormonal changes, leading to inflammation, pain, and scar tissue formation. The exact cause is unknown, but theories include retrograde menstruation (when menstrual blood flows backward through the fallopian tubes), immune system dysfunction, and genetic predisposition. Hormonal imbalances, particularly excessive estrogen, can stimulate further growth.

Emerging Science

Recent studies link endometriosis to altered gut microbiota and systemic inflammation, suggesting that targeting gut health may provide new therapeutic avenues.[8] This is what Ayurveda has been doing for years through strengthening Agni. Research has also highlighted the role of oxidative stress and its contribution to the disease's progression. Anti-inflammatory diets (such as a Pitta-pacifying diet) and antioxidant-rich foods are being explored as therapies.

The Ayurvedic Energetics

In Ayurveda, endometriosis is often viewed as tri-doshic, involving all three doshas. The erratic nature of Vata may manifest as chronic pain, while Pitta's heat can drive inflammation and intensify symptoms, and Kapha stimulates endometrial growth. But metaphysically, endometriosis may reflect something deeper: grief that has not been released or frustration that has been stifled.

For example, Sarah came to me after years of debilitating endometriosis disrupted her life. She described feeling she had to carry the weight of everyone's expectations—her family, her partner, even herself. She was an overachiever who always felt the need to "do more" but rarely paused to honor her emotions. Through Ayurvedic practices, we worked on calming her Vata with grounding routines and reducing Pitta through cooling herbs like shatavari and Gotu Kola and an anti-inflammatory diet. But it wasn't until we delved into the grief she carried—from a childhood where she felt unseen—that her healing truly began.

8   Gua, C & Zhang, C., 2024, "The Role of Gut Microbiota in Endometriosis and Systemic Inflammation," *Frontiers in Microbiology*, https://www.frontiersin.org/journals/microbiology/articles/10.3389/fmicb.2024.1363455/full.

FIBROIDS: UNPROCESSED CREATIVITY AND SUPPRESSED EMOTIONAL WOUNDS

Western Medical Understanding

Fibroids are benign tumors that grow in or around the uterus. They are influenced by hormones like estrogen and progesterone and tend to grow during reproductive years. Genetic predisposition, African ancestry, and lifestyle factors such as diet and stress increase risk. Symptoms can include heavy menstrual bleeding, pelvic pain, and infertility, though many women remain asymptomatic.

Emerging Science

Research shows that insulin-like growth factors play a role in fibroid growth, opening the door to new therapeutic interventions. Additionally, environmental toxins, including endocrine-disrupting chemicals like BPA, have been linked to fibroid development, leading to a focus on reducing toxin exposure. Advances in minimally invasive treatments, such as uterine artery embolization (UAE), are offering more options for women.

The Ayurvedic Energetics

Fibroids, benign growths in the uterus, reflect stagnant energy—unfulfilled potential or emotions that have been suppressed rather than expressed. In Ayurveda, fibroids are often linked to an imbalance in Kapha, the dosha of stability and structure, while TCM associates them with qi stagnation and blood stasis.

Laura told me she felt "stuck" in her job, her marriage, and even her body. Her diagnosis of uterine fibroids coincided with a period when she felt creatively blocked and emotionally burdened. Through Ayurvedic therapies like castor oil packs to stimulate circulation in the pelvic region, a Kapha-pacifying diet, and herbal formulas like Kanchanar Guggulu, we addressed her physical symptoms.

Simultaneously, we worked to unlock her creative energy. Laura set aside fifteen minutes each day to color a beautiful picture. As she reconnected with her creativity, her emotional state shifted, and her physical symptoms began to improve.

HYPOTHYROIDISM: THE VOICE UNHEARD

Western Medical Understanding

Hypothyroidism occurs when the thyroid gland doesn't produce enough thyroid hormones, leading to a slowdown in metabolism. Common causes include Hashimoto's thyroiditis (an autoimmune condition), iodine deficiency, and certain medications. Symptoms include fatigue, weight gain, depression, and hair loss.

Emerging Science

Autoimmune thyroid conditions like Hashimoto's have been linked to gut permeability (leaky gut) and dysbiosis, highlighting the importance of gut health in thyroid management. Selenium and zinc supplementation have been shown to support thyroid function. Additionally, new insights suggest that chronic stress and cortisol dysregulation can impair thyroid hormones, making stress management a critical part of treatment.[9]

Ayurvedic Energetics

The thyroid, often referred to as the "butterfly gland," sits in the throat chakra, or *Vishuddha* in Ayurveda, which governs communication and self-expression. Hypothyroidism, or an underactive thyroid, can reflect a blockage in expressing your truth or feeling unheard in your relationships or environment. From an Ayurvedic perspective, hypothyroidism correlates with Kapha imbalances, leading to stagnation, fatigue, and weight gain. The

---

9   Ben Reebs, "Cortisol and Thyroid: How Stress Affects Your Health," Modern Vital, July 9, 2018, https://www.drreebs.com/cortisol-thyroid-stress/.

heaviness of Kapha mirrors the emotional burden of unspoken words or suppressed desires. Women with hypothyroidism may feel stifled, undervalued, or afraid to use their voice. This condition can also emerge when one sacrifices their needs for others, losing connection to their own purpose and self-expression.

Megan, came to me exhausted and feeling invisible in her marriage. She had spent years catering to her family, putting their needs before her own. Through a combination of Ayurvedic herbs like Kanchanara (to stimulate thyroid function), a lighter Kapha-pacifying diet, and journaling prompts to explore her truth, she reconnected with her voice. Megan found joy in speaking up, and as she made space for herself, her energy and health transformed.

HYPERTHYROIDISM: THE VOICE OVEREXERTED

Western Medical Understanding

Hyperthyroidism results from excessive production of thyroid hormones, often due to Graves' disease (an autoimmune condition) or thyroid nodules. Symptoms include weight loss, heart palpitations, anxiety, and heat intolerance.

Emerging Science

Recent research has explored the role of antibodies in Graves' disease, with advanced antibody therapies under investigation. Vitamin D deficiency has been found to worsen autoimmune thyroid conditions, leading to a greater focus on optimizing vitamin D levels (so get some sunshine, ladies! That's nature's source of vitamin D).[10] Stress reduction techniques like yoga and meditation are studied for their potential to reduce thyroid hyperactivity as well.[11]

---

10 Wentz, I, "The Benefits of Vitamin D for Your Thyroid," Thyroid Pharmacist, February 14, 2025, https://thyroidpharmacist.com/articles/vitamin-d-benefits-thyroid/.

11 Wentz, 2025.

Ayurvedic Energetics

In Ayurveda, hyperthyroidism typically reflects a Pitta-Vata imbalance. Pitta drives the heat, intensity, and urgency; Vata fuels the anxiety, overstimulation, and mental overactivity. It's a pattern of doing too much, giving too much, or speaking too much—often at the expense of grounding and inner peace. The throat chakra, associated with self-expression and truth, may become energetically overcharged when we feel the need to constantly prove ourselves, speak louder to be heard, or overexplain our worth.

Elise came to me in her late thirties. She had been recently diagnosed with Graves' disease after months of unexplained weight loss, racing thoughts, and sleep disturbances. A high-achiever and mother of two, she admitted she hadn't taken a day off in years. She was the "go-to" person at work, the friend who always said yes, and the emotional anchor in her family. Her voice was always in use—teaching, emailing, comforting others—but when I asked her when she last sat in stillness, she paused. "I don't think I ever have," she whispered. Her body was crying out for rest, but her deeper healing came when she began claiming silence—not as a void, but as a form of power. Slowly, she learned to speak less, listen more, and honor her need for stillness.

Women with hyperthyroidism may struggle to set boundaries or feel they are constantly "on," unable to relax or delegate. This overexertion reflects a need for validation or a fear of being irrelevant.

Hyperthyroidism invites us to reflect: Where have I been overextending myself? What am I afraid will happen if I stop? What part of me is asking for quiet?

INFERTILITY: CREATIVITY BLOCKED

Western Medical Understanding

Infertility is defined as the inability to conceive after one year of trying (or six months for women over thirty-five). Causes include ovulatory dysfunction (e.g., PCOS), tubal blockages, endometriosis, and age-related decline in egg quality. Male-factor infertility, often due to low sperm count or motility, also plays a role in many cases.

Emerging Science

Advances in assisted reproductive technology, such as in-vitro fertilization (IVF), are improving success rates. Antioxidant supplementation has shown promise in enhancing egg and sperm quality by reducing oxidative stress. Additionally, research into the impact of environmental toxins, stress, and diet on fertility is growing, with evidence suggesting that a Mediterranean-style diet can boost fertility outcomes.

In a systematic review and meta-analysis published in *Nutrition Reviews*, researchers examined eleven studies involving over thirteen thousand individuals and found that greater adherence to the Mediterranean diet was associated with improved live birth and pregnancy rates, as well as enhanced sperm quality in men.[12] Similarly, research published in Human Reproduction indicated that women who adhered to the Mediterranean diet had higher rates of pregnancy and birth after IVF treatment compared to those with other diets.[13]

These findings suggest that incorporating a Mediterranean-style diet, rich in fruits, vegetables, whole grains, legumes, and healthy fats, may significantly boost fertility outcomes.

---

12 Muffone, de Oliveira, Paola, and Rabito, 2023. "Mediterranean Diet and Infertility: A Systematic Review with Meta-analysis of Cohort Studies," *Nutrition Reviews* 81 (7): 775–789.
13 Muffone et al., 2023.

Ayurvedic Energetics

Infertility is one of the most emotionally charged conditions women face, as it touches the very essence of creation and femininity. Both Ayurveda and TCM view infertility as a blockage in the creative flow, whether it's due to physical stagnation, emotional trauma, or unaligned energy.

Ayurvedic Perspective

Infertility can arise from imbalances in all three doshas:

+ **Vata:** Irregular cycles, stress, or anxiety

+ **Pitta:** Inflammation or hormonal imbalances

+ **Kapha:** Excess weight, sluggish metabolism, or stagnation in the reproductive organs

Infertility often reflects unresolved grief or feelings of inadequacy. It may also emerge when a woman feels disconnected from her feminine power or creative energy in other areas of her life.

Rachel came to me after years of trying to conceive. She admitted she felt unworthy of motherhood due to unresolved guilt from a past decision to have a termination when she fell pregnant at the age of twenty-one years old with her verbally abusive partner. Through Ayurvedic cleansing therapies like Panchakarma, herbal support (Dashamoola and ashoka), and guided meditation to release guilt, Rachel reconnected with her creative energy. Her journey to motherhood became a spiritual awakening as much as a physical one.

PCOS: STAGNATION AND THE LOSS OF FLOW

Western Medical Understanding

Polycystic Ovary Syndrome (PCOS) is a common hormonal condition characterised by irregular or absent menstrual cycles, elevated levels of androgens (often referred to as "male" hormones, though all women produce them in smaller amounts), and the presence of ovarian cysts. A primary driver of PCOS is insulin resistance, which can lead to elevated insulin levels in the blood. This, in turn, stimulates the ovaries to produce more androgens, disrupting ovulation and menstrual rhythm. Chronic low-grade inflammation and metabolic factors, such as excess weight in some women, may also contribute to the development or persistence of symptoms.

Emerging Science

Recent studies emphasise the gut microbiome's role in PCOS, with evidence suggesting that gut dysbiosis can worsen insulin resistance and androgen imbalances. Supplements that improve insulin sensitivity have shown promising results in clinical trials, as has Gymnema, an Ayurvedic herbal medicine. Furthermore, mindfulness-based interventions are gaining attention for their ability to reduce stress and improve PCOS symptoms through cortisol regulation.[14]

Ayurvedic Energetics

PCOS is a common condition I see in my practice. It's a condition deeply connected to Kapha imbalances in Ayurveda—characterised by stagnation, heaviness, and excess—while TCM identifies it as qi stagnation with dampness and phlegm accumulation. Beyond the physical, PCOS often reflects the energetic loss of flow in one's life.

Vanessa described herself as "frozen" in a pattern of self-doubt and overthinking. She was so overwhelmed by her responsibilities that she felt unable to take meaningful action in any area of her life. Her cycles were irregular, her energy was low, and she felt disconnected from her feminine power. Vanessa's treatment plan included dietary adjustments to reduce Kapha (like cutting down

---

14 Han, Q., Wang, J., Li, W., Chen, Z.-J., and Du, Y., 2021, "Androgen-induced Gut Dysbiosis Disrupts Glucolipid Metabolism and Endocrinal Functions in Polycystic Ovary Syndrome," *Microbiome* 9 (1): 101.

on dairy and refined carbs), movement practices like beach walks to rekindle her inner fire, and Ayurvedic herbs to balance her hormones. But just as importantly, we explored the emotional aspects of her stagnation. She began a journaling practice where she asked herself daily, "Where am I holding back?" Over time, Vanessa began to release her fear of failure and take small steps toward her dreams, restoring both her menstrual cycle and her vitality.

PMS (PREMENSTRUAL SYNDROME): IMBALANCES IN SELF-CARE

Western Medical Understanding

Premenstrual syndtome (PMS) refers to a collection of emotional, physical, and behavioral symptoms that arise in the luteal phase, typically easing once menstruation begins. These symptoms, which may include bloating, breast tenderness, mood fluctuations, fatigue, irritability, and food cravings, are thought to be triggered by hormonal shifts—particularly in estrogen and progesterone—as well as changes in neurotransmitters like serotonin.

Emerging Science

Research has shown that lifestyle changes such as regular exercise, improved sleep, mindfulness, and balanced nutrition can significantly reduce PMS symptoms. Key nutrients like calcium, magnesium, and vitamin D have been found to support hormonal stability and reduce discomfort. While PMS is a common experience for many women, it is also a valid and important indicator of how well we are nourishing and caring for our bodies during the premenstrual window. In contrast, conditions like Premenstrual Dysphoric Disorder (PMDD) go beyond the scope of typical PMS, involving severe emotional and physical symptoms that require specific support and intervention.

Ayurvedic Energetics

PMS typically reflects a Vata-Pitta imbalance. Vata aggravation contributes to anxiety, bloating, and irregular cravings, while Pitta manifests as irritability, anger, and breast tenderness. A Kapha imbalance may also contribute to symptoms like water retention and lethargy.

PMS may symbolize unacknowledged emotional needs or imbalances in self-care. It can point to areas in life where a woman feels overextended, undervalued, or out of alignment with her true desires. Focus on warm, nourishing foods like kitchari, root vegetables, and herbal teas with fennel, ginger, or cinnamon. Reduce salt to minimize bloating and favor foods that are easy to digest. Incorporate gentle movement like yoga or walking and practice alternate nostril breathing (Nadi Shodhana) to calm the nervous system.

PMDD (PREMENSTRUAL DYSPHORIC DISORDER): DEEP NEED TO SET BOUNDARIES

Western Medical Understanding

PMDD has been described as a severe form of PMS characterized by debilitating emotional and physical symptoms that usually occur in the luteal phase (post-ovulation) but can occur from ovulation through to menstruation. These symptoms, which often include severe mood swings, irritability, anxiety, depression, and extreme physical discomfort, are thought to stem from abnormal sensitivity to hormonal fluctuations, particularly estrogen and progesterone.

Emerging Science

Recent research highlights the role of serotonin in PMDD, as hormonal changes during the luteal phase affect serotonin levels. Selective Serotonin Reuptake Inhibitors (SSRI's) are now a common treatment in western medicine. Evidence also suggests that magnesium and vitamin B6 supplementation can reduce symptoms.[15]

Ayurvedic Perspective

PMDD is seen as a severe imbalance of Vata and Pitta, however, depending on one's individual constitution, it can certainly involve Kapha dosha too. The unpredictable emotional swings and heightened sensitivity reflect aggravated Vata, while the intense anger, irritability, and frustration point to Pitta excess. The feeling of low moods, depression, and inertia are indicative of Kapha's involvement. Poor Agni and elevated ama exacerbate hormonal dysregulation and emotional instability.

PMDD reflects suppressed emotions, such as unresolved anger, frustration, or sadness, that rise to the surface during the luteal phase. It symbolizes a deep need for emotional expression and boundary-setting, pointing to areas in life where a woman feels unsupported or unheard.

If you suffer with PMDD, try to favor grounding and cooling foods like cooked vegetables, especially root vegetables, as well as ghee and warm milk with spices like nutmeg and saffron. Avoid caffeine, alcohol, and spicy or fried foods.

Some herbs that provide support are shatavari (balances hormones and nourishes Ojas), Brahmi (calms the mind), St. John's-wort (supports low mood), and ashwagandha (reduces stress).

Take time for nourishment through restorative yoga, grounding meditation, and journaling to process emotions. Create a calming evening ritual with warm tea and oil massage.

---

15 Sacher et al., 2023, "Increase in Serotonin Transporter Binding in Patients with Premenstrual Dysphoric Disorder across the Menstrual Cycle: A Case-control Longitudinal Neuroreceptor Ligand PET Imaging Study," *Biological Psychiatry*.

A CLIENT'S JOURNEY: BELLE'S JOURNEY WITH PMDD

Belle, a forty-two-year-old marketing consultant, came to me feeling exhausted and frustrated. She described her PMDD as a "monthly storm" that completely disrupted her life. "It feels like I'm losing control for two weeks out of every month," she said, her voice tinged with both anger and resignation. The symptoms were more than just physical discomfort—intense mood swings, irritability, and a sense of overwhelming sadness began about two weeks before her period and persist until a few days after. "It's like I'm a different person," she explained. "I snap at my partner for no reason, and I can't concentrate at work. It's as if everything feels ten times harder."

As the head of a busy marketing department, Belle was used to managing high-pressure situations, but during the days leading up to her period, she found herself avoiding important meetings and struggling to complete projects on time. "I'd be sitting at my desk, staring at the screen, and I'd feel this wave of hopelessness," she confessed. Colleagues noticed her withdrawal, and she feared it was affecting her reputation at work. At home, her relationship was strained; her partner, who tried to be supportive, often felt helpless during her emotional lows. "I feel guilty for pushing him away," she said. "I know it's not fair, but I don't know how to stop."

Belle's situation was more than a hormonal imbalance; it was a cycle of physical symptoms intertwined with emotional struggles. Through the higHERself™ Method, we identified her Prakriti as Vata-Pitta, with a significant Vata imbalance exacerbating her PMDD. This imbalance contributed to her emotional volatility and low energy. We began with Ayurvedic self-care practices tailored to calm Vata, such as Abhyanga, and incorporating nourishing foods that provided grounding and stability. Acupuncture sessions helped regulate her hormonal cycles, targeting the emotional symptoms as much as the physical. Alongside these treatments, we introduced breathwork exercises to manage stress and guided journaling to process her emotions. We also incorporated a supplement that contained ashwagandha, saffron, and shatavari—three powerful Ayurvedic herbs known for their ability to support hormonal balance, emotional well-being, and stress resilience.

Ashwagandha helped calm her nervous system, reducing anxiety and improving Belle's ability to manage stress. Its adaptogenic properties made it an ideal choice for balancing Vata-related symptoms, promoting overall stability and inner strength.

Shatavari supported hormonal regulation and nourished reproductive health. It provided a deeply grounding effect, helping to stabilize Belle's emotions and restore her vitality.

Saffron, often called the "golden elixir," played a key role in uplifting mood and enhancing emotional balance. With its potent antioxidant and antidepressant properties, it helped Belle combat feelings of overwhelm, supporting a sense of joy and inner radiance.

Belle also started taking Vitamin B6 and Magnesium, which played crucial roles in alleviating her PMDD symptoms. Vitamin B6 is known for regulating mood and supporting neurotransmitter function. It reduces symptoms of irritability and low mood, which were particularly severe during her premenstrual phase. Magnesium, a vital mineral for muscle relaxation and nervous system health, reduces tension, eases cramps, and improves sleep quality. It also contributed to calming Vata, which was an important factor in Belle's overall treatment plan.

As Belle began to integrate these practices daily, she noticed gradual shifts. Her PMDD symptoms became less intense, and the emotional highs and lows evened out. She found herself more in control during the premenstrual phase. "It's like I can finally breathe through it instead of being suffocated," she shared.

The most significant change came in her relationship and work life. She felt more present at home and communicated her needs to her partner with less guilt. At work, she regained her focus and confidence. Belle's journey highlighted that while her hormonal cycle was a major factor, it was the holistic approach of addressing her emotional landscape alongside the physical symptoms that made the real difference.

PMDD DEEP DIVE: THE SILENT STRUGGLE AND THE NEED FOR A HOLISTIC APPROACH

Premenstrual Dysphoric Disorder (PMDD) is more than "bad PMS." It is a severe, often debilitating condition that affects approximately 3 to 8 percent of women of reproductive age, yet for decades, it was misunderstood, misdiagnosed, or dismissed entirely. Only in the last ten to twelve years has PMDD gained proper medical recognition, but awareness and effective treatment options remain limited. For too long women experiencing the intense mood swings, depression, and rage associated with PMDD were labeled as "hysterical" or "overly emotional," with little understanding of underlying biological and psychological factors at play.

Historically, the medical system did not have a name for what we now call PMDD. Instead, women suffering from extreme mood disturbances around their menstrual cycles were often diagnosed with "hysteria"—a term derived from the Greek word *hystera*, meaning uterus. This outdated and deeply misogynistic view led to countless women being institutionalized or subjected to unnecessary hysterectomies, believing that removing the uterus would cure their distress. While we have progressed in medical understanding, many women today still struggle to have their PMDD symptoms taken seriously, often facing years of misdiagnoses before receiving proper support.

PMDD DEEP DIVE: THE STARK REALITY
OF PMDD SUICIDES

PMDD is not solely about discomfort—it is a disorder that significantly increases the risk of suicide, particularly in the luteal phase (the week or two before menstruation begins). Research shows that women with PMDD are at a four-time higher risk of suicidal ideation compared to those without the condition.[16]

In Australia, suicide is the leading cause of death among women aged fifteen to forty-four, and studies suggest that up to 30 percent of women who attempt suicide may have undiagnosed PMDD.[17] In the United States, research indicates that 34 percent of women with PMDD report suicidal thoughts, and 19 percent have attempted suicide at least once.[18]

These statistics highlight why PMDD requires urgent awareness and a comprehensive, individualized approach to treatment. PMDD is not just a hormonal disorder—it is a mind-body-spirit imbalance that requires a multifaceted approach. Conventional treatments, such as SSRI's and hormonal birth control, may provide symptom relief for some, but they often come with side effects or fail to address the root cause. A holistic approach is essential for long-term healing, integrating

+ **diet and nutrition**: anti-inflammatory foods, balanced blood sugar, and herbal support

+ **nervous system regulation**: breathwork, meditation, and stress management

---

16 Osborn et al., 2021.
17 Black Dog Institute, 2025.
18 Osborn et al., 2021; Prasad et al., 2021.

- **hormonal balance:** Ayurvedic herbal formulas tailored to each woman's constitution
- **acupuncture and bodywork:** to regulate Prana/qi, reduce stress, and improve mood
- **community, emotional, and psychological support:** PMDD is isolating—having a support system is vital. Ayurvedic psychology counselling sessions have helped many of my clients navigate PMDD

I have witnessed the profound transformation that is possible when women are met with compassion, knowledge, and a truly integrative approach. Many who once felt overwhelmed by emotional cycles and disconnected from their bodies have rediscovered a sense of rhythm, balance, and inner resilience. PMDD is real. It is not simply a more intense form of PMS—it is a deeply affecting condition that can alter daily life and well-being. It deserves more than acknowledgment; it deserves meaningful support and healing that considers the full physical, emotional, and spiritual spectrum of a woman's experience.

If you are struggling with PMDD, you are not alone. There is hope, there is healing, and there is a way forward. Reach out for support—your cycle does not have to define your life.

Reflection on Reproductive Health

1. What beliefs or messages did I receive about my reproductive health growing up, and how have they shaped my relationship with my body today?

_____

_____

_____

_____

_____

2. Are there any menstrual or reproductive symptoms I tend to overlook or suppress? What might they be trying to communicate?

_____

_____

_____

_____

3. In what ways do I honor or ignore the natural rhythms of my cycle or hormonal changes throughout the month?

_____

_____

_____

_____

4. Have I ever felt disconnected from my womb, voice, or feminine expression? If so, what might have caused that disconnect?

_____

_____

_____

_____

_____

_____

5. What emotions tend to surface around my menstrual cycle, fertility, or hormonal shifts—and how do I typically respond to them?

_____

_____

_____

_____

_____

_____

6. What would it look like to trust the wisdom of my reproductive system and approach it with compassion rather than control?

_____

_____

_____

_____

_____

CHAPTER 13

Biohacking Your Hormones: What Research Reveals

Hormones are often thought of as chemical messengers, regulating everything from our energy and sleep to our menstrual cycles and mood. But through the lens of Ayurveda and Traditional Chinese Medicine, they can also be understood as the physiological expression of our energetic blueprint. Where the ancients speak of doshas, qi, and Ojas, modern science now offers us insight into cortisol, insulin, estrogen, and progesterone—reminding us that these worlds are not in conflict but are, in fact, reflections of one another.

To work with your hormones is to engage with your inner ecosystem. The glands that produce them—thyroid, ovaries, adrenals, pituitary—are not isolated machines. They are responsive to your environment, your thoughts, your nourishment, and your pace of life. This is where the East and West converge: both systems tell us that imbalance does not begin in the body alone. It begins in the relationship we have with ourselves.

Biohacking, then, is not about hacking the body in a cold or mechanical sense. It is about tuning in, making conscious

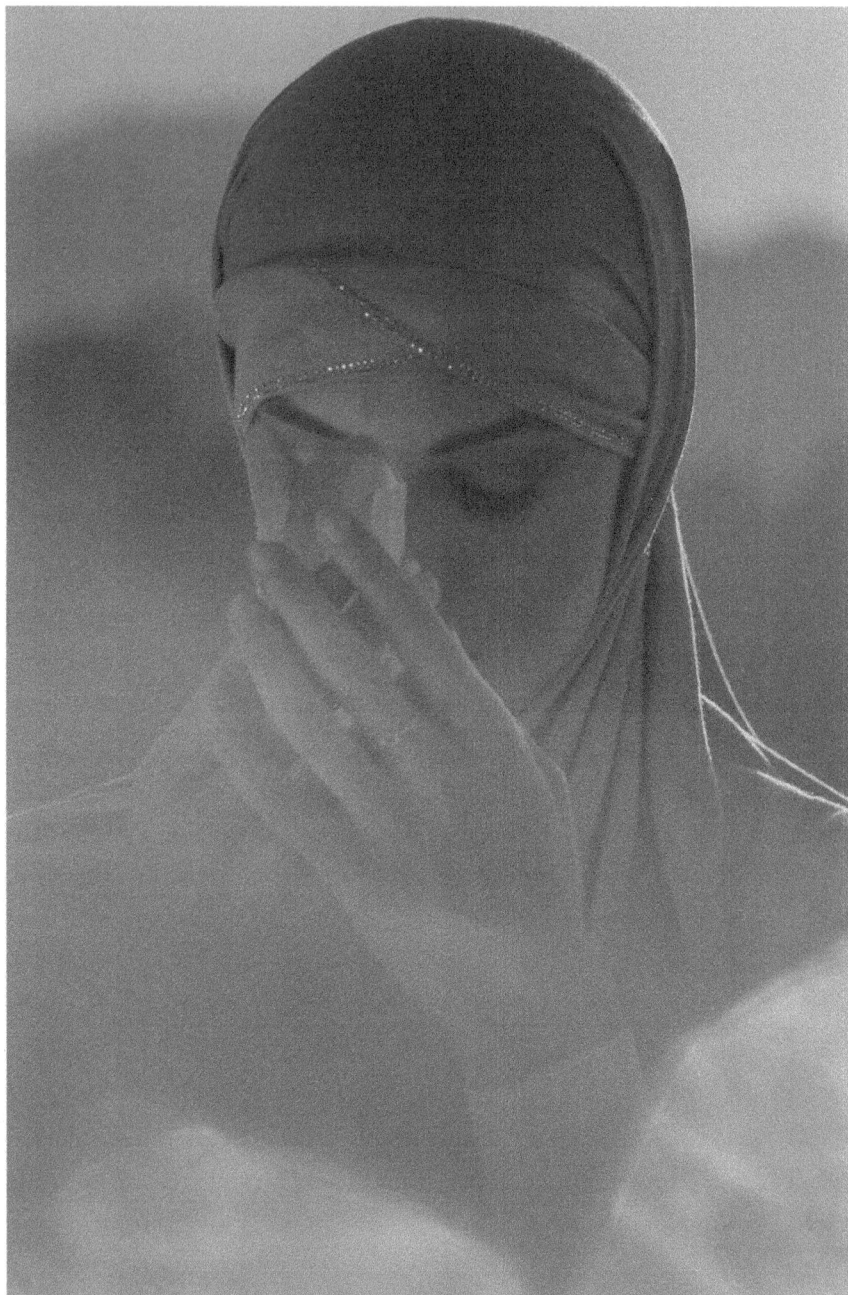

"KNOWLEDGE IS POWER. SELF-KNOWLEDGE IS EMPOWERMENT."

microadjustments, and claiming agency over your health using both ancient wisdom and evidence-based strategies. We are not separate from our biology. We are in constant dialogue with it.

Research continues to confirm what ancient wisdom has known for thousands of years: what we eat, how we manage stress, and the quality of our sleep all play critical roles in regulating hormones.

But here's the issue: hormonal imbalances are on the rise.

✦ 1 in 3 women experiences symptoms of estrogen dominance, leading to issues like fibroids, PCOS, and endometriosis.[19]

✦ 80% of women report sleep disturbances during perimenopause due to erratic progesterone and cortisol levels.[20]

✦ Stress-related hormonal imbalances have skyrocketed, with chronic stress being a major driver of infertility, cycle irregularities, and thyroid disorders.[21]

So, let's break down what's really happening inside the body and how we can work with our hormones, not against them.

In classical Ayurveda, health is supported by three foundational pillars—food (*ahara*), sleep (*nidra*), and regulated energy or moderation (*brahmacharya*). These pillars are seen as the essential supports of vitality and long life. When one is weakened or neglected, the entire system begins to wobble.

While your own healing journey may include different

---

19 Endocrine Society, 2022; US Department of Veterans Affairs, 2025.

20 National Sleep Foundation, "How Can Menopause Affect Sleep?," January 18, 2024, https://www.sleepfoundation.org/women-sleep/menopause-and-sleep.

21 Harvard Medical School, "How Does Exercise Reduce Stress? Surprising Answers to This Question and More," Harvard Health Publishing, July 7, 2021, https://www.health.harvard.edu/mind-and-mood/exercising-to-relax.

touchstones, understanding this traditional framework offers insight into how deeply rest, nourishment, and conscious living are intertwined.

1. Nutrition: The Food-Hormone Connection

Food is more than fuel. It is information. Every bite carries messages to your hormones—either signaling balance or disruption. Both Ayurveda and modern science agree: the quality, timing, and energetics of what you consume shape your internal landscape.

In Ayurveda, food is medicine, and each ingredient carries a vibrational imprint that influences the doshas and the body's subtle channels. Western research echoes this truth through a biochemical lens, showing how nutrients modulate inflammation, influence hormone receptor function, and support cyclical regulation.

Let's explore how certain foods and nutrients can support hormonal harmony in everyday life.

PHYTOESTROGENS AND HORMONAL BALANCE

Compounds known as phytoestrogens, found in flaxseeds, tofu, lentils, and sesame seeds, have been shown to mimic estrogen in the body. For women navigating perimenopause, these plant-based allies can gently ease symptoms like hot flushes and mood swings by modulating hormonal activity in a safe, natural way.[22]

On the other hand xenoestrogens, which are synthetic compounds that mimic estrogen in the body, are found in plastics, pesticides, and cosmetics and contribute to hormonal imbalances.

THE BLOOD SUGAR–HORMONE LINK

When we consume refined sugars or ultraprocessed carbohydrates, insulin levels spike, setting off a hormonal ripple effect. This can

---

22   Chen et al., 2023; Desmawati and Sulastri, 2019.

disrupt the delicate balance between estrogen, progesterone, and testosterone. Women with PCOS are especially sensitive to this cascade, as insulin resistance affects nearly 70 percent of those diagnosed.[23] Balancing blood sugar isn't just about energy; it's a foundational act of hormonal self-care.

NUTRIENTS THAT SUPPORT HORMONAL STABILITY

+ **Magnesium** supports progesterone production, calms the nervous system, reduces PMS-related mood changes, and promotes restful sleep. It's found in dark chocolate, leafy greens, almonds, and pumpkin seeds.

+ **Vitamin B6** helps regulate cortisol and supports the production of serotonin, easing symptoms of stress and irritability. Chickpeas, bananas, and salmon are excellent sources.

+ **Omega-3 fatty acids** are powerful anti-inflammatories that enhance hormone receptor sensitivity and support brain and reproductive health. These are found in fatty fish, chia seeds, and walnuts.

Rather than following restrictive diets or fleeting trends, true hormonal nourishment invites you to eat with intention.

A CLIENT'S JOURNEY: SOPHIE

Sophie was thirty-six and working full-time as a high school teacher when she came to see me. She told me she was exhausted but couldn't slow down. Her periods were irregular, PMS made her short-tempered and teary, and she hadn't had a full night's sleep in months. "I feel like I'm falling apart," she said during our first session.

She was living on caffeine and skipping meals, grabbing

---

23 The Endocrine Society, 2022.

something quick between classes, and collapsing into bed at night wired but unable to settle. Her lab results showed high cortisol, low progesterone, and signs of hormonal stress—nothing surprising, but confirmation that her body was overwhelmed.

We didn't overhaul everything at once. We started small. A proper breakfast—something protein-rich and warm—became her nonnegotiable. Eggs with avocado, or porridge with almond butter and seeds. She began taking a magnesium supplement to help with sleep and mood, and once she felt more balanced, we shifted toward food-based sources like leafy greens, tahini, and dark chocolate. She made space for three meals a day at regular times and swapped her afternoon coffee for herbal tea.

It wasn't a dramatic overnight change. But within three months, her cycle stabilized, her sleep improved, and she told me, "I feel like I'm finally alive again." What helped wasn't just what she ate or took— it was that she started paying attention and responding with care.

2. Stress: The Silent Hormone Saboteur

"Stress is not a mental state—it's a full-body experience."

When the nervous system is stuck in a chronic state of fight-or-flight, the body shifts into survival mode. An early response is the release of cortisol, the primary stress hormone. While short bursts of cortisol help us stay alert and focused in a true emergency, long-term elevation wreaks havoc on hormonal balance.

Chronic stress interferes with communication between the brain, ovaries, thyroid, and adrenals—known as the HPA axis. Over time, this can lead to

+ estrogen dominance, due to impaired detoxification and blood sugar imbalances

+ progesterone depletion, as the body prioritises cortisol over reproductive hormone production

✦ thyroid suppression, which slows metabolism and contributes to fatigue, hair loss, and weight gain

The body doesn't distinguish between being chased by a tiger or rushing to meet a deadline, skipping meals or scrolling through emotionally charged news at midnight. Every stressor—physical, emotional, or energetic—adds to the same internal load.

In women, stress often shows up subtly at first. Irregular periods. Sleep disturbances. Feeling overwhelmed by things that once felt manageable. Over time, these whispers grow louder if not addressed.

WHAT THE SCIENCE SAYS

✦ **Cortisol and cycle disruptions:** Women with high cortisol levels are more likely to experience irregular periods, severe PMS, and difficulty conceiving.[24]

✦ **The burnout cycle:** When cortisol is elevated for too long, the body steals progesterone to keep up with stress demands—this is why many women feel anxious and "wired but tired" and struggle with sleep before their period.

HORMONAL STRESS RESILIENCE TOOLS

✦ **Breathwork and meditation:** A study from Stanford University found that five minutes of deep breathing reduces cortisol levels by 22 percent.

✦ **Adaptogens:** Herbs like ashwagandha and shatavari have been clinically shown to lower stress hormones and support reproductive health.[25]

✦ **Movement:** Exercise is a double-edged sword. Overexercising

---

24 Harvard Medical School, 2021.

25 Chesak, Jennifer, 2022, "The No BS Guide to Adaptogens for Hormonal Balance and Stress," Healthline, September 9, https://www.healthline.com/health/stress/smart-girls-guide-to-adaptogens.

(especially HIIT and long-distance cardio) spikes cortisol, while restorative movement (yoga, strength training, and walking) helps regulate it.

A CLIENT'S JOURNEY: BARBARA

Barbara lived off caffeine, overexercised, and constantly felt exhausted. Despite eating "healthy," her hormonal symptoms worsened. When she switched to low-impact workouts, started daily meditation, and incorporated adaptogenic herbs, her body responded within weeks—her energy returned, her PMS disappeared, and she no longer felt like she was running on fumes.

3. Sleep: The Underestimated Hormonal Regulator

Sleep is one of the most overlooked yet potent forms of hormonal support. Poor sleep affects nearly every system in the body: the brain, the gut, the reproductive organs, and the stress response. Both modern science and Ayurvedic wisdom state this truth—when we sleep well, we heal better, think more clearly, and regulate hormones with greater ease.

WHAT THE SCIENCE SAYS

✦ **Melatonin and hormonal harmony**: Melatonin doesn't only help us fall asleep—it also supports the regulation of estrogen and progesterone. Studies show women who don't get sufficient sleep often experience cycle irregularities and worsened menopause symptoms.[26]

✦ **Growth hormone and metabolism**: During deep sleep, the body releases growth hormone, which supports tissue repair and

---

26 National Sleep Foundation, 2022.

metabolic function. Research links sleep deprivation (especially under six hours per night) to increased risk of insulin resistance, weight gain, and estrogen dominance.[27]

ALIGNING WITH NATURAL RHYTHMS

Ayurveda teaches that going to bed before 10:00 p.m. allows us to enter the Kapha phase of the night, when the body is primed for deep, restorative sleep. After 10:00 p.m., Pitta energy increases again, which can stimulate the mind and make it harder to wind down. Aligning with this natural rhythm helps stabilise cortisol levels and support your body's overnight healing processes.

PRACTICAL TIPS FOR BETTER SLEEP

+ Avoid pushing through late nights. Aim to start winding down around 9:00 p.m. so you're ready to sleep by 10:00.

+ Reduce caffeine after midday to support natural melatonin release.

+ Turn off screens 60–90 minutes before bed to minimize blue light exposure.

+ Drink a warm, calming sleep tonic. Try moon milk made with turmeric, nutmeg, and honey.

+ Create a bedtime ritual. Light stretching, journaling, herbal tea, or breathwork can signal to your body that it's safe to rest.

+ Massage the soles of your feet with warm oil (like brahmi or sesame) to ground excess energy and soothe the nervous system.

---

27   Prasad et al., 2021

THE TAKEAWAY: BALANCE IS BUILT THROUGH DAILY CHOICES

Your hormones are not your enemy. They are your body's messengers, responding to the food you eat, the stress you carry, and the lifestyle you live. When we stop fighting against our body and start working with it, we unlock hormonal harmony, energy, and long-term well-being.

✦ **Eat with intention:** Fuel your body, don't deprive it.

✦ **Stress less:** Protect your nervous system like you protect your skin from the sun.

✦ **Prioritize sleep:** Your hormones depend on it.

Exercise for Health

THE POWER OF MOVEMENT: FLEXIBILITY, STRENGTH, AND RESILIENCE

As women move through their thirties, forties, and fifties, and the years beyond, movement becomes more than a health habit— it becomes a tool for emotional balance, mental clarity, and hormonal resilience. These transitions often bring shifts in estrogen, progesterone, and cortisol, which affect everything from energy and sleep to joint health and metabolism.

Ayurveda and TCM have long seen movement as a way to balance energy and support circulation of qi or prana. Today, science is catching up. Regular, intentional movement—especially when it includes strength, flexibility, and mindful awareness—helps prevent many physical changes that arise during midlife hormonal shifts, such as reduced bone density, joint stiffness, and muscle loss.

THE DECLINE OF ESTROGEN AND ITS EFFECTS

Estrogen supports more than reproductive health. It plays a critical role in maintaining

+ bone strength, by supporting the activity of bone-building cells (osteoblasts)

+ muscle mass and metabolism, by preserving lean tissue

+ joint lubrication and mobility, reducing stiffness and risk of injury

As estrogen declines, especially during and after menopause, women may experience increased risk of osteoporosis, sarcopenia (age-related muscle loss), and joint issues like frozen shoulder. But these effects are not inevitable. Movement is medicine—and it works best when it's consistent and aligned with your body's needs.

THE IMPORTANCE OF STRENGTH TRAINING

Strength training is a key component of hormone-supportive movement in midlife and beyond. It helps

+ preserve muscle mass and improve metabolic function

+ support bone density, reducing the risk of fractures

+ enhance joint stability, easing stiffness and improving posture

Simple practices like bodyweight squats, Pilates, resistance bands, and weightlifting can be powerful. And everyday actions—like carrying groceries, walking up and down stairs, or gardening—also count, especially when done with intention.

FLEXIBILITY, BALANCE, AND ENERGY FLOW

Incorporating movement that enhance flexibility, balance, and nervous system regulation is equally essential. Practices like yoga, tai chi, and qigong combine breath, awareness, and gentle movement to

+ reduce stress and calm the nervous system

+ improve coordination and reduce the risk of falls

+ increase circulation and energy flow through joints and muscles

+ restore connection to the body in a grounded, feminine way

These forms of movement offer more than physical benefits—they support emotional regulation and help cultivate presence, especially during hormonal transitions.

How to Add More Movement to Your Life

You don't need to overhaul your life or commit to hours in a gym to experience the benefits of movement. What your body truly responds to is consistency, intention, and enjoyment. Movement becomes medicine when it's integrated into your everyday life with ease and awareness.

Start by asking yourself: *What kind of movement brings me pleasure, not pressure? Where in my day can I create spaciousness, not strain?* The goal is not perfection; it's presence.

Here are five ways to gently invite more movement into your rhythm.

1. Infuse Movement into Daily Activities

Sometimes the simplest shifts can have the biggest impact.

+ Take the stairs instead of the elevator.

+ Park farther from the entrance when running errands.

✦ Use a standing desk and take short stretch breaks between tasks.

✦ Walk while listening to a podcast or watching your favourite show—yes, even a walking pad in front of the TV counts.

These aren't only time-savers—they're energy boosters and hormone-supportive moments of motion.

2. Make Movement a Ritual, Not a Task

Movement doesn't have to be intense to be meaningful. Choose forms of exercise that nourish your body and your nervous system.

✦ Try restorative yoga, tai chi, or qigong in the evening to promote calm and release tension.

✦ Pair light stretching with breathwork or meditation to transition out of your workday and prepare for sleep.

These forms of movement not only support flexibility and balance— they help regulate cortisol and soothe the mind.

3. Stack Movement onto Existing Habits

Gently make exercise part of your routine without adding more to your to-do list.

✦ Stretch while the kettle boils or coffee brews.

✦ Do a few squats or calf raises while brushing your teeth.

✦ Walk around the house during phone calls or meetings.

This approach helps build momentum and removes the mental barrier of "finding time."

4. Let Movement Be a Source of Connection

When movement becomes social, it becomes joyful.

✦ Walk with a friend after school drop-off.

✦ Join a local class or online group to stay accountable.

✦ Make weekend hikes or swims a family ritual.

When we move together, we reinforce the message that our bodies are worth showing up for at every stage of life.

5. Start Small, Stay Consistent

You don't need to begin with sixty-minute workouts. In fact, aiming for just ten to fifteen minutes a day can be transformational—especially when done with mindfulness. Ideally, we want to work up to thirty minutes of intentional movement most days, but your progress should feel supportive, not stressful.

The key is to meet yourself where you are. Honor your energy. Celebrate your effort. Let movement be an act of devotion, not discipline.

An Example Weekly Routine for Movement and Exercise

Here's a simple yet effective weekly routine that combines strength, flexibility, and cardiovascular health while aligning with Ayurvedic principles.

Day	Morning	Evening
Monday	20-minute brisk walk or light jogging to invigorate circulation.	Gentle yoga focusing on hip openers and spinal twists to release tension.
Tuesday	Bodyweight strength exercises (e.g., squats, lunges, and push-ups for 20 minutes) followed by stretching	Self-massage with warm sesame oil (Abhyanga) followed by a hot shower to relax the muscles.
Wednesday	30-minute Pilates session or resistance band workout to build core strength.	Breath awareness and mindfulness meditation to calm Vata energy.

Thursday	Outdoor activity such as hiking or cycling to connect with nature.	Tai chi or gentle stretches to support joint mobility.
Friday	Strength training with weights (e.g., dumbbells or kettlebells) for 30 minutes.	Restorative yoga or guided relaxation to ground Pitta energy.
Saturday	Dance or Zumba for 30-60 minutes—something joyful and energizing.	Reflective journaling and foot massage with calming essential oils like lavender or sandalwood.
Sunday	Long walk in nature or a slow, meditative yoga flow.	Reflection and gratitude practice to reset for the week ahead.

By weaving movement into your everyday life, you can create a routine that not only supports physical health but also nurtures emotional balance and spiritual growth. Whether lifting weights, practicing yoga, or taking a brisk walk, each movement becomes a step toward embodying your higHERself™.

The key is consistency and intention. Choose movements that align with your dosha and bring you joy, and let this commitment to yourself serve as a reminder that this phase of womanhood is not about slowing down—it's about showing up for yourself in new and empowered ways.

CHAPTER 14

Dinacharya: Your Daily Routine for Success

In Ayurveda, the concept of *dinacharya,* or daily routine, is not only a list of tasks to check off, it's a profound practice of aligning body and mind with nature's rhythms. When you establish a dinacharya tailored to your dosha, you create physical health, mental clarity, and emotional stability. It's a system of self-care that nurtures your entire being, allowing you to step into your higHERself™ with intention and grace.

The beauty of dinacharya lies in its simplicity.

While the modern world often glorifies productivity at the expense of well-being, Ayurveda reminds us that success stems from consistency and balance.

The most accomplished individuals know this truth. As author Robin Sharma says, "The secret of your success is found in your daily routine."

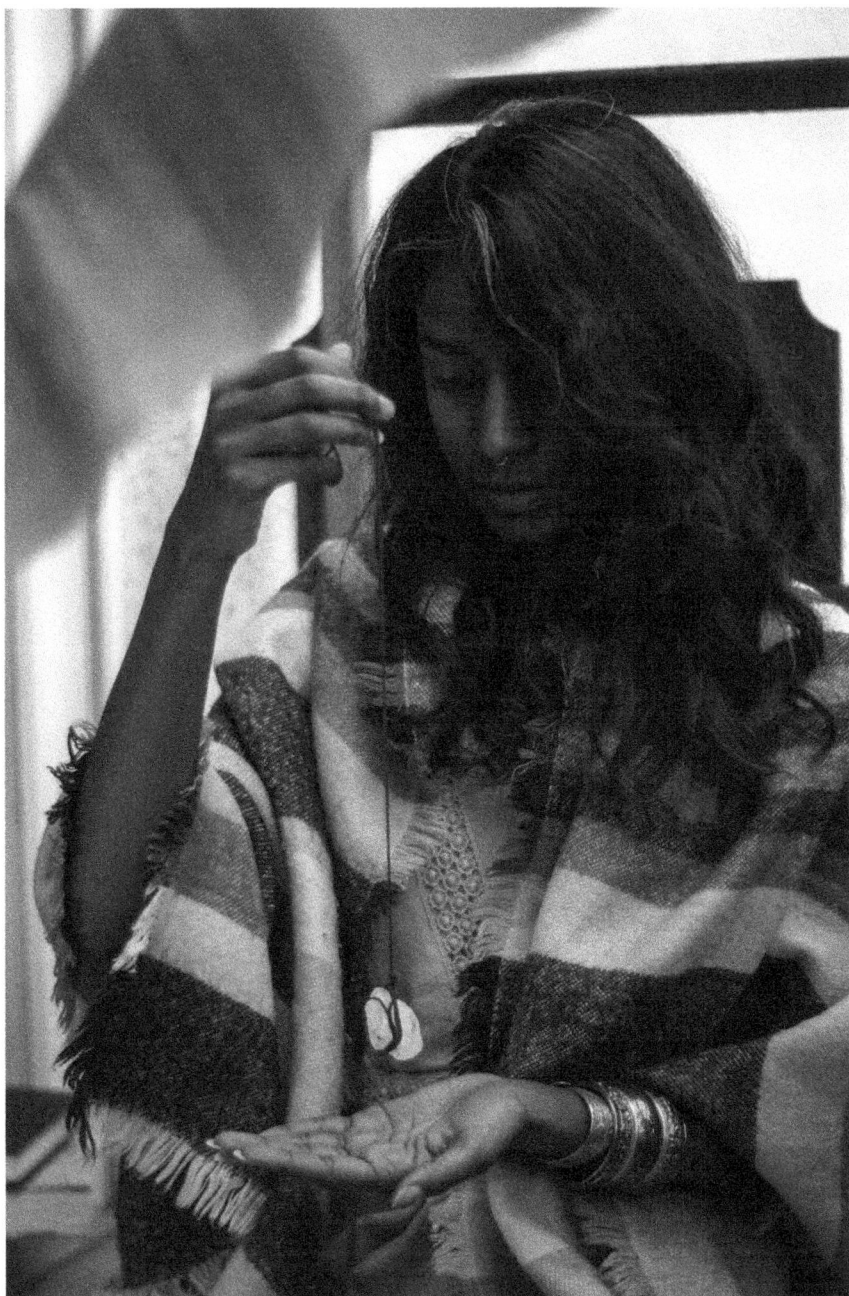

"YOUR HABITS WILL EITHER MAKE YOU OR BREAK YOU—CHOOSE THEM WISELY."

The Power of Dinacharya and Rituacharya

In Ayurvedic culture, *dinacharya* (daily routine) and *rituacharya* (seasonal routines) are essential practices that harmonize the individual with the greater cosmos. Our bodies are microcosms of the universe, influenced by cycles of the sun, moon, and seasons. By aligning your routine with these natural rhythms, you can prevent disease, optimize energy, and cultivate a sense of inner peace.

Rituacharya, for example, teaches us to adapt our diet and lifestyle as the seasons change. In summer, we favor cooling foods and activities to balance the heat of Pitta. In winter, we embrace warming practices to counteract the cold qualities of Vata. This cyclical wisdom is the ultimate preventative medicine, keeping the doshas in balance year-round.

When you combine seasonal awareness with a consistent daily routine, you create a solid foundation for success—not only in your health but in every area of your life.

Understanding the Doshas in Dinacharya

Each dosha has its own tendencies, strengths, and challenges when it comes to establishing a daily routine. By understanding what pacifies your dosha and what you may resist but need most, you can create a routine that feels both supportive and achievable.

VATA DOSHA: THE FREE SPIRIT

Vata types are creative, energetic, and spontaneous, but they thrive on grounding and consistency—even if it feels counterintuitive.

✦ **What pacifies Vata:** Regularity, warmth, and nourishment. A predictable routine with grounding meals and calming activities helps Vata find balance.

✦ **What Vata resists:** Sticking to a schedule or slowing down. The

Vata mind loves to flit from one thing to the next, but this often leads to burnout or anxiety.

Dinacharya for Vata

1. **Morning rituals:** Wake up at the same time each day, ideally around 6:00 a.m. or with the sunrise, and drink warm water with lemon to stimulate digestion.

2. **Abhyanga:** Use warm sesame oil to calm the nervous system and soothe dry skin.

3. **Mindful movement:** Choose gentle, grounding exercises like yoga, tai chi, or walking in nature.

4. **Meals:** Eat warm, cooked meals at regular intervals. Avoid skipping meals, as this can aggravate Vata's erratic tendencies.

5. **Evening wind-down:** Limit screen time before bed and engage in calming activities like journaling or meditation.

PITTA DOSHA: THE ACHIEVER

Pitta types are driven, focused, and goal-oriented, but they often push themselves too hard, leading to burnout or irritability.

+ **What pacifies Pitta:** Cooling, calming, and relaxing practices that balance their intensity.

+ **What Pitta resists:** Taking breaks or letting go of control. Pittas need to learn that rest is productive.

Dinacharya for Pitta

1. **Morning rituals:** Begin the day with meditation or pranayama (breathwork) to set a calm tone.

2. **Exercise:** Opt for moderate activities like swimming or Pilates. Avoid overheating with intense workouts.

3. **Cooling foods:** Favor fresh fruits, salads, and hydrating beverages like coconut water.

4. **Midday pause:** Schedule a lunch break away from work. Eat your largest meal at this time, as digestion is strongest at midday.

5. **Evening rituals:** Unwind with cooling teas like peppermint or chamomile. Incorporate moon-gazing or gentle yoga to release stress.

KAPHA DOSHA: THE NURTURER

Kapha types are steady, caring, and grounded, but they can become stuck in inertia or resistant to change.

✦ **What pacifies Kapha:** Stimulation, movement, and lightness. Kapha thrives with invigorating routines that get them out of their comfort zone.

✦ **What Kapha resists:** Starting new habits or engaging in vigorous exercise. Once momentum is established, however, Kapha finds it easier to maintain.

Dinacharya for Kapha

1. **Morning rituals:** Wake up early, ideally by 5:30 a.m., to avoid sluggishness. Begin the day with dry brushing to stimulate circulation.

2. **Energizing movement:** Engage in vigorous activities like jogging, dance, or strength training to shake off stagnation.

3. **Light meals:** Focus on warm, spiced foods with bitter and astringent flavours. Avoid heavy or oily meals.

4. **Stay active:** Incorporate regular breaks throughout the day to avoid lethargy.

5. **Evening rituals:** Spend time journaling about goals and accomplishments to keep motivation high.

The Science Behind Daily Routines: Why They Matter

In our fast-paced world, it's easy to underestimate the profound impact of a consistent daily routine. Yet, science continually affirms that living in harmony with our natural rhythms is an effective way to enhance overall well-being.

Take circadian rhythms, for example. These internal twenty-four-hour cycles govern everything from sleep to metabolism. Research published in *Nature* highlights how disruptions to circadian rhythms—like irregular sleep patterns or eating late at night—contribute to metabolic and hormonal imbalances, increasing the risk of conditions like obesity, diabetes, and mood disorders. Aligning your daily activities, such as meals and sleep, with these rhythms significantly improves your energy, focus, and overall health.

Exercise, too, plays a key role in maintaining mental and physical health. According to findings from Harvard Medical School, regular physical activity not only reduces symptoms of anxiety and depression but also boosts mood and cognitive function. A brisk morning walk or yoga practice sets a positive tone for your day, grounding your mind and energizing your body. Even consistency yields profound benefits. A study published in *Psychological Science* reveals that it's not sporadic bursts of motivation that lead to long-term success, but rather the steady foundation of consistent habits. Whether it's waking up at the same time each day or carving out moments for meditation or journaling, small acts compound over time to create a life of purpose and balance. Daily routines aren't simply about discipline—they creating space for your higher self to thrive.[28]

---

28 Lally, P., van Jaarsveld, C. H., Potts, H. W., & Wardle, J., 2010, "How Are Habits Formed: Modelling Habit Formation in the Real World," *European Journal of Social Psychology* 40 (6): 998–1009.

Routines Are Not Only for A-list Famous People

Daily habits are not merely small actions; they are the foundation upon which extraordinary lives are built. Many successful and inspiring figures of our time swear by their routines—not because they are rigid or monotonous, but because these rituals anchor them in purpose, energy, and clarity.

Take Oprah Winfrey, for example. One of the most influential women in the world, Oprah begins her day with a sacred trifecta of meditation, movement, and gratitude journaling. It's not about ticking off a checklist for her; it's about starting from a place of grounded presence. She says, "When you are grateful, it allows you to be fully present in your own life." This simple act of reflecting on gratitude transforms the energy she carries into the rest of her day, making her a force of positivity and intention.

Tony Robbins, the dynamic and larger-than-life motivational coach, has a different approach. His mornings are a nonnegotiable time for "priming"—a powerful practice that blends breathwork, visualization, and gratitude. Tony believes that starting his day by visualizing success, acknowledging the blessings he already has, and energizing his body sets the tone for peak performance. He says, "The only thing keeping you from getting what you want is the story you keep telling yourself." By choosing a story of empowerment each morning, he primes his mind and heart for action.

Then there's Ariana Huffington, a trailblazer in media and wellness. After experiencing burnout herself, Ariana shifted her priorities to focus on balance and restoration. Her day starts with a commitment to sleep—yes, sleep! She's a firm advocate for its power, calling it "the ultimate performance enhancer." Ariana also prioritizes journaling and disconnecting from technology to create space for creativity. Her transformation proves that self-care is not indulgent—it's essential.

Building Your Dinacharya: A Simple Weekly Plan

Monday–Friday

✦ Wake up at the same time each day.

✦ Begin with a morning ritual: drink warm water, meditate, and move your body.

✦ Schedule meals at consistent times to support digestion.

✦ Incorporate a midday pause to reset your energy.

✦ End the day with reflective journaling, breathwork, or meditation.

Weekends

✦ Use weekends to deepen your practices—try longer yoga sessions, nature walks, or self study through reading.

✦ Reflect on the week and set intentions for the days ahead.

Dinacharya is more than a routine—it's a ritual of self-connection and empowerment. When you align your daily actions with your dosha and the rhythms of nature, you cultivate a life that is not only productive but deeply fulfilling. As you weave these practices into your life, remember that small, consistent steps are the key to lasting transformation. Your routine becomes your superpower, grounding you in the present while propelling you toward your highest self.

Your Daily Clocks:
The Ayurvedic Clock and TCM Clock

Ayurveda and TCM both include a set of guidelines about energy cycles throughout the day to help us manage our time and activities for our best individual outcomes.

Harmony Inspired *Health*

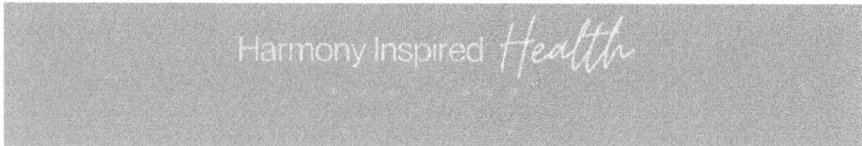

Ayurvedic Clock

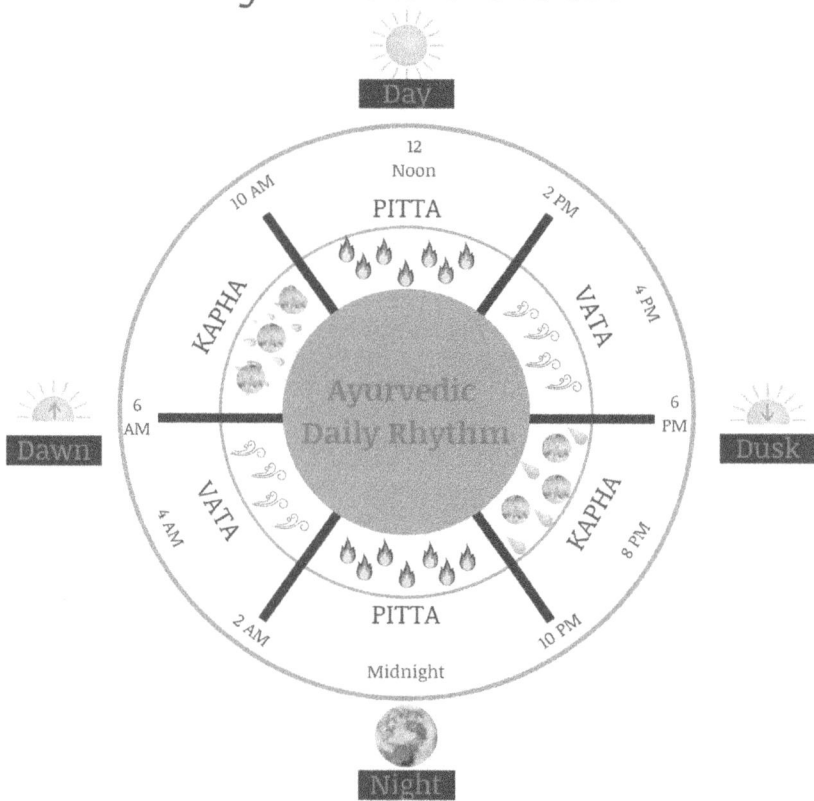

Day

12
Noon

PITTA

10 AM

2 PM

KAPHA

4 PM

VATA

6
AM

Ayurvedic
Daily Rhythm

6
PM

Dawn

Dusk

VATA

4 AM

KAPHA

8 PM

2 AM

PITTA

10 PM

Midnight

Night

THE AYURVEDIC CLOCK

The Ayurvedic Clock is a guiding framework that aligns daily activities with the natural rhythms of the doshas (Kapha, Pitta, and Vata) to optimize well-being. Each dosha is dominant during specific times of day, influencing our energy, digestion, and mental clarity. By living in harmony with these cycles, we can enhance physical vitality, emotional balance, and productivity.

EXPLAINING THE AYURVEDIC CLOCK

1. Kapha Time (6 a.m.–10 a.m. and 6 p.m.–10 p.m.)

+ *Morning (6 a.m.–10 a.m.):* Kapha energy is heavy, slow, and steady, making this the best time for activities like exercise, elimination, and a light breakfast. The body is naturally primed for movement, which counteracts Kapha's tendency toward lethargy.

+ *Evening (6 p.m.–10 p.m.):* As the day winds down, Kapha's nurturing energy supports relaxation and connection. Time to slow down, have a light dinner, and prepare for sleep.

2. Pitta Time (10 a.m.–2 p.m. and 10 p.m.–2 a.m.)

+ *Midday (10 a.m.–2 p.m.):* Pitta, with its fiery and transformative qualities, governs digestion and productivity. This is when digestion is strongest, making it ideal for eating your largest meal of the day. It's also a time for focus and action.

+ *Midnight (10 p.m.–2 a.m.):* Pitta governs the body's metabolic and repair processes during sleep. Eating too late interferes with this cycle, so it's essential to avoid heavy meals before bed to allow Pitta to work efficiently on internal restoration.

3. Vata Time (2 a.m.–6 a.m. and 2 p.m.–6 p.m.)

✦ *Early Morning (2 a.m.–6 a.m.):* Vata's light and creative energy is dominant, making this the ideal time for meditation, visualization, and spiritual practices. Waking up early during this phase promotes clarity and creativity.

✦ *Afternoon (2 p.m.–6 p.m.):* Vata energy inspires communication and creativity, making it a great time for brainstorming or social interactions. However, it can also lead to scattered energy, so grounding practices are helpful.

THE TCM CLOCK AND THE ZANG-FU ORGANS

In Traditional Chinese Medicine (TCM), the body is viewed as a dynamic, interconnected system of energy, and the twenty-four-hour TCM clock maps how qi energy flows through the body's organs in a cyclical rhythm. This clock is divided into 12 two-hour intervals, each corresponding to a specific Zang-Fu organ system. Each organ pair takes turns being the "energetic focus," receiving the most qi during its designated time. Understanding this clock helps us align our lifestyle with our body's natural rhythms, optimizing health and preventing disease.

THE FLOW OF ENERGY: THE TCM ORGAN CLOCK

3 a.m.–5 a.m.: Lung (Yin)

The lungs are associated with breath, renewal, and grief. This is the time when qi is at its peak in the lungs, making early morning an ideal time for breathwork, meditation, or gentle yoga to awaken the body. Those who wake during this time may have unresolved grief or lung imbalances.

Harmony Inspired *Health*

TCM Clock

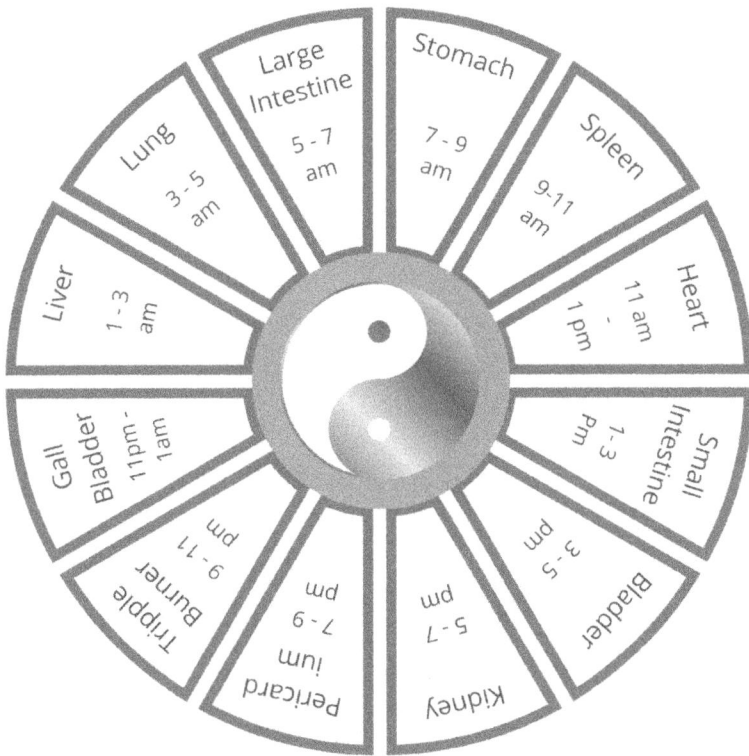

TCM Clock wheel showing organ times:
- Large Intestine 5 - 7 am
- Stomach 7 - 9 am
- Spleen 9-11 am
- Heart 11 am - 1 pm
- Small Intestine 1 - 3 pm
- Bladder 3 - 5 pm
- Kidney 5 - 7 pm
- Pericardium 7 - 9 pm
- Tripple Burner 9 - 11 pm
- Gall Bladder 11pm - 1am
- Liver 1 - 3 am
- Lung 3 - 5 am

www.harmonyinspiredhealth.com.au

5 a.m.–7 a.m.: Large Intestine (Yang)

The large intestine governs elimination, both physical and emotional. This is the best time for detoxification and bowel movements. Drinking warm water upon waking supports this process. Imbalances may manifest as constipation or difficulty letting go, emotionally or mentally.

7 a.m.–9 a.m.: Stomach (Yang)

The stomach thrives on nourishment and digestion. Eating a balanced, nourishing breakfast sets the tone for the day. If you experience indigestion or nausea during this time, it could indicate a stomach imbalance.

9 a.m.–11 a.m.: Spleen (Yin)

The TCM spleen transforms food into qi and blood. This is the prime time for mental focus and productive work, as the spleen is also linked to intellectual thought. Imbalances may show as fatigue, poor digestion, or overthinking.

11 a.m.–1 p.m.: Heart (Yin)

The heart, the body's "emperor" in TCM, governs blood circulation and emotional balance. This is an ideal time for connection, whether through lunch with loved ones or meaningful conversations. Heart imbalances may lead to anxiety, insomnia, or palpitations.

1 p.m.–3 p.m.: Small Intestine (Yang)

The small intestine sorts the pure from the impure, both physically (digestion) and mentally (decision-making). This is a good time for tasks that require discernment. Symptoms like bloating or indecisiveness may indicate imbalances.

3 p.m.–5 p.m.: Bladder (Yang)

The bladder governs the storage and excretion of fluids. Mid-afternoon is a good time to hydrate and recharge. If fatigue hits, it may signal stagnant qi or overwork.

5 p.m.–7 p.m.: Kidney (Yin)

The kidneys, the source of vital life energy (Jing), are deeply tied to longevity, reproduction, and fear. Early evening is a time for nourishment and restoration. Weak kidneys may show as low back pain, premature aging, or burnout.

7 p.m.–9 p.m.: Pericardium (Yin)

The pericardium protects the heart and governs joy and intimacy. This is a time to relax, connect emotionally, or engage in light-hearted activities. Imbalances may manifest as social anxiety or lack of joy.

9 p.m.–11 p.m.: Triple Burner (Yang)

The Triple Burner regulates the body's three energy centers (upper, middle, and lower). This is the time for winding down, supporting qi flow throughout the body. Difficulty sleeping may indicate blockages or overstimulation.

11 p.m.–1 a.m.: Gallbladder (Yang)

The gallbladder governs courage and decision-making. Sleep during this time allows the body to recover and detoxify. Waking often signals unresolved decisions or suppressed frustration.

1 a.m.–3 a.m.: Liver (Yin)

The liver detoxifies and replenishes blood. It is linked to anger and planning. Waking during this time may reflect unresolved anger, frustration, or resentment. It can also be a sign of stagnation of qi, chronic stress or pushing oneself too hard.

DAILY RHYTHMS: COMPARISON OF AYURVEDA, TCM, AND MODERN SCIENCE

	Ayurveda	TCM	Modern Science	Practice Suggestions
2–6 a.m.	*Vata time:* clarity, lightness, ideal for meditation & spiritual practice	Liver (1–3 a.m.) detox unprocessed emotion Lung (3–5 a.m.) breath, Qi cycle starts, grief Large Intestine (5–7 a.m.) elimination, letting go	Melatonin declines, cortisol begins rising. Body shifts from rest to alertness. Ideal for mindfulness and setting circadian rhythm.	Wake early, journal, meditate, gentle movement, bowel elimination, warm water
6–10 a.m.	*Kapha time:* slow, steady, grounded energy; ideal for movement & light food	Stomach (7–9 a.m.) nourishment Spleen (9–11 a.m.) digestion & focus	Cortisol peaks. Body temp & alertness rise.	Morning walk or workout, nourishing breakfast, avoid sluggishness
10 a.m.–2 p.m.	*Pitta time:* strong digestion, productivity, focus	Heart (11 a.m.–1 p.m.) connection & joy Small Intestine (1–3 p.m.) sorting truth	Insulin sensitivity peaks. Brain sharpness optimal.	Eat main meal, do focused work, have social or heart-led conversations
2–6 p.m.	*Vata time:* energy disperses, creativity rises but can feel scattered	Bladder (3–5 p.m.) energy reserve Kidneys (5–7 p.m.) Jing, rest to restore vitality	Cortisol drops, mental fatigue common. Energy dips in many people.	Hydrate, gentle movement, walk in nature, finish demanding tasks by 4 p.m.
6–10 p.m.	*Kapha time:* calm, nurturing, slow down, prepare for sleep	Pericardium (7–9 p.m.) intimacy, laughter Triple Burner (9–11 p.m.) Prepare for sleep	Melatonin rises, Body cools, digestion slows.	Light dinner by 7 p.m., connect with others, gentle stretching, no screens after 9 p.m.
10 p.m.–2 a.m.	*Pitta time:* internal repair, detox, metabolism	Gallbladder (11–1 a.m.) Courage, rest, decisions Liver (1–3 a.m.) detox, unprocessed emotions	Deep sleep enables hormonal reset. Body detoxifies, restores tissues.	Be asleep by 10 p.m., avoid late meals. Deepest sleep, growth hormone released, repair and fat metabolism occur. Essential for hormonal and cognitive balance.

Why Aligning These Cycles Matters

Both systems emphasise the importance of syncing with natural rhythms to prevent disease, improve digestion, support our hormonal changes and enhance mental clarity.

By integrating Ayurvedic dosha principles with TCM's organ-specific insights, you create a truly holistic approach to daily living.

Whether it's the grounding of Kapha, the transformational energy of Pitta, or the creativity of Vata, honoring these cycles cultivates balance and well-being.

Reflection on Daily Routines (Dinacharya)

Both Ayurveda and Traditional Chinese Medicine remind us that healing doesn't happen in grand gestures—it happens in the quiet rhythm of our days. This is the essence of Dinacharya: the conscious alignment of your daily routines with the natural cycles of time, energy, and light.

Imagine your day like a river. When it flows with purpose—guided by intention, not pressure—it gradually carves a path of clarity, steadiness, and self-trust. The small things you do consistently—waking before sunrise, sitting in stillness, moving your body, or pausing to exhale—become acts of devotion that reconnect you to your center.

Your routine doesn't have to be perfect, it just needs to be yours.

JOURNAL PROMPTS FOR REFLECTION

1. Which part of my daily rhythm feels most aligned with my body and which part feels rushed or disconnected?

_____

_____

_____

_____

_____

_____

2. What is the first message I give myself when I wake up? How would I like to rewrite it?

_____

_____

_____

_____

_____

_____

3. How do my energy levels shift throughout the day? Can I notice a pattern that mirrors the Ayurvedic or TCM clock?

_____

_____

_____

_____

_____

4. What small ritual could I add (or return to) that would help me start or end the day with more intention?

_____

_____

_____

_____

_____

5. Where do I resist routine, and what might that resistance be protecting me from?

_____

_____

_____

_____

_____

6. If my day was a sacred ceremony, what would I begin with, honor, and release?

_____

_____

_____

_____

_____

CHAPTER 15

Gut Wisdom: The Alchemy of Digestion and Detox

The health of your body, mind, and spirit is intricately tied to the state of your digestion. In Ayurveda, digestion is considered the cornerstone of health, and the concept of Agni—your digestive fire—is revered as the inner flame that governs not only the breakdown of food but the assimilation of life itself. When Agni burns brightly, it supports physical vitality, mental clarity, and emotional stability. But when it becomes weak or erratic, it allows ama, or toxins, to accumulate, leading to sluggishness, imbalances, and even disease.

This chapter dives deep into the sacred alchemy of digestion and detoxification, offering practical wisdom to rekindle your Agni, cleanse your body, and ultimately tranform your health from the inside out. Through stories, ancient Ayurvedic principles, and modern insights, we'll explore how nurturing your digestive health can transform not only your body but your mind and soul.

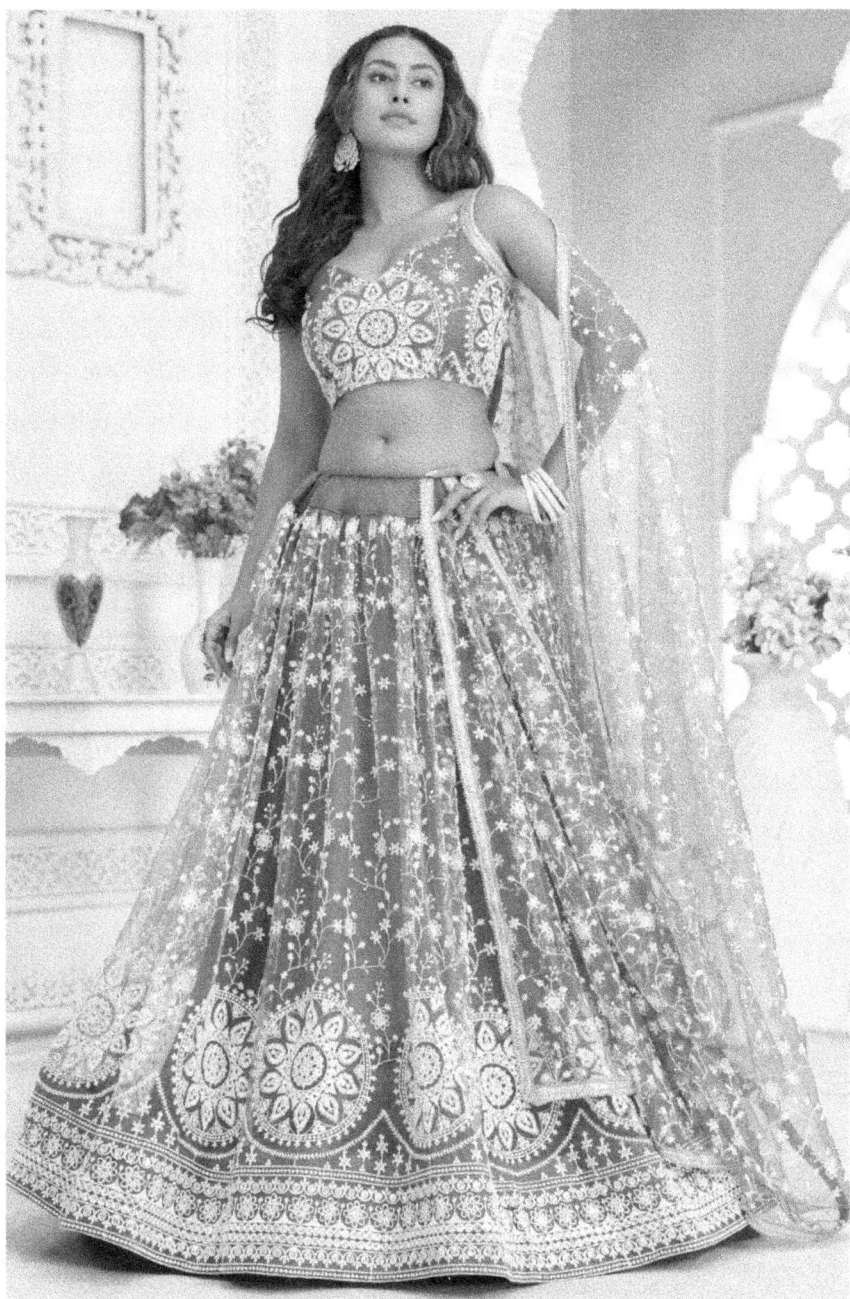

"THE GUT IS THE SECOND BRAIN, AND WHAT YOU FEED YOUR
BODY, YOU FEED YOUR MIND."

The Flame of Agni: The Guardian of Health

In Ayurveda, Agni is more than your physical digestion—it's the fire of transformation, the force that metabolizes food, thoughts, and emotions into energy. When Agni is strong and balanced, you feel light, energised, and clear-minded. Your skin glows, your body maintains its natural weight, and your hormones hum in harmony.

However, if Agni becomes weakened by stress, poor food choices, or erratic routines, undigested food and emotions turn into Ama, clogging your system and dampening your vitality. Ama isn't just physical—it clouds the mind, fuels negative emotions, and disconnects you from your intuition.

I often tell my clients that digestion is like a campfire. If you overfeed it with heavy logs (too much food at once) or starve it (skip meals), the fire will smolder. But with the right fuel—timely meals, wholesome foods, and supportive habits—Agni burns brightly, sustaining you on every level.

Optimizing Digestion: Dosha-Specific Nutrition and Rituals

Ayurveda teaches that no single diet fits everyone. Your unique dosha determines not only what you should eat but how and when you should eat.

✦ **Vata Digestion:** Vata's irregularity often manifests as gas, bloating, or constipation. To balance this, favor warm, grounding foods like stews, root vegetables, and healthy fats like ghee. Avoid raw salads and cold drinks, which aggravate Vata. Eating at regular times is key to soothing Vata's unpredictability.

✦ **Pitta Digestion:** Pitta's fiery digestion can lead to acidity, inflammation, or loose stools. Cooling foods like cucumbers, leafy greens, and coconut are ideal. Avoid overly spicy, sour, or oily foods that stoke Pitta's flames. Eating in a calm environment can help reduce Pitta's intensity.

✦ **Kapha Digestion:** Kapha's slow metabolism benefits from light, spiced foods and smaller portions. Ginger, black pepper, and turmeric help stoke Kapha's Agni, while heavy, sugary, creamy or fried foods should be minimized. Movement before or after meals, like a brisk walk, helps stimulate digestion.

In addition to dosha-specific nutrition, mindful eating is universal. Chew slowly, savor the flavors, and eat without distractions to enhance your body's ability to absorb nutrients.

Sarah came to me with chronic bloating and fatigue. She felt emotionally stuck, constantly craving sugar but never feeling satisfied. Together, we identified her Kapha imbalance, which weighed down her Agni. By introducing lighter, spiced foods and herbal teas with ginger and turmeric, Sarah began to feel her energy return.

Dosha	Common Imbalance Symptoms	Favor These Tastes	Best Foods	Rituals to Support Digestion
Vata	Gas, bloating, constipation, dryness, irregular appetite	Sweet, sour, salty *(grounding and moistening)*	Warm stews, root vegetables, ghee, oats, cooked apples, soaked nuts	Eat at regular times, sit to eat, sip warm ginger tea.
Pitta	Acidity, inflammation, heartburn, loose stools, irritability	Sweet, bitter, astringent *(cooling and calming)*	Leafy greens, cucumber, coconut, rice, mung dal, coriander, fennel	Eat in a calm setting, avoid multitasking, avoid spicy/oily food.
Kapha	Slow digestion, heaviness, lethargy, sluggish metabolism	Pungent, bitter, astringent *(stimulating and drying)*	Light soups, legumes, steamed greens, ginger, turmeric, barley	Movement before/after meals, avoid naps post-eating, drink warm water with lemon, dry brushing.

Seasonal Cleansing: Releasing Ama, Reclaiming Vitality

Ayurveda recognises the cyclical nature of life and offers seasonal cleansing practices to reset the body and mind. Unlike harsh detoxes or extreme diets, these rituals are gentle and nurturing, designed to support Agni while eliminating ama.

AMA: THE ROOT CAUSE OF IMBALANCE

Ama, the toxic residue of undigested food and emotions, is a major contributor to poor health. When Agni is weak, ama builds up in the body, creating stagnation, inflammation, and even disease. Signs of ama include fatigue, bad breath, coated tongue, and a lack of mental clarity.

During the transition of seasons, particularly from winter to spring and summer to autumn, cleansing practices like Panchakarma or simple mono-diets with kitchari (a spiced mung bean and rice dish) can rejuvenate the system. These rituals help women maintain hormone balance, reduce inflammation, and rekindle vitality.

For women in perimenopause or menopause, seasonal cleansing can be particularly beneficial, helping to balance fluctuating hormones and ease symptoms like fatigue, mood swings, and weight gain.

WHAT IS AMA?

Ama is often described as undigested matter, but it goes beyond food. It includes undigested experiences, suppressed emotions, and mental residue. In simple terms, ama is anything the body or mind has not been able to process or eliminate—physically, emotionally, or energetically.

When left unchecked, ama creates sluggishness in the system, blocking the channels (*srotas*), dampening Agni, and setting the stage for imbalance or disease.

Common signs of ama include

+ a coated tongue

+ bloating or heaviness after meals

+ brain fog or mental dullness

+ low motivation or lethargy

+ bad breath or body odor

+ mucus or congestion

+ cravings for heavy, oily, or cold foods

METABOLISM AND THE BODY IMAGE NARRATIVE

Metabolism is a key expression of Agni—your digestive fire—impacting how your body uses energy, regulates hormones, and maintains balance. But for many women, metabolism becomes a loaded topic, tangled in years of diet culture and body image conditioning.

In my early teens, I struggled with bulimia. It wasn't driven by social media—it didn't exist back then. It came from a deep inner disconnect and an attempt to cope with emotions I didn't yet have the tools to process. The binging and purging became a way to feel in control, to escape, and to punish myself for emotions I didn't know how to hold.

I thought it was a solution at the time. But it only made everything worse. It didn't give me the confidence I was seeking. It didn't make life easier. It left me with lasting damage—disrupted gut motility, dysbiosis, weakened Agni, and years of metabolic instability. I lost trust in my body. I didn't feel connected to hunger or fullness. And more than that, I didn't feel safe in who I was. Studies show that up to 50 percent of individuals with a history of bulimia experience long-term gastrointestinal complications such as gastroparesis, chronic constipation, and irritable bowel symptoms—even decades later.[29] Recovery didn't happen overnight, and it didn't begin with Ayurveda. It began with a shift in mindset—recognizing that my body wasn't the problem. That I didn't need to control my way into worthiness. Slowly, I began to rebuild my relationship with food, with self-image, and with safety. I started nourishing instead of restricting. Listening instead of silencing.

Ayurveda came into my life later, but when it did, it gave structure and language to what I had already started to feel—that health isn't built on discipline alone but on respect. That Agni isn't something to override but something to support. That true metabolic health is less about appearance and more about energy, clarity, and ease in the body.

Disordered eating doesn't only harm the gut—it creates long-term hormonal disruption, immune dysregulation, and emotional patterns that can take years to unlearn. But healing is possible. I've lived it, and I continue to support other women through it. Because no diet, restriction, or behavior rooted in shame will ever create real health. That only comes through honesty, self-respect, and connection.

Even now, as a practitioner, I see women in their sixties who still wrestle with body image issues, punishing themselves with diets and exercise that only deplete their Agni further. Ayurveda teaches us to approach the body with love and reverence, to see it as a temple rather than a project.

---

29 Norris M. L., Harrison M. E., Isserlin L., Robinson A., Feder S., Sampson M., March 2016, "Gastrointestinal Complications Associated with Anorexia Nervosa: A Systematic Review," *International Journal of Eating Disorders* 49 (3): 216–37, doi: 10.1002/eat.22462.

Metabolism is not fixed. It thrives when nurtured with dosha-aligned eating, daily movement, and rest. The body is always seeking balance—it's our job to listen and support it.

WHAT IS AGNI?

Agni, meaning *fire* in Sanskrit, is the sacred flame of digestion—not just of food, but of thoughts, emotions, and experiences. It is the transformational force within us that breaks down, assimilates, and eliminates what we take in from the outer world.

When Agni is strong, we feel

+ energized and light after meals

+ clear-headed and focused

+ emotionally steady

+ resilient to stress and seasonal changes

When Agni is weak or disturbed, digestion slows, toxins accumulate (ama), and we may feel bloated, foggy, irritable, or sluggish.

In Ayurveda, nearly all healing begins with restoring Agni because without strong digestion, nothing in the body can function optimally, including hormone regulation, immunity, and emotional well-being.

THE TYPES OF AGNI

While Agni is often discussed as a single force, Ayurveda recognizes multiple forms of this internal fire.

✦ **Jatharagni:** The central digestive fire in the stomach and small intestine. This is the master Agni, responsible for breaking down food and preparing nutrients for absorption.

✦ **Bhutagni:** The elemental Agnis, responsible for metabolising the five elements (earth, water, fire, air, space) within the body.

✦ **Dhatvagni:** The tissue-level Agnis, each one governs the transformation and nourishment of a specific tissue (*dhatu*), such as blood, muscle, fat, or bone.

Together, these forms of Agni ensure that what we take in becomes who we are—physically, mentally, and energetically.

Stop Fighting Your Natural Composition

Lisa came to me utterly depleted after years of battling her own body. She was a Pitta-Kapha constitution, naturally curvy and strong, but had spent most of her adult life chasing a thin, Vata-like figure that her body was never designed to achieve. The pursuit of an ideal that didn't align with her natural constitution left her burned out, with irregular cycles, mood swings, and a deep sense of frustration.

Ayurveda teaches us that our natural constitution—our Prakriti— is a gift, not a flaw. Each dosha embodies a unique strength: Vata's lightness and creativity, Pitta's intensity and focus, and Kapha's stability and endurance.

When we fight against our Prakriti, we not only exhaust ourselves physically but also disconnect from our true essence. For Lisa, striving for a body that wasn't hers was more than exhausting—it was self-sabotaging.

Women, like Lisa, who grew up in the 1990s and early 2000s might remember the relentless glorification of ultra-thin bodies. The fashion runways were dominated by the "heroin chic" aesthetic—models with hollow cheeks, protruding bones, and waif-like frames. Victoria's Secret models with flat stomachs, large perky breasts, and endless legs became the gold standard of beauty. Magazine covers and diet culture sent one loud, clear message: smaller was better. But it wasn't simply about thinness. Many women internalized the belief that only certain features were "feminine enough"—from breast size to hair texture, height, skin tone, and even the absence of body hair in "unacceptable" places. For some, it was the pressure to be curvy and petite at the same time. For others, having small breasts or broad shoulders became a quiet source of shame. These conflicting ideals imprinted deeply, leaving behind body stories that still whisper, shape-shift, and sometimes shout in the mirrors of adulthood.

For Lisa, we had to quiet these echoes and change her behaviors.

We began her healing journey by focusing on balance rather than restriction. Lisa had been overexercising, thinking she could "burn off" her Kapha tendencies. I encouraged her to replace punishing workouts with exercise that she *enjoyed*, allowing her body to rebuild rather than break down. Instead of extreme diets that left her Agni weak and erratic, we introduced nourishing, meals and herbal teas to stabilize her digestion and hormones.

But the biggest transformation came when Lisa began to reframe her relationship with her body. We worked on cultivating body gratitude, replacing harsh self-criticism with appreciation for her strength, resilience, and the ways her body carried her through life. I reminded her that Ayurveda doesn't see curves or softness as imperfections but as natural expressions of Kapha's nurturing, grounding energy.

Lisa's journey wasn't only about weight; it was about coming home to herself. "For the first time in decades," she told me, "I feel at peace with my body. I'm not trying to shrink myself anymore—I'm learning to honor what makes me strong and unique."

This is not to say that striving for a healthy body weight isn't important, but health isn't about conforming to a singular ideal—it's about finding balance and vitality within the body you were born into. For some, this may mean embracing curves and working with Kapha's grounding energy; for others, it might involve tempering Pitta's intensity and muscular physique or nourishing Vata's lightness.

The key is to honor your body's natural composition, knowing that alignment with your Prakriti will lead to true wellness. When you stop fighting against your nature and instead work with it, you not only heal your body but also reconnect with your higher self.

Dosha-Specific Food Lists

Ayurveda places significant emphasis on food as medicine, teaching us that the right diet can balance the doshas and support overall health. Below are the foods to favor and avoid based on your dosha. These guidelines take into account the inherent qualities of each dosha—light and dry for Vata, hot and sharp for Pitta, and heavy and moist for Kapha—and aim to bring balance by choosing opposing qualities in food.

Dosha	Qualities	Goal	Foods to Favor	Foods to Avoid
Vata	Light, dry, cold, irregular	Ground, nourish, warm	**Grains:** Cooked oats, rice, quinoa, wheat **Vegetables:** Sweet potatoes, carrots, beets, squash, zucchini (cooked and lightly spiced) **Fruits:** Mangoes, bananas, dates, figs, cooked apples or pears **Proteins:** Lentils, mung beans, tofu, chicken (in warm, moist forms) **Dairy:** Whole milk, ghee **Oils:** Sesame, almond, olive oil **Spices:** Ginger, cinnamon, cardamom, cumin, fennel, black pepper	**Dry/raw foods:** Crackers, chips, raw salads, popcorn **Cold foods:** Ice cream, cold drinks, leftovers **Bitter/astringent:** Cranberries, pomegranate, excess raw greens **Light/airy foods:** Rice cakes, puffed cereals, soda
Pitta	Hot, sharp, light, oily	Cool, calm, stabilize	**Grains:** Barley, oats, quinoa, basmati rice **Vegetables:** Leafy greens, cucumber, asparagus, broccoli, zucchini, green beans **Fruits:** Melons, apples, pears, pomegranate, cherries **Proteins:** Tofu, chickpeas, mung beans, turkey **Dairy:** Milk, ghee, unsalted butter (cooling) **Oils:** Coconut, sunflower, olive (in moderation) **Spices:** Coriander, fennel, turmeric, cardamom	**Hot/spicy foods:** Chili, garlic, onions, hot sauces **Sour foods:** Citrus, tomatoes, vinegar, pickles **Fried/oily foods:** Fries, chips, greasy meats **Salty foods:** Processed snacks, salted nuts, cured meats
Kapha	Heavy, moist, cool, stable	Lighten, invigorate, energize	**Grains:** Barley, millet, rye, buckwheat, quinoa **Vegetables:** Kale, spinach, Brussel sprouts, peppers, cauliflower **Fruits:** Apples, cranberries, pears **Proteins:** Lentils, mung beans, chicken, eggs **Dairy:** Low-fat milk (in moderation), avoid cold prep **Oils:** Mustard or flaxseed oil (light, moderate use) **Spices:** Ginger, black pepper, mustard seed, cloves	**Heavy/oily foods:** Cheese, cream, butter, fried foods **Sweet/salty foods:** Desserts, sweetened drinks, snacks **Cold foods:** Ice cream, cold drinks, frozen desserts **Dense grains:** Wheat, rice, oats (in excess)

PRACTICAL TIPS FOR DOSHA-SPECIFIC EATING

1. **Balance is key:** No food is inherently "bad" or "good;" it's about moderation and timing.

2. **Seasonal adjustments:** Adapt your diet to align with seasonal influences on your dosha (e.g., favoring cooling foods for Pitta in summer).

3. **Mindful eating:** Sit down to eat in a calm environment, chew thoroughly, and listen to your body's hunger and fullness cues.

This tailored approach ensures your diet nourishes not just your body but also aligns with your inherent constitution.

Rewriting the Narrative of Weight and Worth

As women, we've been conditioned to equate weight with worth, chasing an ideal that often comes at the expense of our health. Ayurveda offers a different perspective: Your body is your partner in life, deserving of care, compassion, and nourishment.

When we honor our Agni, detoxify our systems, and nourish ourselves with love, we naturally align with our healthiest, most vibrant selves. True transformation comes not from fighting the body but from befriending it.

The Connection Between Digestion, Mood, and Mental Clarity

One of the most profound lessons Ayurveda offers is the intimate relationship between digestion and the mind. Modern science affirms this connection, revealing that the gut is not just a digestive organ but also a "second brain," home to the enteric nervous system and a vast network of neurons and microbes that influence mood, cognition, and overall mental well-being.

When Agni is strong, the gut produces neurotransmitters like serotonin and dopamine in abundance, contributing to feelings of happiness and focus. But when ama clogs the digestive system, it can lead to mental fog, anxiety, and even depression. Ayurveda recognized this connection long before the term "gut-brain axis" entered the modern lexicon.

I remember working with a client named Jan, who came to me struggling with persistent brain fog and low energy. She described feeling "mentally stuck," unable to focus on even simple tasks. Her diet was a jumble of convenience foods eaten on the go, and she had irregular bowel movements—a clear sign of disrupted Agni.

Through Ayurveda, we focused on rekindling her digestive fire. Jan began eating warm, freshly prepared meals at regular times, starting her day with ginger tea to stimulate digestion. We incorporated digestive herbs like cumin, coriander, and fennel and encouraged her to chew her food slowly and mindfully. Within weeks, Jan reported feeling clearer and more energized, saying, "It's like my mind and body are finally speaking the same language."

This story illustrates a powerful truth: when we nurture our digestion, we nourish our mind. A clear mind begins with a balanced gut, and healing starts from the inside out.

Reflection on Your Gut and Health Connection

Use the prompts below to explore your relationship with food, digestion, and inner balance.

1. What are the most common messages your body sends you after eating?

_____

_____

_____

_____

2. Are there specific foods that leave you feeling clear, energized, or grounded?

_____

_____

_____

_____

3. When do you tend to feel most bloated, heavy, or sluggish—and what might be contributing to that?

_____

_____

_____

_____

_____

_____

4. How do your eating habits reflect your current emotional state or stress level?

_____

_____

_____

_____

_____

_____

5. Have you ever ignored a gut feeling—literally or metaphorically—and what happened?

_____

_____

_____

_____

_____

_____

6. What small change can you commit to this week to honor your digestion more fully?

_____

_____

_____

_____

_____

_____

CHAPTER 16

Align, Embody, Rise: higHERself™ Evolution

The journey of health alchemy is not about striving for perfection; it's about integration. True health extends far beyond the physical—it's a harmony of mind, emotions, spirit, and actions aligned with your highest purpose.

When all five aspects of health—physical, mental, emotional, spiritual, and dharmic—come together, the transformation is profound. It is here that you meet your higHERself™, the most radiant, aligned, and authentic version of you.

The Power of Alchemy in Everyday Life

Throughout this section, we've explored the pillars of health alchemy, from nurturing your digestive fire to balancing hormones, honoring your emotions, and living in alignment with your unique dharma. Each puzzle piece connects to create well-being that is deeply personal and incredibly powerful.

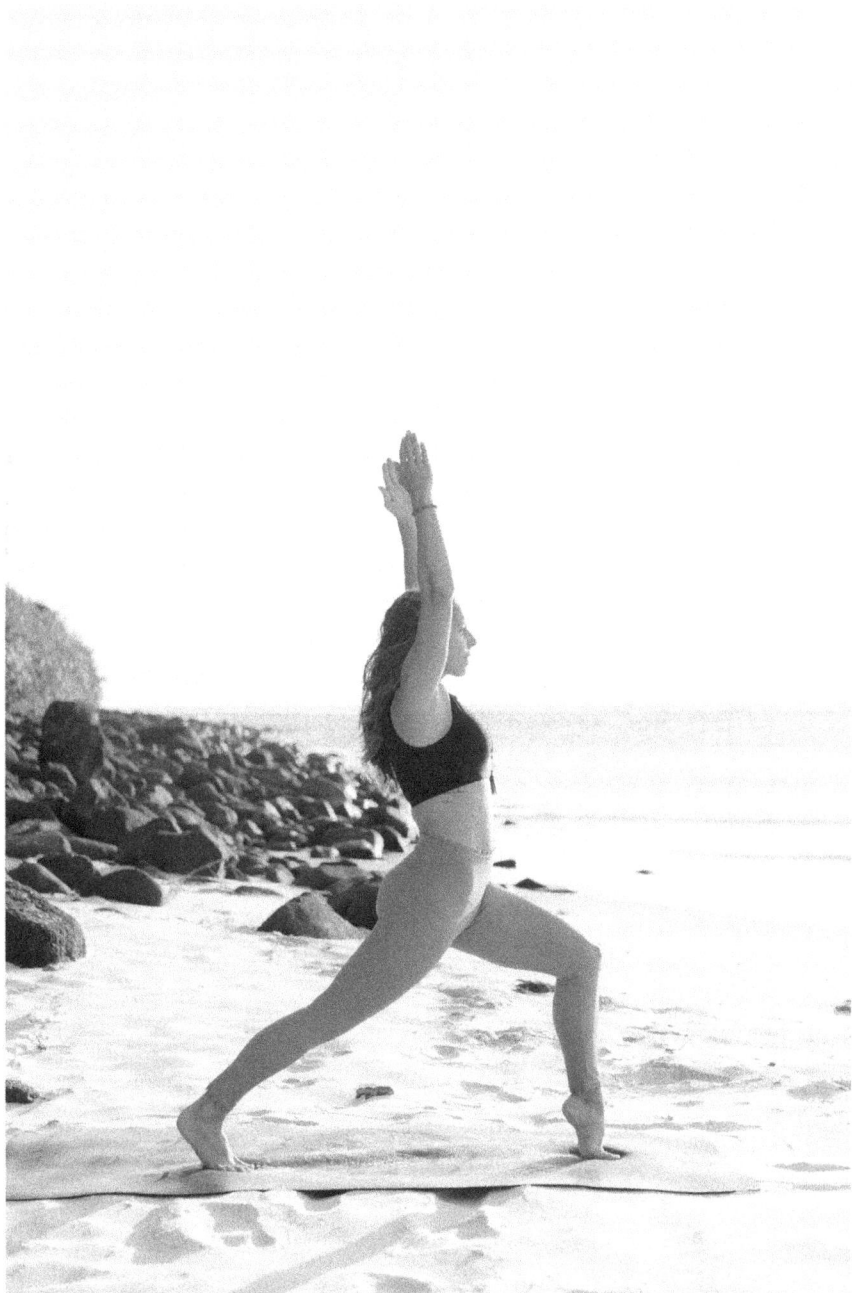

""THE BODY IS YOUR TEMPLE. KEEP IT PURE AND CLEAN FOR THE
SOUL TO RESIDE IN." – B.K.S. IYENGAR

Ayurveda teaches us that health is not the absence of disease, but the presence of vitality, clarity, and purpose. It is living in flow with your body's natural rhythms, the cycles of nature, and the truth of your spirit. When we honor this holistic approach, we unlock the ability to live fully— not just surviving but thriving.

This journey is not linear. There will be times when imbalance creeps in, when life's challenges disrupt your flow. But with the tools of health alchemy, you will always have a way to recalibrate and reconnect to your center. Every step you take toward balance, no matter how small, brings you closer to your higHERself™.

A Client's Journey to Wholeness: Finding Alchemy

When Ashley first walked into my clinic, she was a bundle of emotions—teary-eyed and unsure of what she wanted from life. At thirty-three years old, Ashley worked as a receptionist in a high-pressure office environment. She felt stuck, with no clear vision for her future. While she knew she wanted to have children one day, she didn't have a boyfriend, and her struggle with PCOS (polycystic ovary syndrome) had left her doubting whether pregnancy would even be possible.

Her symptoms were classic: irregular periods, weight gain, cystic acne, and a sense of emotional overwhelm that often left her crying at night. But beyond her physical symptoms, Ashley's spirit seemed dimmed. She described herself as "just existing," feeling unworthy and disconnected from any sense of purpose. Together, we began the process of piecing her back together—not fixing her but helping her rediscover her inner balance and inherent power.

PHYSICAL ALCHEMY: REKINDLING HER AGNI

PCOS is often linked to Kapha imbalances, with stagnation in metabolism and insulin resistance playing significant roles. Ashley's diet was erratic, filled with processed convenience foods, and she often skipped meals, leading to blood sugar crashes and binge eating later in the day.

We worked to rekindle her Agni by introducing warm, light, and spiced foods to pacify Kapha and regulate her blood sugar. She also began incorporating Ayurvedic herbs to support her reproductive health and to gently detoxify and improve digestion.

For exercise, Ashley transitioned from sporadic intense workouts that drained her energy to fun and invigorating exercise with her bestie, consistency being key.

MENTAL ALCHEMY: REWIRING HER MIND

Ashleys mind was consumed with self-doubt and negative narratives about her body and her worth. She constantly compared herself to others, fueling feelings of inadequacy.

Through Ayurvedic psychology, we worked to cultivate Sattva— the clarity and purity of mind. I introduced her to mantra meditation, encouraging her to repeat affirmations like, "I am whole, just as I am," and "I honor my unique path."

Ashley also began a journaling practice, writing each evening about three things she was grateful for and one small win from her day. Over time, these practices rewired her thought patterns, replacing criticism with compassion.

EMOTIONAL ALCHEMY: ALLOWING HER TEARS TO HEAL

Ashley's tears were not a weakness—they were a sign that her emotions needed space to flow. In Ayurveda, the Kapha dosha governs emotional holding, and excess Kapha often leads to feeling stuck or burdened by unexpressed grief.

One transformative practice for Ashley was writing letters to herself. She wrote to the girl she had been at thirteen, the woman she was now, and the mother she hoped to become. These letters became a safe space to honor her pain, release her fears, and acknowledge her resilience.

SPIRITUAL ALCHEMY: RECONNECTING WITH HER INNER LIGHT

Ashley admitted that she had lost touch with her sense of spirit. Her days felt like a repetitive grind, leaving little room for connection or inspiration.

I encouraged her to start small, lighting a candle each morning as a symbolic gesture of inviting light into her day. She also began a practice of gazing at the moon each evening, aligning herself with its cycles and finding comfort in its quiet, constant presence.

As Ashley deepened her connection to her spiritual self, she began to trust the timing of her life. She stopped comparing herself to friends who were married with children and started embracing the beauty of her own path.

DHARMIC ALCHEMY: LIVING WITH PURPOSE

When we first discussed Ashley's dharma, she hesitated. "I'm just a receptionist," she said. But as we explored further, Ashley realised her dharma wasn't tied to her job title—it was about how she showed up in the world. She had a gift for making others feel seen and valued, whether it was through a kind smile or a thoughtful gesture.

Over time, Ashley began to align her daily actions with her values. She would randomly offer acts of kindness such as buying people in line behind her their morning coffee. This act of service reignited a sense of purpose, helping Ashley see the profound impact she could have, even in small ways.

She also began to see the beauty of her full-time job allowing her to take six weeks off per year for pure fun and travel. Her job afforded her to do this, something that was very important to her. She looked forward to planning her trips and immersing herself in different cultures and taking her acts of kindness overseas.

THE TRANSFORMATION

Within six months, Ashley's periods became more regular, her acne improved, and she began to lose weight—not because she was dieting, but because her body was finding balance. More importantly, she felt alive again. She described feeling a sense of hope and possibility that had been absent for years.

Ashley's journey is a testament to the power of health alchemy. By addressing all five aspects of her being—physical, mental, emotional, spiritual, and dharmic—she was able to step into her higHERself™.

Your Own Alchemy Awaits

Ashley's story is one example of what's possible when we embrace health alchemy. Each of us has the power to transform, to heal, and to thrive. The key is integration—seeing yourself as a whole, honoring every aspect of your being, and trusting that the journey is as important as the destination.

To fully embrace the essence of health alchemy, we must understand that our mindset, mental well-being, and the alignment of our lives with our values and purpose are not separate from our health—they are its foundation. These elements influence every choice we make, every habit we build, and how we show up for ourselves and the world around us. These elements are so integral that they have become pillars of their own: the Empowered Mind Paradigm and Dharmic Impact.

In the next sections of this book, we will delve into these final two pillars. Section 3 will explore the Empowered Mind Paradigm, revealing how your mindset shapes your reality, while section 4 will uncover Dharmic Impact, guiding you to live a life of purpose and alignment. Together, these pillars complete the higHERself™ Method, offering a comprehensive framework to rise into your most radiant, empowered, and aligned self.

Reflection: Your Own Health Alchemy

As you reflect on this chapter, ask yourself:

1. What area of your life feels out of balance?

2. How can you nurture your physical, mental, emotional, spiritual, and dharmic health today?

You, too, have the power to create alchemy in your life. This is your time to rise.

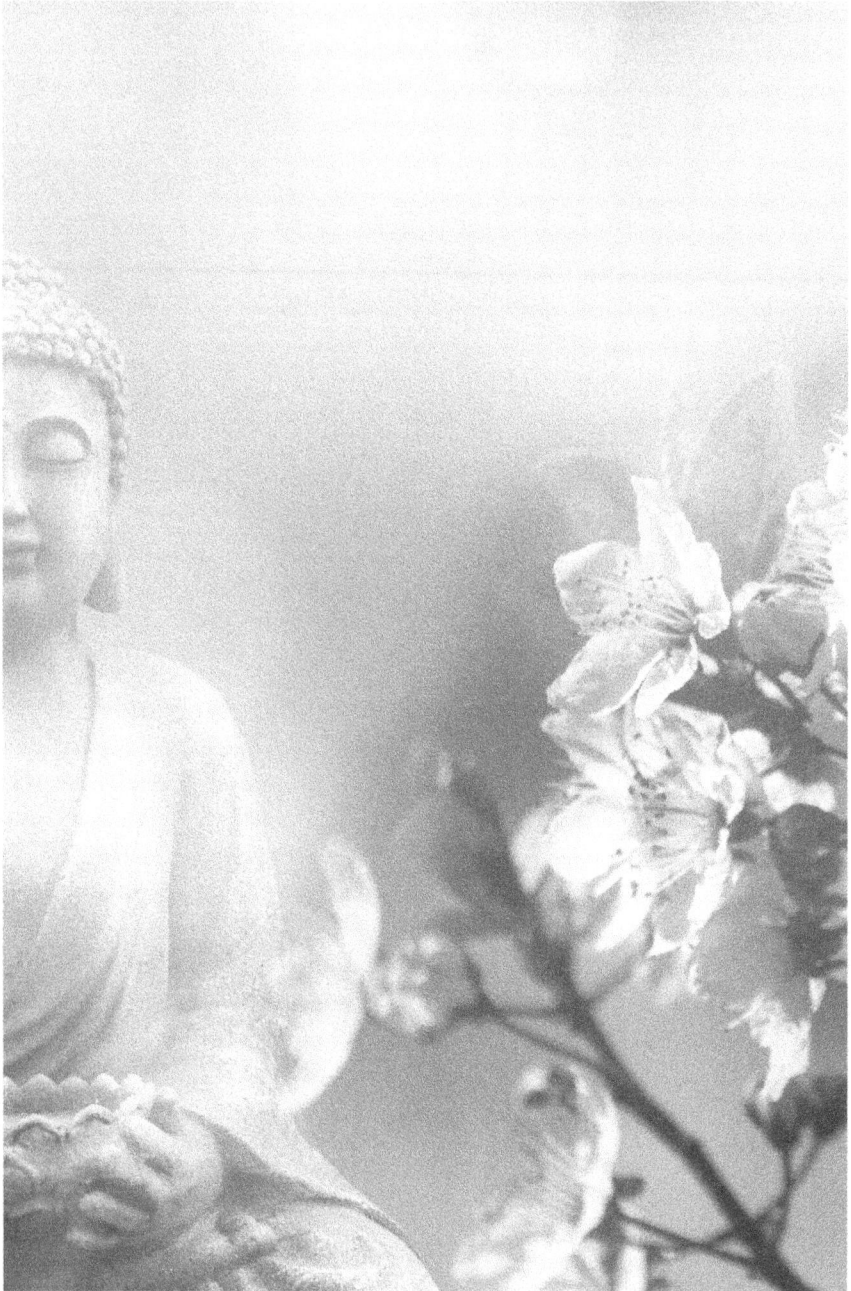

"THE MIND IS EVERYTHING. WHAT YOU THINK, YOU BECOME."
BUDDHA

PART 3

The Empowered Mind Paradigm

Unlocking the Power of Your Mind to Step into Your higHERself™

The mind is both the architect of our reality and the greatest barrier to our transformation. In this section, we explore how an empowered mindset is essential for stepping into your higHERself™. Without mastering the mind, no amount of physical health, lifestyle changes, or external achievements create lasting fulfillment.

For women in their power years, this becomes even more crucial. This phase of life brings immense change—physically, emotionally, and spiritually. It is often a time of deep reflection, where old identities are shed, and new possibilities arise. However, stepping into this new phase requires dismantling the limiting beliefs and conditioned patterns that have kept us small, uncertain, or fearful.

This section combines Ayurvedic psychology, modern neuroscience, and practical mindset strategies to help you rewrite your internal narrative, strengthen mental resilience, and cultivate the confidence and clarity to move forward with purpose.

CHAPTER 17

The Mindset Code: Unlocking Your True Potential

Why Mindset Is the Key to Your higHERself™

WHAT IS THE EMPOWERED MIND PARADIGM?

The mind is the foundation of everything. It is the filter through which we experience life, the architect of our beliefs, and the driving force behind our actions. When the mind is aligned, clear, and empowered, it becomes a force of transformation. When it is clouded by doubt, fear, and limiting beliefs, it keeps us stuck in patterns of self-sabotage.

For many women in their thirties, forties, and fifties, this is a time of profound transition. Children grow up, careers shift, relationships evolve, and the body undergoes its own metamorphosis. It is easy to feel lost or untethered, as if the identity that once defined you no longer fits. This is where the Empowered Mind Paradigm becomes essential.

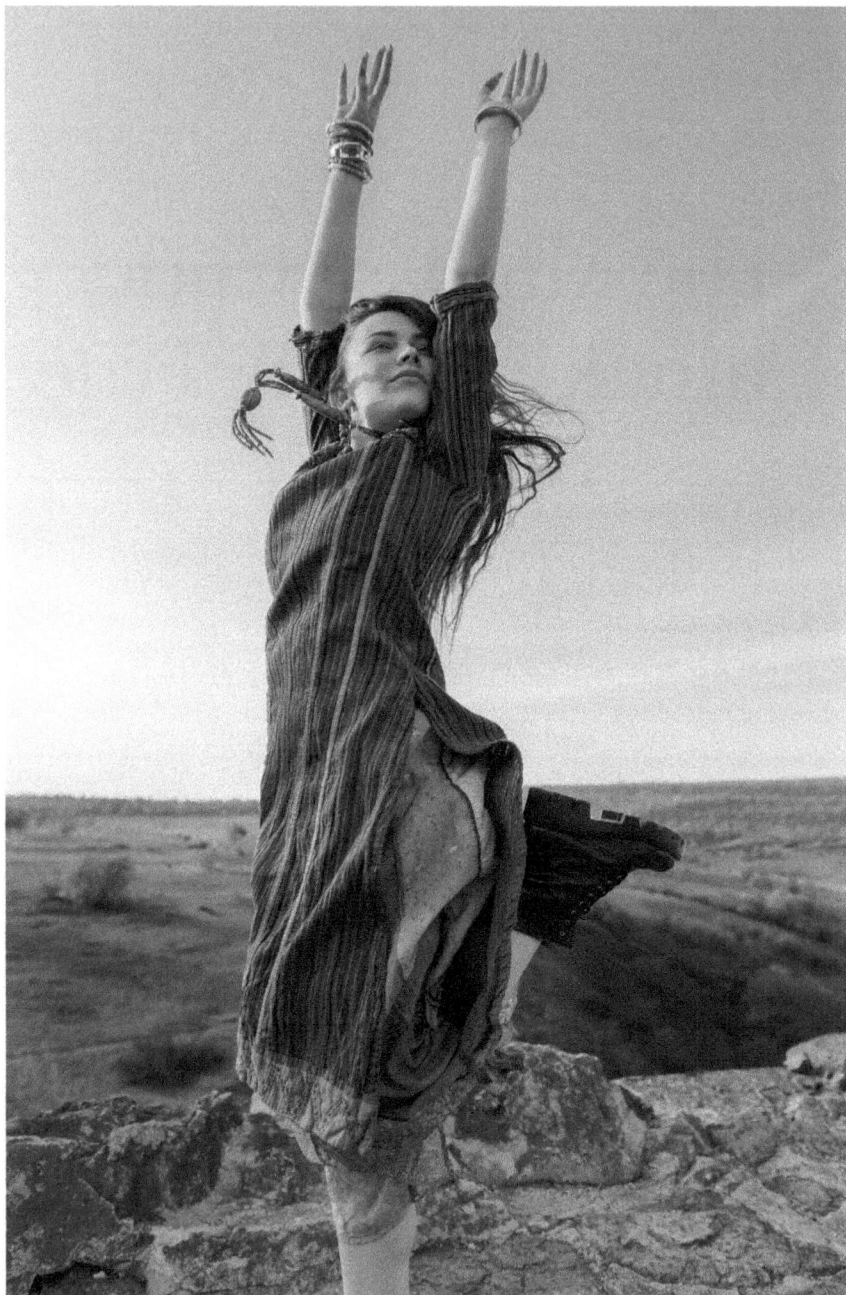

"WHEN WE ARE LIFTED, WE RISE. WHEN WE RISE, WE LIFT."
– OPRAH WINFREY

The Empowered Mind Paradigm is about taking conscious control of your thoughts, beliefs, and perceptions. It is about stepping into the role of cocreator of your life rather than being a passive observer.

This isn't about forced positivity or ignoring life's challenges—it's about recognizing the immense power of your mind to shape your reality.

At forty-six, my client Amelia had built an impressive career as a financial advisor—structured, respected, and predictable. But inside, she felt like a fraud.

"I can tell people how to manage their investments, how to grow their wealth, but I can't seem to convince myself that I'm allowed to start over," she admitted, her voice tight with hesitation. "I've spent years dreaming about running cacao ceremonies and women's circles, hosting retreats, helping other women step into their power after having personally benefited from the ones that I have attended. But who would take me seriously? I don't have a background in wellness. I'm too old to start from scratch."

Amelia's mind had become a fortress of self-doubt, built brick by brick with expectations—what a successful woman should do, how a career should unfold, when it was too late to pivot. She was paralyzed, not because she lacked ability, but because she was trapped by the belief that reinvention at her age wasn't an option.

I asked her a question that shifted something inside her: "As a financial advisor, if a forty-six-year-old woman sat across from you, saying she had spent all her inheritance and was in debt but dreamt of being debt-free and starting over with financial literacy and freedom, would you tell her she is too old and it's too late?"

She exhaled sharply, almost laughing at the obvious answer. "I'd tell her she owes it to herself to become financially free and provide her with the strategy to do it."

That moment cracked the foundation of her old beliefs. Together, we worked to dismantle the internalized fears keeping her small. Amelia used Ayurvedic practices to strengthen her mindset— morning journaling to quiet her inner critic, pranayama to calm the nervous energy that kept her stuck, and mantra meditation to rewire the way she spoke to herself.

Slowly, she started putting her dream into motion. She led her first women's circle in her living room, heart pounding as she guided a group of five women through a cacao ceremony and self-reflection. It wasn't perfect, but it was real. She threw herself into courses on health, wellness and spirituality, including the Ayurveda Alchemist Program, which helped her move her business from an idea to a reality. Over time, her circles grew. She pursued training, built a website, and, a year later, hosted her first weekend retreat, which sold out within days.

One afternoon, months after she left finance, she sent me a message. "I just realized—I haven't questioned myself in weeks. I'm actually doing this."

Amelia hadn't changed overnight, and the doubts hadn't disappeared entirely. But she had learned to override the voice that told her she wasn't capable. She stepped into her calling not because she was fearless, but because she chose to move forward despite the fear.

This is what happens when we stop believing the lie that reinvention is reserved for the young. The mind is not fixed; it is adaptable, expansive, and powerful. When we align our thoughts with our higher self, we open the door to possibilities that once seemed out of reach.

And just like Amelia, we all have the power to walk through that door.

How the Mind Shapes Our Reality

Every thought we think creates a ripple. The way we perceive ourselves, others, and the world determines the choices we make and the opportunities we recognize.

In Ayurveda, the mind is seen as Manas, the seat of perception and cognition. A Sattvic mind is clear, peaceful, and discerning, while an imbalanced mind, clouded by Rajas (restlessness) or Tamas (inertia), leads to confusion and suffering.

Modern neuroscience confirms what Ayurveda has taught for thousands of years:

+ **Your thoughts shape your brain:** Every repeated thought strengthens neural pathways, making it easier to think that thought again.

+ **Your beliefs filter reality:** The Reticular Activating System in the brain ensures that you notice what aligns with your beliefs. If you believe "I am not good enough," your brain will seek out evidence to confirm it.

+ **Your emotions follow your thoughts:** Negative thoughts trigger stress hormones like cortisol, while positive thoughts boost serotonin and dopamine, creating a sense of well-being.

The Influence of Beliefs, Thoughts, and Conditioning in Women's Evolution

From a young age, we are conditioned by our environment— our families, culture, and experiences shape the beliefs we carry into adulthood. By midlife, many of these beliefs are running on autopilot, dictating our decisions without us even realizing it.

+ "I'm too old to start something new."

+ "I have to put others first."

✦ "Success means financial achievement, not personal fulfillment."

These are not truths—they are mere beliefs that have been repeated so often they feel like reality. The Empowered Mind Paradigm teaches us that we can challenge and change these beliefs.

Carrie a mother of three, struggled with self-worth after years of prioritizing her family over herself. "I don't even know who I am anymore," she admitted. Understanding her mindset through Ayurvedic psychology, she began to rewrite her story. She began to see herself as worthy of her own attention.

A woman's evolution isn't about external change—it begins in her mind. When we rewrite our beliefs, we change the trajectory of our lives.

Rewiring the Mindset of Abundance

I grew up in a tiny house on a hill—a house with no internal walls. My parents, my brother, and I each had our own space, but those spaces were shaped not by walls but by cupboards positioned to mimic them. There was no flushing toilet, just a small camping toilet tucked into a corner. My Dad had to manually carry the toilet out and empty it every day. Some days it was too late, and the smell of sewage would infiltrate the house as the toilet began to overflow. It was a house that was more function than form—a house where I learned resilience but also limitation. And in that house, I developed another kind of cycle. A cycle of purging. When my external world felt small and uncontrollable, I tried to create control within my own body. Bulimia became my outlet, a way to grasp at power over something, anything, when everything else felt constrained. It was destruction disguised as discipline.

As a child, I remember feeling embarrassed when friends would come over. I hated that our house looked nothing like theirs, that it didn't have polished, cozy spaces. I longed for something bigger, something nicer—something that didn't make me feel so small. But at the same time, I learned to suppress that longing. Somewhere along the way, I absorbed the idea that wanting more was selfish, that desiring abundance meant I wasn't grateful for what I had. I told myself I should be happy with what I was given, and that it was enough.

But deep down, I wasn't yearning for a different home—I was yearning for a sense of security, a sense of belonging within myself. What I didn't realize was that my environment wasn't only shaping my external perception of scarcity—that perception was seeping into my internal world, wiring me to believe I wasn't allowed to want more. That played out in ways I didn't understand back then. I denied myself nourishment, then punished myself for it. I told myself I was in control, when in reality, I was trapped in a cycle of deprivation—one that mirrored the subconscious limitations I placed on my own worth.

Years later, when I found Ayurveda, I finally understood what was missing. I had spent years controlling my body, but I had never learned how to truly nourish it. I had mistaken restriction for strength, when real strength came from learning to receive— whether that was food, abundance, or self-love. It was only through this deeper healing that I was able to rewrite the story I had told myself for so long.

Because wanting more isn't selfish. It's human.
And it's safe to step into the fullness of who we are.

My subconscious shaped my money mindset for years. When I got older and began to create my own life, I found myself unconsciously holding back—resisting success, undercharging for my work, and feeling guilty anytime I did allow myself to indulge in something luxurious. I was stuck in a loop of scarcity, believing that too much desire meant too little gratitude.

But here's the thing: I never felt abundant in that little house. I never felt that so-called humility brought me joy. And yet, I have felt deeply abundant staying in small, simple villas all over the world—because abundance is not about size or luxury, it's about mindset. The difference was how I felt.

Abundance is not about having more; it's about feeling worthy of more. It took years of deep inner work, unlearning old beliefs, and rewriting my narrative to shift into a mindset of abundance. I had to recognize that my childhood environment had wired me to associate scarcity with virtue and desire with selfishness. But I now understand that wanting more—whether it's more joy, more love, more financial freedom, or more space to breathe—is not selfish. It is expansive.

Ayurveda teaches us that the mind holds *samskaras*—impressions from our past experiences that shape how we see the world. My childhood home left deep samskaras of lack, which in turn influenced my self-worth, my financial decisions, and even my ability to dream big. But just as the body can heal so can the mind.

We have the power to rewire our beliefs, to step out of scarcity and into a space of receiving. If you've felt guilty for wanting more, if you've believed that success means you've abandoned humility, if you've felt stuck in patterns of lack—know that it is not a reflection of your worth, but of your conditioning. And conditioning can be rewritten.

You are worthy of abundance. You are allowed to desire more. And most importantly, you are capable of creating it.

How a Disempowered Mindset Holds You Back: The Inner Critic, Fear-Based Thinking, and Self-Sabotage

The biggest obstacle to transformation isn't external circumstances—it's the voice in our own heads. We all have an inner critic—a voice that whispers (or shouts) doubts and fears. This voice is not your true self; it is a collection of past experiences, societal conditioning, and unprocessed fears.

✦ "You're not smart enough."

✦ "You'll fail, so why even try?"

✦ "People will judge you."

When left unchecked, this voice can hold us back from growth. It keeps us playing small, afraid to take risks, and stuck in familiar (but unfulfilling) cycles.

Ayurveda teaches that when the mind is dominated by Tamas (inertia and fear), it resists change. The key to breaking free from this cycle is awareness. Once you recognize the inner critic is not your truth, you gain power to reframe those thoughts.

And when you do—it changes everything.

As I sit writing this section, sipping on chai at my favourite café on the Gold Coast after a grounding Pilates class, two messages land in my inbox. They're from students of Ayurveda Alchemist Academy, both expressing deep gratitude. These women—at different stages of life, from different parts of the world—shared how overcoming imposter syndrome through this work has changed their lives' trajectories.

One wrote, "Thank you for helping me see what's possible. I never thought I could do something like this, but now I'm running workshops and helping women through Ayurvedic holistic health coaching." The other said, "You helped me believe in myself. That voice in my head told me I wasn't qualified—but I chose not to listen. And now I'm living my dharma through Vedic breathwork."

These moments are the reason I continue this work.

They are a reminder that transformation doesn't happen by silencing the inner critic entirely—but by choosing not to believe it. By aligning with your truth, your dharma, your inner clarity.

If these women—once held back by doubt—can rise, so can you. Your higher self is not something you have to become. She's already within you. Sometimes, all it takes is one decision to listen to her instead of the fear.

How Societal Conditioning and Past Experiences Shape Our Beliefs

Women, especially, are conditioned to prioritize others, seek external validation, and play it safe. We absorb subtle messages from childhood—messages about what is "appropriate" for us to want, pursue, or dream about.

But what if those old beliefs no longer serve you?

Michelle, always put her family first, dismissing her own needs. When I asked her, "What do *you* want?" she burst into tears—she had never considered it. Through deep inner work, she began dismantling the belief that prioritizing herself was selfish. Today, she is thriving, having started her own book club for mothers. Your beliefs can either empower or imprison you. The choice is yours.

Reframing Your Thoughts: The Thought Alchemy Method

If your mindset is the lens through which you experience life, then reframing your thoughts is like adjusting the focus—shifting from a blurred, fearful perspective to one of clarity and empowerment.

One effective tool for breaking free from the grip of a disempowered mindset is what I call the Thought Alchemy Method. It's a simple yet profound three-step process rooted in both Ayurvedic psychology and modern cognitive reframing techniques.

STEP 1: CATCH THE THOUGHT

The first step is awareness. You can't change what you don't acknowledge. Start paying attention to the inner dialogue that runs on autopilot. Write down the thoughts that arise when you face a challenge or hesitate to take action.

For example, let's say you dream of launching your own business, but the moment you consider it, a thought creeps in: "I'm too old to start over. No one will take me seriously."

Instead of accepting this as truth, recognize it for what it is—a conditioned belief, not a fact.

STEP 2: CHALLENGE THE THOUGHT

Now, question its validity. Ask yourself:

✦ Is this thought absolutely true? Where's the proof?

✦ Would I say this to a friend in the same situation?

✦ Has anyone like me succeeded at this before? (Hint: the answer is always yes!)

Most of our limiting beliefs crumble when we examine them. If someone else has succeeded despite similar circumstances, why not you?

STEP 3: CHOOSE A NEW THOUGHT

Here's where the real magic happens. Instead of letting the old belief dictate your actions, reframe it into a more empowering perspective. Aim to shift any limiting belief into an empowered, positive and proactive belief.

Limiting Belief	Empowered Shift
"I'm too old to start over."	"I bring decades of wisdom and experience— people will trust me because of it."
"I'll fail, so why even try?"	"Every expert was once a beginner. Growth comes from action, not perfection."

By consistently shifting your thoughts, you rewire your brain's neural pathways (this is backed by neuroplasticity research) and replace fear-based conditioning with empowered thinking.

Your Mind as Your Ally

Your thoughts create your reality. If you master the art of reframing, you will no longer be at the mercy of self-doubt—you'll be in control. With practice, this becomes second nature, and instead of your mind working against you, it becomes your greatest ally.

Start today. The next time your inner critic whispers something limiting, pause. Catch it. Challenge it. Reframe it. Watch how your world begins to shift.

CHAPTER 18

Science of Mindset and Mental Resilience: How Thoughts Shape Brain Chemistry and Create Neural Pathways

Modern neuroscience validates what Ayurveda has known for centuries—your thoughts shape your brain. This is known as neuroplasticity, the brain's ability to rewire itself based on repetitive thoughts and behaviors.

✦ If you constantly think, "I am not good enough," your brain strengthens that neural pathway, making it easier to believe.

✦ If you start replacing it with, "I am growing, learning, and worthy," over time, this new pathway becomes dominant.

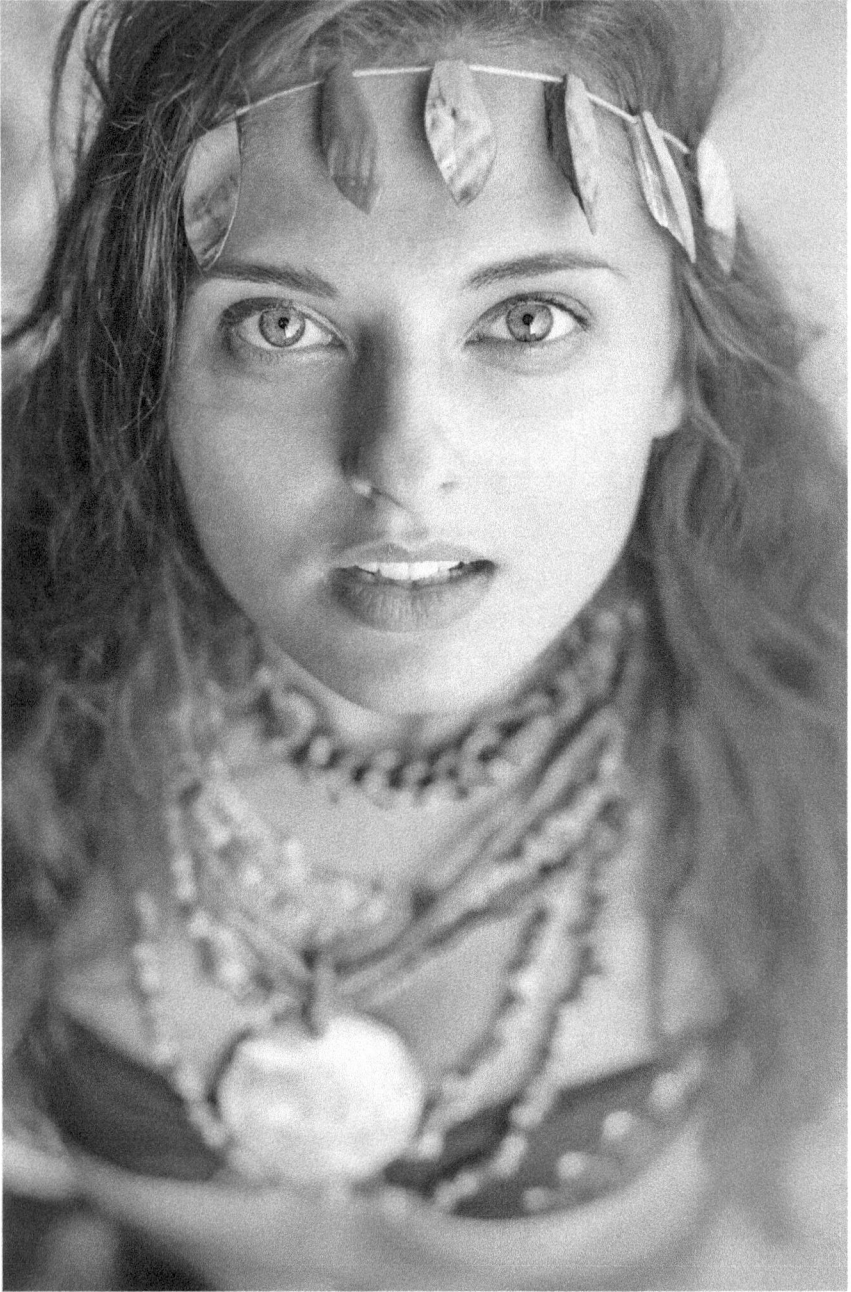

"WHAT LIES BEHIND US AND WHAT LIES BEFORE US ARE TINY
MATTERS COMPARED TO WHAT LIES WITHIN US."
– RALPH WALDO EMERSON

The Power of Positive Affirmations and How They Rewire the Brain

Studies in psychology have shown that self-affirmation practices can reshape brain activity, particularly in the prefrontal cortex, the area responsible for decision-making and self-regulation. A study in *Social Cognitive and Affective Neuroscience* found that affirmations activate the brain's reward centers, increasing feelings of self-worth.[30] Self-affirmation activates brain systems associated with reward and is reinforced by repetition.[31] Another study in *Psychological Science* showed that people who used affirmations were more likely to persist in challenges and problem-solving.[32] Self-affirmation also improves problem-solving under stress.[33]

This is why mantras and affirmations are so powerful in Ayurvedic psychology. By repeating truthful, empowering statements, you are literally reprogramming your brain.

Mantras and Affirmations for an Empowered Mindset

To fully embrace the power of neuroplasticity and Ayurvedic psychology, let's turn knowledge into practice. For the next thirty days, I invite you to repeat one affirmation seven times upon waking and before bed—the moments when your subconscious mind is most receptive.

Set a reminder on your phone to stay consistent and watch how your mindset transforms.

---

30 Cascio, C. N. et al., 2016, "Self-affirmation Acivates Brain Systems Associated with Self-related Processing and Reward and Is Reinforced by Future Orientation," *Social Cognitive and Behavioral Neuroscience* 11 (4): 621–629, doi: 10.1093/scan/nsv136.

31 Cascio et al., 2016.

32 Creswell, J. D. et al., 2013, "Self-affirmation Improves Problem-Solving Under Stress," *PLoS ONE* 8 (5): e62593.

33 Crewell et al., 2016.

If one of these affirmations resonates with you, use it. If not, create your own that aligns with your highest self and the reality you want to step into.

10 MANTRAS AND AFFIRMATIONS FOR TRANSFORMATION

1. "I am stepping into my highest self with confidence and grace."

2. "I trust that my path is unfolding exactly as it is meant to."

3. "I release fear and embrace limitless possibilities."

4. "I am worthy of abundance, love, and success in all areas of my life."

5. "Every day, I grow stronger, wiser, and more aligned with my truth."

6. "My mind is clear, my heart is open, and my soul is at peace."

7. "I honor my past, embrace my present, and trust my future."

8. "I choose thoughts that empower, uplift, and support me."

9. "I am resilient, adaptable, and capable of handling anything that comes my way."

10. "I radiate confidence, wisdom, and inner peace in all that I do."

WHY THIS PRACTICE WORKS

These affirmations are more than simple words—they are a tool for rewiring your subconscious mind. By repeating them daily, you are literally programming your brain to shift from fear to empowerment, from doubt to self-trust.

The invitation is simple:

✦ Choose one mantra.

✦ Commit to thirty days.

✦ Say it aloud seven times in the morning and seven times before bed.

✦ Set a daily reminder so you don't forget.

Transformation doesn't happen overnight, but with consistency, your brain will start to believe these words as truth. And once your mind believes, your reality follows.

I have used this method many times. One recent example is when I noticed I would get anxious at the thought of tackling my inbox, which is inundated with tasks set by others, requests and notifications, and emails waiting for replies. I started envisioning this experience of opening my inbox as exciting, full of opportunities, with beautiful emails from clients or students and emails that reflected an abundant cash flow. Every morning and every night I repeated, "I am excited to open my inbox, which is full of love, opportunities, and reminders of the impact I am making in the world." At first, it felt like I was trying to convince myself of something that wasn't true. But with repetition, something shifted, and *now*, I truly get excited to see what beautiful messages await me.

This experience reinforced a powerful truth: our reality is shaped by the meaning we give to it. By consciously shifting the way we think, we transform even the smallest, most mundane aspects of life into something empowering and positive.

Stronger Mind, Longer Life: The Science of Resilience and Health

Resilience is not about avoiding difficulties—it's about how we rise after we fall.

The ability to navigate challenges with grace and adaptability is what sets apart those who merely survive from those who truly thrive.

Science strongly supports the link between mental resilience and overall well-being:

✦ Women with high mental resilience have significantly lower rates of anxiety, depression, and chronic disease.

✦ A 2019 study published in the *American Journal of Lifestyle Medicine* found that individuals with a resilient mindset were more likely to maintain healthy habits, such as regular exercise and balanced nutrition, even under stress.

✦ The Harvard Study of Adult Development, one of the longest-running studies on human happiness and longevity, found that a positive mindset and emotional resilience were stronger predictors of a long, fulfilling life than genetics, wealth, or even physical health.[34]

How to Build Mental Resilience

Resilience is not something you either have or don't have—it's a skill that can be cultivated. Here's how you can strengthen yours.

REFRAME CHALLENGES AS OPPORTUNITIES

Difficulties are an inevitable part of life, but the way you perceive them determines their impact. Instead of seeing challenges as roadblocks, view them as stepping stones. Ask yourself:

✦ What is this experience here to teach me?

✦ How can I grow from this?

✦ What strengths am I developing by navigating this situation?

This mindset shift not only helps you move through difficulties with greater ease but also rewires your brain for long-term resilience.

---

34 McLean, C. P., Asnaani, A., Litz, B. T., & Hofmann, S. G., 2011, "Gender Differences in Anxiety Disorders: Prevalence, Course of Illness, Comorbidity, and Burden of Illness," *Journal of Psychiatric Research* 45 (8): 1027–1035, https://doi.org/10.1016/j.jpsychires.2011.03.006; Vaillant, G. E., 2012, "Triumphs of Experience: The Men of the Harvard Grant Study," Harvard University Press.

BUILD A MENTAL TOOLKIT FOR TOUGH MOMENTS

When stress arises, having reliable tools can make all the difference. Some effective strategies include:

+ **Breathwork (Pranayama):** Deep, controlled breathing helps calm the nervous system and shifts you from a reactive state to a responsive one. Try Nadi Shodhana (alternate nostril breathing) to restore balance.

+ **Mantra Work:** The repetition of affirmations like "I am strong, I am steady, I am capable" can help reprogram limiting beliefs.

+ **Journaling:** Writing out your thoughts provides clarity and allows you to process emotions rather than suppress them.

+ **Gratitude Practice:** Actively acknowledging what is good in your life creates a resilience buffer, helping you shift focus from what's missing to what's thriving.

REGULATE YOUR NERVOUS SYSTEM

Chronic stress keeps your nervous system in a constant state of fight-or-flight, making it harder to think clearly and respond wisely. Ayurveda and modern science both emphasize the importance of nervous system regulation through the following:

+ **Daily movement:** Whether it's a yoga practice, a nature walk, or strength training, movement is essential for emotional resilience.

+ **Consistent sleep cycles:** Sleep deprivation heightens emotional reactivity and impairs problem-solving. Ayurveda recommends being in bed by 10:00 p.m. to sync with the body's natural rhythms.

+ **Mindful pauses:** Throughout the day, take a moment to close your eyes, take a deep breath, and check in with yourself. A simple pause can shift your entire mindset.

SURROUND YOURSELF WITH SUPPORTIVE ENERGY

You are a reflection of the people you spend the most time with. Surround yourself with those who uplift, challenge, and inspire you. Limit exposure to negativity—whether from people, media, or self-talk.

Emotional resilience doesn't happen in isolation—it's nurtured through the relationships that surround us. Studies from the American Psychological Association show that strong social support not only buffers against stress but is one of the most influential predictors of how well someone adapts after adversity. When you're regularly exposed to criticism, negativity, or people who drain your energy, it chips away at your capacity to bounce back. But when you're in the company of people who believe in you, remind you of your strength, and walk beside you through the messy middle, your nervous system finds safety—and that safety becomes the foundation for resilience.

You don't have to do it all alone. Choose relationships that hold space for both your vulnerability and your power. Let go of environments that require you to shrink. Emotional resilience is not about how you face the storm—it's about who's holding your umbrella beside you.

EMBRACE THE POWER OF LETTING GO

Resilient women understand that holding onto past pain, resentment, or failure only weighs them down. Release what no longer serves you, whether it's outdated beliefs, toxic relationships, or self-doubt.

In the Bhagavad Gita, Krishna reminds Arjuna, "You have a right to your actions, but never to your fruits." This wisdom teaches us to focus on what we can control—our mindset, our efforts, and our responses—while letting go of attachment to outcomes. Gabby Bernstein beautifully echoes this teaching with her famous words,

"The Universe has your back." When we align with our dharmic path and step into our higHERself™, we are supported in ways we cannot always see. What is meant for us will find us, and what is not aligned will naturally fall away—if we allow it.

But how often do we resist this natural flow? We grip onto relationships, careers, or identities that no longer serve us out of fear of the unknown. Yet, what if what we hold onto so desperately actually keeps us from stepping into something far greater? When we loosen our grip and trust the unfolding, we create space for what is truly aligned to enter our lives.

True empowerment comes when we embrace this trust— when we release the need to control every outcome and instead anchor ourselves in faith, knowing that every step forward is leading us exactly where we are meant to be.

Resilience Is the Gateway to Your higHERself™

By strengthening your mental resilience, you're not only changing your mind—you're transforming your health, relationships, and future. Resilience allows you to move through life with greater ease, confidence, and inner peace.

You are not your past. You are not your mistakes. You are the strength you cultivate, the wisdom you embody, and the light you share.

Your mind is your greatest tool. Will you use it to empower yourself or hold yourself back? The choice is yours.

Don't Get Stuck in the Healing Loop —Choose Joy as Your Frequency

A word of gentle truth: healing is not a personality trait. It's a sacred part of your evolution, not your entire identity.

So many women begin their self-development journey with the best intentions—seeking clarity, release, growth. But somewhere along the way, the process itself becomes a trap. We can become addicted to digging, fixing, unearthing, endlessly diagnosing what's "wrong" with us. As if the only way to be whole is to constantly be broken first.

But you are not broken—you are becoming. True transformation doesn't live in the constant reactivation of wounds. It lives in the integration of what you've learned. In the choice to rise, even when the world says stay small. In the decision to laugh, dance, and create—even when your healing isn't finished.

You don't need another breakthrough to be worthy of joy.

Your higHERself™ isn't obsessed with perfection—she is devoted to aliveness. She shows up, even in uncertainty. She finds magic in mundane moments. She knows that joy is not a reward for healing—it's part of the medicine.

So, if you've been circling the same inner story, ask yourself: what would it feel like to write a new one? To stop waiting to be fully healed before you start living fully?

You didn't come here to fix yourself.

You came here to become yourself.

And she—your radiant, wild, powerful higHERself™— is already within you.

Reflection on Mental Resilience

1. What does my life look like when I'm living from joy instead of pain?

---

2. Who am I when I no longer need to be "healing" to be worthy of happiness?

Let this be your invitation to stop circling the same story and begin writing the next chapter—from your power, not your past.

CHAPTER 19

Ayurvedic Psychology and the Path to Mental Mastery

For centuries, Ayurveda has taught that the mind is not merely an organ of thought—it is a dynamic, layered system that influences every aspect of our health, emotions, and consciousness. Unlike modern psychology, which often focuses on cognitive patterns and behavior, Ayurvedic psychology (Manas Vidya) views the mind as a multidimensional entity composed of seven layers, each contributing to our perception of reality, our emotional responses, and our ability to step into our highest potential.

Imagine the mind as an ancient temple, with each layer representing a different chamber. As we explore each chamber, we unlock a deeper understanding of ourselves. The goal is to activate all layers, leading to an empowered, clear, and expansive mindset.

The Vedic perspective on cognition teaches us that the mind is influenced by Sattva (clarity and wisdom), Rajas (passion and restlessness), and Tamas (inertia and confusion). A mind that is overactive with Rajas may become obsessive, anxious, or overly ambitious. A mind dominated by Tamas may feel stuck, foggy, or weighed down by self-doubt. But a mind infused with Sattva is calm,

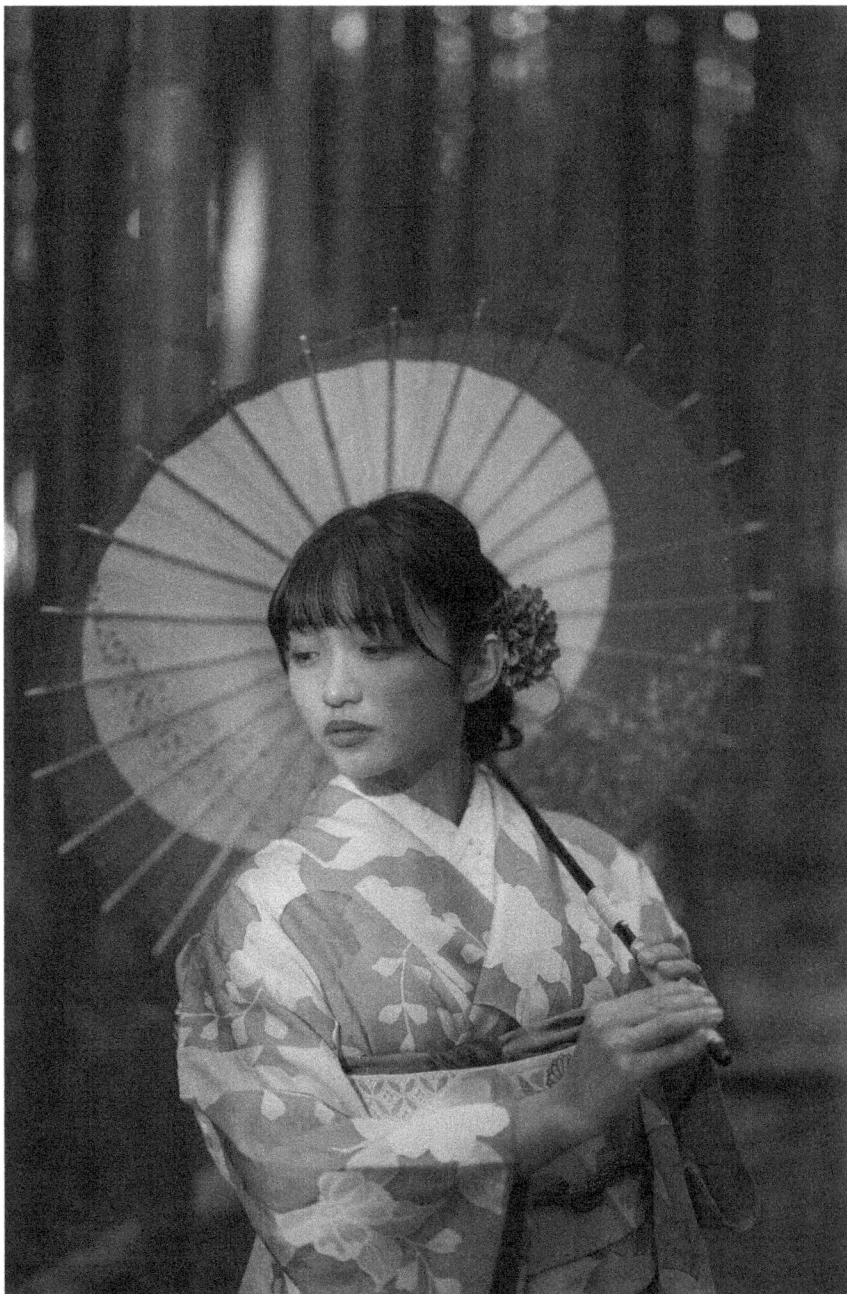

"FALL DOWN SEVEN TIMES, STAND UP EIGHT."
– JAPANESE PROVERB

resilient, and aligned—capable of making wise decisions and seeing life with clarity.

The Seven Layers of Consciousness: Ayurveda's Map to the Mind

Ayurvedic psychology recognizes that the mind is not fixed; it is malleable, conditioned by past experiences, and influenced by our doshic constitution. While Western psychology tends to focus on cognitive functions and mental health conditions, Ayurveda takes a holistic approach—seeing the mind as an evolving, layered structure that connects the physical, mental, emotional, and spiritual dimensions of our being.

The mind's seven layers form the foundation of our thoughts, emotions, decision-making, and spiritual growth. Each layer serves a unique function, but when imbalanced, it can hold us back—creating mental stagnation, self-doubt, or limiting beliefs.

Let's explore each of these layers and how they shape our mindset, identity, and perception of reality.

MANAS: THE SENSORY MIND (THE REACTIVE LAYER)

Manas is the surface layer of the mind—the part that interacts with the external world. It processes sensory input from our five senses, dictating how we respond to stimuli in the moment. This is the mind that reacts when we hear a loud noise, crave something sweet, or feel a surge of irritation in traffic.

When Manas is imbalanced, we become overly reactive, impulsive, and easily distracted. This is common in Vata imbalances, where overstimulation leads to scattered thoughts and anxious energy.

For example, imagine a woman in midlife, juggling work, family, and social obligations. She wakes up and immediately reaches for her phone, scrolling through emails, news, and social media. Before even getting out of bed, her mind is bombarded with information, setting her up for a day of reactive living rather than intentional action.

Balancing Manas

✦ Start the day with silence and mindfulness rather than technology.

✦ Engage in breathwork (Pranayama) to anchor the mind before external distractions take hold.

✦ Practice sensory awareness—savoring a meal, listening deeply, and being present in daily experiences.

AHAMKARA: THE EGO MIND (THE IDENTITY LAYER)

Ahamkara is the sense of self-identity—the part of the mind that says "I am." It helps us form a personal identity but can also create attachment to roles, beliefs, and past experiences.

While Ahamkara is essential for navigating the world, an unchecked ego can lead to comparison, perfectionism, and fear of change.

When Ahamkara is imbalanced, we define ourselves rigidly: "I am a mother, I am a businesswoman, I am not creative, I am too old to change." These beliefs become self-imposed limitations, preventing growth.

Example: A forty-six-year-old financial advisor, dreamed of starting a wellness business but feared she wouldn't be taken seriously at her age. Her Ahamkara was stuck in an outdated version of herself, preventing her from stepping into her next chapter.

Balancing Ahamkara

✦ Shift from ego-driven identity to soul-aligned identity—you are not your job, age, or past mistakes.

✦ Release the need for external validation and embrace inner authenticity.

✦ Use affirmations like "I am evolving. I am limitless. I am more than my past."

BUDDHI: THE DISCERNING MIND (THE WISDOM LAYER)

Buddhi is the intellect, intuition, and higher reasoning. It allows us to step back from emotions, analyze situations clearly, and make aligned decisions. This is where self-awareness and wisdom come into play.

When Buddhi is weak, we act impulsively, driven by emotions rather than discernment. When Buddhi is strong, we make choices that align with our higher self rather than reacting from fear or ego.

For example, a woman struggling with emotional eating recognizes her cravings aren't about hunger but unmet emotional needs. Rather than mindlessly indulging, she pauses and asks, "What do I truly need right now?" That moment of discernment is Buddhi in action.

Strengthening Buddhi

✦ Cultivate self-inquiry through journaling and introspection.

✦ Meditate to separate reaction from response.

✦ Trust inner wisdom—your intuition often knows before your logical mind catches up.

CHITTA: THE SUBCONSCIOUS MIND (THE SAMSKARA LAYER)

Chitta is the storehouse of memories, impressions, and deep-seated beliefs. It holds everything we have ever experienced—both conscious and unconscious. Within Chitta reside samskaras, the mental imprints formed by past experiences that shape our present reality.

When Chitta is imbalanced, we operate on autopilot, replaying old fears, traumas, and limiting beliefs. These unconscious patterns influence our behavior without us realizing it.

For example, a woman who grew up in a household where money was always a struggle may carry a deep-seated samskara of lack, leading to financial self-sabotage in adulthood.

Healing Chitta and Releasing Samskaras

✦ Identify and challenge repetitive negative thought patterns.

✦ Practice forgiveness and self-compassion to reframe painful past experiences.

✦ Engage in guided meditation or hypnotherapy to reprogram subconscious beliefs.

SMRITI: THE MEMORY AND RECOLLECTION MIND (THE WISDOM KEEPER LAYER)

Smriti is the ability to remember, recall, and integrate wisdom. It governs not only short-term memory but also our ability to learn from past mistakes and apply life lessons.

When Smriti is weak, we repeat the same unhealthy cycles—whether in relationships, career, or personal habits. Strengthening smriti helps us retain insights and break patterns.

For example, a woman who has always been drawn to toxic relationships finally remembers her worth and chooses a partner who respects her.

Strengthening Smriti

✦ Reflect on past experiences and extract wisdom rather than shame.

✦ Engage in mantra repetition—repeating spiritual truths to reinforce higher awareness.

✦ Keep a wisdom journal to track insights and lessons learned.

VIJNANA: THE HIGHER KNOWLEDGE MIND
(THE INTUITIVE LAYER)

Vijnana is deep knowing, intuition, and spiritual intelligence. It is the level of perception beyond logic—where we access universal truth. This is where we recognize we are not only the mind; we are consciousness itself.

When Vijnana is blocked, we doubt ourselves and seek external answers rather than trusting our inner guidance.

For example, a woman is offered a promotion that would elevate her career, but it requires long hours and time away from her children. Logically, it looks like the right move—more money, more prestige. But something in her gut says no. She turns it down, trusting her inner knowing. Months later, the entire department is restructured, and the role she would have accepted is made redundant, but not before it caused complete burnout and chaos to the person who accepted it.

Accessing Vijnana

+ Spend time in nature—the quietest place where intuition speaks.

+ Practice meditative stillness to hear your inner wisdom.

+ Follow your gut feelings—intuition is rarely wrong.

ATMAN: THE PURE CONSCIOUSNESS
(THE TRUE SELF LAYER)

Atman is the eternal self, beyond thoughts, emotions, and identity. This is pure awareness, divine connection, and the ultimate truth of who we are. While the other layers fluctuate, Atman remains unchanged. The more we align with this deepest layer, the more we step into our higher self.

For example, after years of searching for identity through external labels—mother, practitioner, partner—a woman sits in deep meditation and experiences a moment of profound stillness. In that silence, she no longer feels the need to be anyone, because she already is. This isn't a thought, it is a conscious knowing and being.

Connecting to Atman

+ Practice self-inquiry: Who am I beyond my roles, fears, and stories?

+ Engage in deep meditation and breathwork to experience stillness.

+ Embrace presence, realizing that you are already whole.

Breaking Free from the Past: Samskaras and Mindset Blocks

The mind is shaped by past conditioning, and negative samskaras (mental imprints) keep us stuck in limiting beliefs. These subconscious patterns affect our confidence, relationships, and ability to step into our highest potential.

How to Reprogram the Mind and Clear Negative Samskaras

1. AWARENESS AND REFLECTION: QUESTIONING THE STORIES YOU TELL YOURSELF

The first step in shifting limiting beliefs is awareness—becoming the observer of your own thoughts and patterns. Ask yourself:

+ Where did this belief come from?

+ Is it even true?

+ What evidence do I have that supports it?

+ What evidence do I have that disproves it?

We often carry stories that were never ours to begin with. Sometimes they stem from a single moment—a comment, a look, a reaction—that burrowed into our subconscious and became truth.

For example, I spent years believing, "I'm not smart enough," and I never questioned where that belief had come from—until one day, I did. I traced it back to a moment in primary school, when a teacher dismissed my answer in front of the class with a tone that implied I was way off track. The kids all burst into laughter. I don't remember exactly what she said. Maybe it wasn't even cruel. But in that moment, something in me decided: You're not as clever as the others. Be quiet. Don't get it wrong again.

That single moment became a samskara—a deep mental imprint. It played on repeat through my life, influencing how I showed up in the world, what I pursued, and how much I trusted my own voice.

But when I finally paused to examine it, the belief unraveled. My lived reality told a very different story: I've earned multiple university degrees with high distinctions. I've built a thriving business. I've coached and empowered countless women. The "not smart enough" story was never about truth—it was about perception, frozen in time.

Your mind will always find evidence for whatever you choose to believe. The question is: What beliefs are you choosing to confirm?

2. MANTRA AND AFFIRMATIONS: EMBODYING YOUR TRUTH

Repeating positive, truthful statements is a powerful way to rewrite old samskaras and reprogram the subconscious mind. But the key isn't just in saying the words—it's in feeling them, embodying them, and allowing them to shift your energy. For example, if your mantra is: "I am love; I am light; I am filled with a world of wisdom and intelligence," then pause for a moment and ask yourself, What would that actually look like? How would it feel to embody that truth?

If I close my eyes, I might see myself draped in a flowing white dress, standing tall with grace, feeling light and radiant, as universal wisdom pulses through my heart. Every word of the mantra resonates in my being, shifting my posture, my energy, my very presence in the world.

For another person, that same mantra might evoke a completely different vision—perhaps a powerful woman in a deep purple suit, confidently standing on stage in front of hundreds, speaking with conviction, her voice strong and unwavering.

The vision you receive is personal to you, but the feeling is what creates the transformation.

When you repeat your mantra, let it ignite that feeling within you. Carry it into your day. Walk, speak, and move as if that truth is already yours—because it is.

3. MEDITATION AND BREATHWORK: ACCESSING THE SUBCONSCIOUS MIND

Meditation and breathwork are powerful tools for accessing the subconscious mind, where samskaras are stored. These practices help you bypass the constant chatter of the conscious mind and tap into the deeper layers of awareness where true transformation happens.

Why is this important? Because limiting beliefs aren't only mental—they are energetically stored in the body. The nervous system holds onto past conditioning, and unless we consciously rewire these patterns, they continue to dictate our actions, reactions, and self-perception.

One of my clients struggled with a fear of speaking up. She traced this fear back to an experience in childhood when she was shamed for expressing her thoughts. Every time she had an idea to share at work, her body would tighten, her breath would become shallow, and her throat would close up—a physical response to an emotional wound.

Through breathwork and meditation, we worked on releasing the stored energy in her body. Using practices like box breathing and triangle breathing, she gradually shifted from fear to confidence.

She later told me she finally spoke up in a meeting: "I didn't even plan to speak—it just came out. And afterward, I realised nothing bad happened. No one laughed. No one shut me down. I actually felt... proud. It was such a small thing, but it changed everything for me."

TRY THIS

Box Breathing for Calming the Nervous System

Box breathing (also known as square breathing) helps regulate the nervous system, reduce stress, and improve focus. It's a simple technique used by athletes, military personnel, and high-performing leaders to maintain composure under pressure.

How to Practice Box Breathing

1. Inhale through your nose for four counts.

2. Hold your breath for four counts.

3. Exhale slowly through your nose for four counts.

4. Hold your breath again for four counts.

5. Repeat this cycle five to ten times, focusing on the steady rhythm of your breath.

Imagine tracing the sides of a square in your mind with each phase—inhale, hold, exhale, hold—creating a sense of balance and control. This technique is especially useful before stressful situations, like public speaking, difficult conversations, or moments of self-doubt.

Triangle Breathing for Emotional Release

Triangle breathing helps release stored emotions, creating space for clarity and emotional regulation. Unlike box breathing, which is even and steady, triangle breathing encourages a longer exhale, which activates the parasympathetic nervous system (your "rest and digest" mode).

How to Practice Triangle Breathing

1. Inhale deeply through your nose for four counts.

2. Hold your breath at the top for four counts.

3. Exhale slowly through your nose for six to eight counts.

4. Repeat this cycle for five to seven minutes, allowing your body to fully release tension with each long exhale.

5. This technique is especially powerful for letting go of negative emotions, reducing anxiety, and restoring inner balance.

4. ACTION AND REPETITION: CREATING NEW SAMSKARAS

The final and most crucial step: You cannot simply think your way out of limiting beliefs—you have to act differently to create new samskaras. Every time you step out of your comfort zone and take action that contradicts an old belief, you weaken the old samskara and strengthen a new one. This is how neuroplasticity works in the brain—repetition rewires pathways.

Imagine a forest path: If you keep walking the same route every day, the path becomes well-worn and easy to follow. If you stop walking that path and start forging a new one, the old path grows over, and the new path becomes clearer.

The same is true for your thoughts and beliefs. The more you practice empowered thinking, the more natural it becomes.

One of my clients wanted to start a wellness business but believed, "I'm not qualified enough. Who would take me seriously?" Through our work together, she identified this as a deeply rooted samskara from growing up in an environment where she was compared to others.

What did we do? We paired affirmations with action.

✦ Every day, she wrote, "I have knowledge and wisdom that is valuable to others."

✦ She took action by offering free community wellness workshops, proving to herself that she was capable and respected in her field.

Within months, she started charging for her services, and today, she runs a thriving wellness business. Her mindset shift happened not just through thinking but through doing.

TRY THIS

The 1% Rule—Each day, take one small action that contradicts an old limiting belief. If you believe you're "not creative," spend five minutes drawing, writing, or creating. If you believe you "can't speak in public," practice reading out loud.

Small daily actions create massive change over time.

Reflection: Seven Layers of Consciousness, Your Past, and Your Goals for Reprograming Your Mind

You cannot think your way into a new mindset—you must embody it. Meditation and breathwork create internal shifts, while action and repetition solidify new patterns in the real world. Which belief will you challenge today?

1. Which layers of my mind am I currently operating from?

_____

_____

_____

_____

2. Where am I stuck?

_____

_____

_____

_____

3. How can I activate more Sattva to access my highest wisdom?

_____

_____

_____

_____

_____

CHAPTER 20

Mind by Design: Understanding Your Dosha's Influence

In Ayurveda, the mind and body are deeply interconnected—you cannot fully understand one without considering the other. Just as your dosha influences your physical health, digestion, and energy levels, it also plays a profound role in your mindset, thought patterns, and emotional tendencies.

Your mental constitution is shaped by Vata, Pitta, and Kapha, and understanding how each dosha influences your thoughts can help you recognize both your strengths and your challenges. When out of balance, your dosha can create mental roadblocks—overthinking, perfectionism, self-doubt, or stagnation. But when in balance, each dosha brings unique gifts that help you step into your higHERself™.

Let's explore how each dosha shapes your mindset, how imbalances show up, and how you can work with your mental constitution to cultivate clarity, confidence, and resilience.

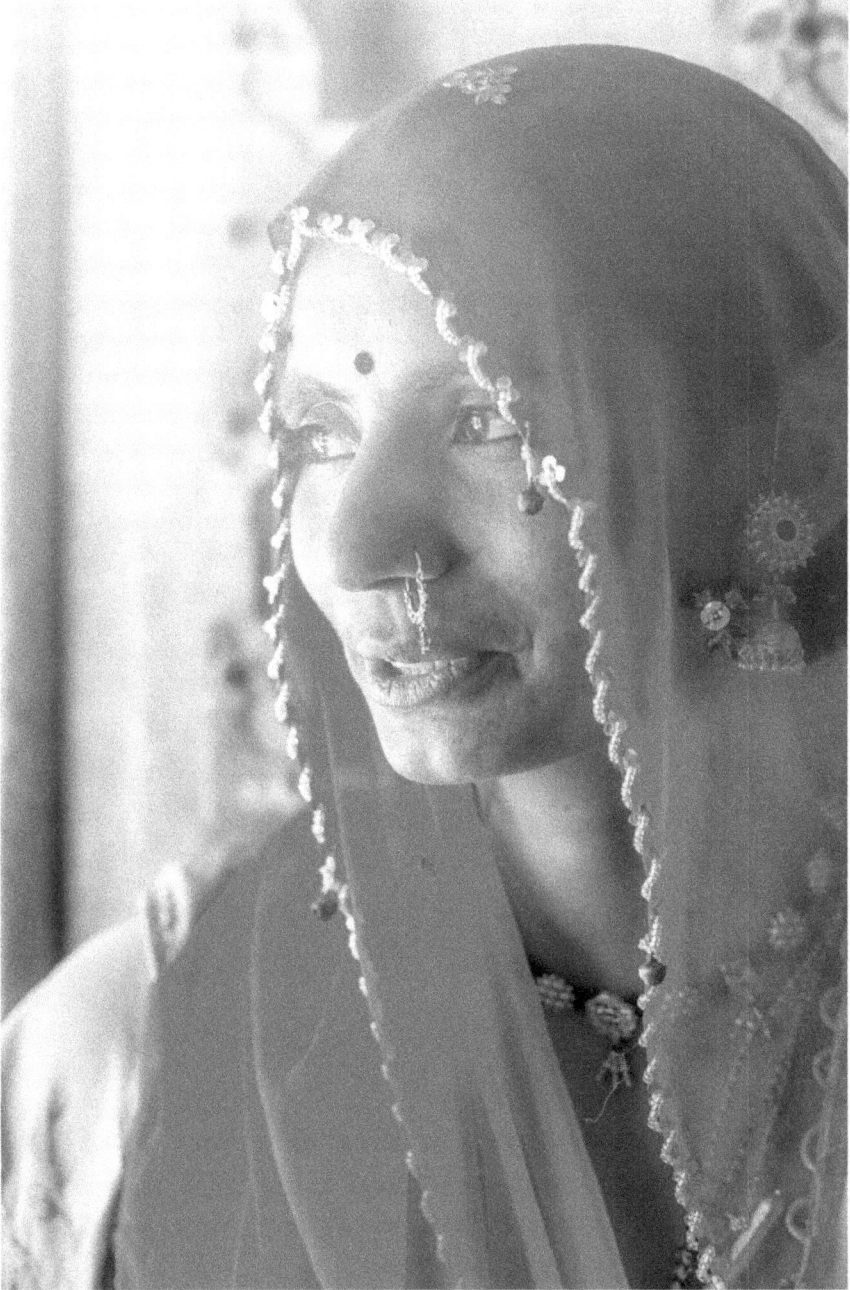

"MASTERING THE MIND IS THE KEY TO MASTERING YOUR LIFE."
— VEDIC WISDOM

Vata Mindset: The Creative but Anxious Thinker

Vata is the air and ether dosha, associated with movement, creativity, and imagination. If you have a Vata-dominant mind, your thoughts are fast, expansive, and always seeking newness. You are a visionary, full of inspiration and intuitive insights.

VATA STRENGTHS (WHEN IN BALANCE)

+ **Imaginative:** You think outside the box and generate creative solutions.

+ **Intuitive:** Your mind naturally connects to deep spiritual insights.

+ **Inspired:** You have bursts of enthusiasm and excitement for new projects.

VATA CHALLENGES (WHEN OUT OF BALANCE)

+ **Overthinking and self-doubt:** You analyze everything, leading to decision fatigue.

+ **Scattered and distracted:** You start projects but struggle to finish them.

+ **Anxiety and worry:** Your mind races ahead, creating fear about the future.

A VATA MIND IN ACTION: THE OVERWHELMED ENTREPRENEUR

Eve was a yoga teacher with a dream of expanding her business. Every week, she had a new idea—online courses, in-person retreats, a wellness membership. But instead of taking action, she found herself paralyzed by overthinking. She second-guessed her decisions and feared failure.

Through Vata-balancing practices, we worked on grounding her energy and creating structure in her mindset. Instead of chasing every idea, she focused on one goal at a time. Being clear on her main goal and communicating it with confidence gave Eve a newfound sense of leadership. Her students began to see her not only as a teacher but as an authority in her field. She channeled her creativity into marketing her one signature offering in engaging and dynamic ways rather than creating entirely new offers each month. This shift not only reduced her overwhelm but amplified her results.

If you're a Vata-minded entrepreneur, I highly recommend reading *The ONE Thing* by Gary Keller and Jay Papasan. It's a game-changing book that teaches you how to focus on what truly matters so you can achieve more by doing less. Its core question helps you cut through the noise and find clarity: "What's the *one* thing you can do such that by doing it everything else will be easier or unnecessary?"

By applying this concept, Eve stopped chasing every opportunity and started making intentional choices. This not only brought her business success but also restored a sense of grounded confidence in her purpose.[35]

HOW TO BALANCE THE VATA MINDSET

+ **Create routine:** Structure stabilizes your thoughts. Set dedicated times for planning and decision-making.

+ **Grounding practices:** Warm, nourishing foods, Abhyanga, and time in nature calm Vata energy.

+ **Breathwork for stability:** Try box breathing or slow, deep belly breathing to anchor your mind.

+ **Journaling:** Write down your thoughts before bed to quiet the mental chatter.

35 Keller G, Papasan J., *The ONE Thing: The Surprisingly Simple Truth Behind Extraordinary Results*, Bard Press, 2013.

Pitta Mindset: The Driven but Self-Critical Perfectionist

Pitta is the fire and water dosha, associated with drive, focus, and discipline. If you have a Pitta-dominant mind, you are goal-oriented, ambitious, and thrive on structure. You love learning, analyzing, and improving—but this sharp intellect can turn inward as self-criticism if left unchecked.

PITTA STRENGTHS (WHEN IN BALANCE)

+ **Focused and determined:** You set clear goals and take action.

+ **Passionate and motivated:** You bring intensity and big vision to everything you do.

+ **Disciplined and productive:** You follow through and get things done.

PITTA CHALLENGES (WHEN OUT OF BALANCE)

+ **Perfectionism and self-judgment:** You are hard on yourself and never feel "good enough."

+ **Frustration and irritability:** You expect others to match your intensity and get frustrated when they don't.

+ **Burnout and overwork:** You push yourself too hard, leading to exhaustion.

A PITTA MIND IN ACTION: THE HESITANT WELLNESS COACH

Alice, a thirty-six-year-old medical receptionist, had always been the go-to person in her circle for health tips, natural remedies, and calming advice. Her true passion lived in wellness—particularly Ayurveda—and she often dreamed of becoming an Ayurveda holistic health coach. But when it came time to step into that identity, her mind flooded with doubt:

"I need another certification first."

"What if no one takes me seriously—receptionist to health coach?"

"I don't have a perfect plan yet. How would I even launch this business?"

This is classic Pitta overdrive: intelligent, ambitious, and capable but paralyzed by perfectionism. Instead of using her fire to lead, she turned it inward as self-criticism and hesitation.

Pitta minds often believe they need a flawless roadmap before starting. But in truth, that need for control is often rooted in fear, not logic. For Alice, the fear of being seen as inexperienced or "not enough" kept her in analysis paralysis.

When we began working together, I introduced her to the idea of imperfect action. Instead of waiting until she felt "ready," she chose to simply start with what she had, where she was. She enrolled in the Ayurveda Alchemist Academy, and instead of waiting until graduation, she began taking practice clients, sharing simple Ayurvedic tips on social media, and hosting wellness chats with women in her community.

To her surprise, she was met with curiosity and trust, not criticism. Women didn't need her to be perfect—they needed her to be real, relatable, and willing to help.

With every small step, her confidence grew. She built a coaching practice that reflected her values—intentional, empowering, and authentic. And perhaps more importantly, she redefined what success looked like—not perfection, but progress.

For the Pitta-driven woman who thinks she needs all the answers first: you don't. Start now. Refine as you go. Your clarity will come through action, not before it.

HOW TO BALANCE THE PITTA MINDSET

✦ **Practice self-compassion:** Speak to yourself as you would a friend.

✦ **Cool the fire:** Spend time in water, practice moon-gazing, and incorporate cooling herbs like mint and aloe.

✦ **Prioritize rest:** Avoid overworking; incorporate breaks and walks in nature.

✦ **Let go of control:** Perfectionism keeps you stuck. Start before you feel ready.

Kapha Mindset: The Loyal but Resistant-to-Change Thinker

Nina, a mother of three with a heart as generous as her hands were skilled, had always been the one her family turned to for comfort. Her world revolved around home, her children, and the quiet rhythms of family life. She had a natural gift for care and healing—something that led her to study Ayurvedic massage and body therapies.

By the time she graduated, she had a clear vision: to offer deeply nourishing treatments to women in her community, helping them reconnect with their bodies, their nervous systems, and themselves. And when she was in session—hands moving with intention, oils warmed to perfection, soft music in the background—she felt completely aligned. "This is my happy place," she told me.

But when the treatment ended, so did the momentum.

Between school pick-ups, meal planning, and the endless to-dos of motherhood, Nina struggled to show up for her business. Social media felt foreign. Promoting her offerings felt like boasting. Even telling friends about her new practice felt like a stretch.

"I don't want to come across as salesy," she said. "And honestly, by the time the kids are in bed, I'm exhausted."

This is classic Kapha mindset—deeply nurturing, devoted, and steady but also prone to inertia and resistance when stepping out from the familiar.

We didn't overhaul her life. Instead, we anchored her in small, consistent steps—what I call Kapha activation. She committed to one story a week on Instagram. She told three close friends about her work. She wrote a list of local mothers who might benefit from her therapies and gently reached out.

And slowly, things began to shift.

Not only did clients start to come, but her confidence grew.

She realized she didn't have to "be" a marketer—she simply had to share from her heart. Her business became an extension of her caregiving, and her community responded. By staying grounded in who she was and choosing to stretch beyond her comfort zone, Nina found the rhythm that worked for both her family and her dharma.

For Kapha minds, it's not about hustling—it's about igniting. One intentional spark at a time.

KAPHA STRENGTHS (WHEN IN BALANCE)

+ **Calm and emotionally resilient:** You stay steady during stressful times.

+ **Compassionate and loyal:** You build deep, meaningful relationships.

+ **Trustworthy and grounded:** You are the person others turn to for wisdom and support.

KAPHA CHALLENGES (WHEN OUT OF BALANCE)

+ **Resistance to change:** You cling to comfort zones and struggle with new beginnings.

+ **Lack of motivation:** You procrastinate and feel stuck in old routines.

✦ **Emotional holding:** You suppress emotions, leading to emotional eating or fatigue.

HOW TO BALANCE THE KAPHA MINDSET

✦ **Movement is key:** Exercise energises Kapha. Try dance, brisk walks, or heated yoga.

✦ **Lighten your diet:** Favor spiced foods, greens, and warming herbs like ginger and cinnamon.

✦ **Change your environment:** Rearrange your space, try something new, or travel to break stagnation.

✦ **Challenge yourself:** Kapha thrives when gently pushed outside comfort zones.

Your Dosha, Your Superpower

Your dosha doesn't have to be an obstacle—it is your greatest gift. It holds the key to your mindset, your unique brilliance, and your path to empowered living.

When you understand your mental constitution, you stop trying to fit into someone else's version of success. You start designing a life that honors your strengths and supports your evolution.

✦ Vata minds thrive in creativity, innovation, and inspired vision, but they need grounding and focus to bring their ideas to life.

✦ Pitta minds are natural leaders, strategists, and catalysts for change, but they need softness, compassion, and rest to avoid burning out.

✦ Kapha minds offer stability, depth, and heart-centered connection, but they need momentum, stimulation, and belief in their own voice to keep moving forward.

Reflection on Balanced Mind/Dosha

Your mind is beautifully designed. But like any elemental force, it needs to be supported, balanced, and aligned with your dharma.

Ask yourself:

1. Do you find yourself overanalyzing and jumping from idea to idea? (Vata)

_____

_____

_____

_____

_____

2. Do you set high expectations for yourself and get frustrated easily? (Pitta)

_____

_____

_____

_____

_____

_____

3. Do you hold onto emotions and struggle with motivation? (Kapha)

_____

_____

_____

_____

_____

_____

4. Which dosha most reflects your mental tendencies right now?

_____

_____

_____

_____

_____

_____

5. Where are you overexpressing or underutilizing its qualities?

_____

_____

_____

_____

_____

_____

_____

6. What small shift could you make today to honor your mind's true nature?

_____

_____

_____

_____

_____

_____

_____

_____

_____

_____

_____

_____

_____

_____

_____

_____

Whether that means grounding your Vata, softening your Pitta, or activating your Kapha—it starts with awareness, followed by intention. And when you choose to embrace your doshic strengths, align with your highest values, and lead your thoughts with intention—you don't just think differently.

You become the woman who lives, leads, and creates from her higHERself™.

CHAPTER 21

The Rituals of an Empowered Mind

WHY RITUALS SHAPE YOUR REALITY

The key to harnessing the power of your mind lies not in willpower alone, but in the rituals and habits that shape your everyday life. What you do consistently, from the moment you wake to how you close your day, defines the thoughts you process, the energy you carry, and the identity you embody.

Throughout this book, we've explored how rhythm is healing. In chapter 12, we looked at the body as an energetic mirror of the soul. In chapter 13, **we unpacked how hormones respond to sleep, food, and stress.** Dinacharya **taught us to align with the cycles of nature,** and in-chapter sections on movement reminded us that our vitality is shaped by consistency, not intensity.

Now, we bring these threads together. Ayurveda teaches that mental clarity and emotional resilience are not random traits, they are cultivated through intentional rituals. A scattered mind can be trained into focus. A self-critical voice can be softened into self-trust. And an anxious heart can be grounded through steady practice.

In this chapter, you'll learn simple daily rituals and mindset practices rooted in Ayurvedic psychology and neuroscience. These

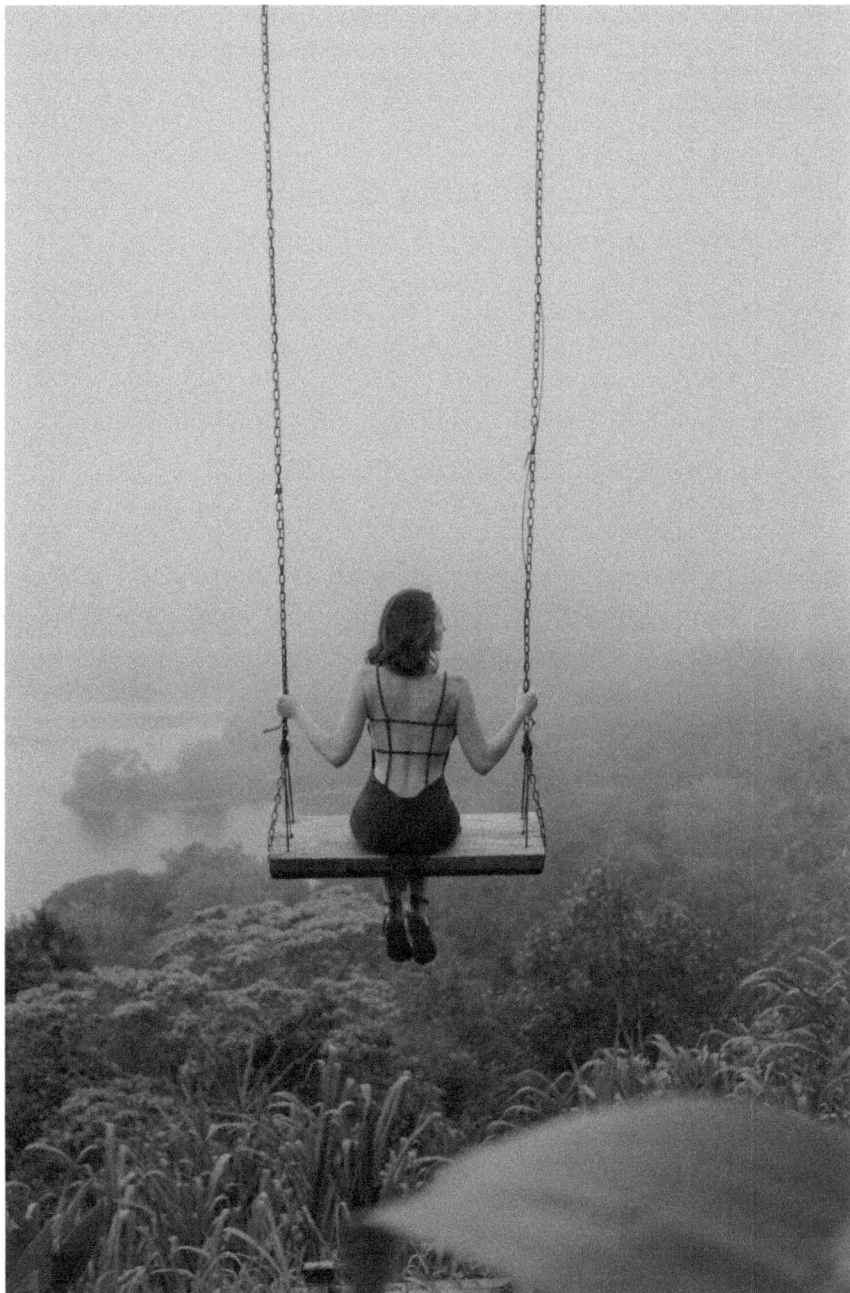

"KNOW YOURSELF AND YOU WILL KNOW THE UNIVERSE."
— SOCRATES

tools are not about achieving perfection but about reinforcing the woman you are becoming—centered, calm, and aligned with your higHERself™.

Cultivating Sattva: The Ayurvedic Path to Mental Clarity

In Ayurveda, the mind is governed by three gunas (mental qualities):

+ **Sattva:** Purity, clarity, wisdom, and balance

+ **Rajas:** Activity, ambition, restlessness, and agitation

+ **Tamas:** Inertia, dullness, heaviness, and fear

A Sattvic mind is calm, focused, and resilient. It does not react impulsively but instead responds with wisdom. The more we cultivate Sattva, the easier it becomes to navigate life's challenges with grace, strength, and self-trust.

HOW TO CREATE A SATTVIC LIFESTYLE

1. Nourish Your Mind with Sattvic Foods

The foods you eat directly impact your mental state. Sattvic foods include

+ fresh fruits and vegetables

+ whole grains like rice and quinoa

+ nuts, seeds, and healthy fats

+ herbal teas and pure water

+ spices like turmeric, cardamom, and saffron

Avoid excessive caffeine, processed foods, and refined sugars, as they increase Rajas (agitation) and Tamas (heaviness).

2. Create a High-Vibrational Environment

Your external space reflects your internal world. Declutter, use natural light, fresh flowers, incense, or essential oils to elevate the energy of your home.

3. Engage in Daily Spiritual Practices

Meditation, breathwork, prayer, and journaling help purify the mind and create a sense of inner stability.

Morning and Evening Rituals for Mental Strength

Successful women don't wait for motivation—they create it through daily rituals. The strongest minds are built in the small, intentional habits practiced every day.

MORNING RITUALS TO EMPOWER YOUR MINDSET

+ **Wake up with intention:** Before checking your phone, take a deep breath and set an intention for your day.

+ **Hydrate and nourish:** Drink warm lemon water to awaken digestion.

+ **Move your body:** Even ten minutes of stretching, yoga, or a short walk activates circulation and clarity.

+ **Meditation and visualization:** Spend a few moments in stillness, visualizing yourself moving through your day with calm confidence.

+ **Affirmations or journaling:** Write down one powerful statement that aligns with the mindset you want to embody. Example: "I trust myself. I am grounded. I attract abundance and ease."

EVENING RITUALS TO DETOX THE MIND

✦ **Digital detox:** Reduce screen time at least one hour before bed.

✦ **Self-massage with oil (Abhyanga):** A few minutes of gentle massage with warm sesame or coconut oil calms the nervous system.

✦ **Gratitude reflection:** Write down three things you are grateful for to shift your mind into positive awareness.

✦ **Breathwork for sleep**—Practice triangle breath (inhale for four, hold for four, exhale for six) to quiet the mind.

Remember: Your morning determines your day, and your evening determines your sleep. Choose wisely. Refer back to the Dinacharya, chapter 14 in the Health Alchemy Section for more on dosha specific routines and rituals.

Reflection on Empowerment and Rituals

1. What daily rituals currently support my mental clarity and emotional balance? Where might I strengthen or refine these practices?

_____

_____

_____

_____

_____

_____

2. How do my mornings shape the tone of my day? What would it feel like to begin each day with greater intention and ease?

_____

_____

_____

_____

_____

_____

3. What limiting thoughts do I replay throughout the day, and what empowering beliefs can I begin to anchor instead?

_____

_____

_____

_____

_____

_____

4. Which rituals feel sacred and personal to me, and which ones do I feel I'm doing out of obligation?

_____

_____

_____

_____

_____

_____

5. In what ways can I cultivate more Sattva in my environment and mind this week?

_____

_____

_____

_____

_____

_____

_____

_____

6. Who am I becoming through the daily practices I choose? Does this version of me reflect my higHERself™?

_____

_____

_____

_____

_____

_____

_____

_____

_____

CHAPTER 22

The Women Who Rise: Stories of Resilience and Strength

The most extraordinary women I've met are not those who have lived an easy life, but those who have endured unimaginable pain and still found a way to rise. Resilience is not something we are simply born with—it is something we build, layer by layer, through every challenge.

I think of Eslana, who witnessed the unthinkable—the tragic loss of her child. The weight of grief could have buried her, but instead, she made a choice: to keep living, to keep loving, to keep creating meaning in a life that would never be the same. It wasn't about "moving on;" it was about moving forward. With time, she allowed herself to feel joy and sorrow, understanding that resilience does not mean the absence of pain but the ability to hold space for both light and dark.

Or Priya, who grew up in Mumbai, where traditional expectations for women often dictated their futures. She dared to challenge that narrative, pursuing her own path, working relentlessly to build a career that gave her independence, even when the odds were against her. Resilience, for her, wasn't only about survival—it was about rewriting her own story.

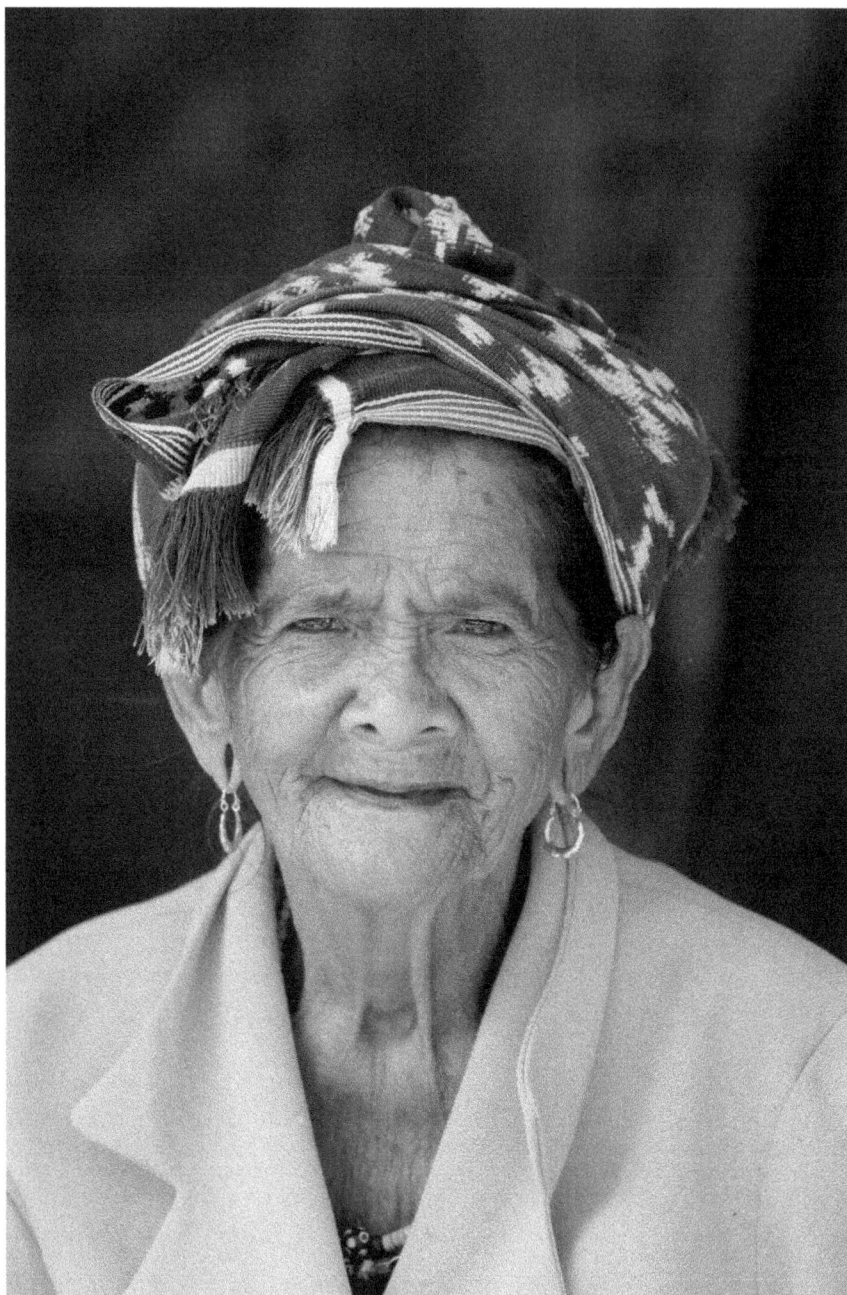

"WE ARE WHAT WE REPEATEDLY DO. EXCELLENCE, THEN, IS NOT AN ACT, BUT A HABIT." – ARISTOTLE

Resilient women are not those who never fall—they are the ones who get up, again and again. They are the women who have lost and still found love, who have struggled and still found success, who have been broken and still found beauty.

You Are Who YOU Choose to Become— The Mindset Shift That Changed Everything

Some people let their past dictate their future. Others refuse.

Melissa is one of those women who refuses. She has lived through experiences that could have broken her—childhood trauma and sexual assault at the hands of those who should have protected her, devastating financial loss, businesses that failed, and dreams that slipped through her fingers time and time again. Yet, she never stops creating. She never stops rising.

Most people see failure as a sign to stop. She sees it as a reason to keep going.

Her life has been a cycle of building, losing, and rebuilding. She has faced the depths of uncertainty, yet she never lets fear dictate her choices. She shows up. She reinvents. She claims her power, again and again. To me she is a true embodiment of graceful resilience.

One day, I asked her, "How do you keep going when everything feels like it's falling apart?"

Her reply:

"You are not what happened to you. You are who YOU choose to become."

This realization came to Melissa after the birth of her third child, which she says was one of the hardest times in her life. Motherhood unearthed something in her—the emotions she had buried, the wounds she had numbed, the pain she could no longer outrun. She hit rock bottom.

One day, while driving—lost in the chaos of her own mind—she had a sudden download, a flash of clarity. A single thought came through so clearly it felt like it was being delivered straight to her soul: "You are not what happened to you. You are who YOU choose to become."

It was like a switch flipped.

For the first time, she realized she had a choice. She was not bound by her past. She was not defined by her pain. She could stay in the story of what had happened to her, or she could choose to rewrite it.

That quote became her activator. A portal from victimhood to empowerment.

Every time she felt herself sinking back into the wounds of her past, she repeated it, over and over again, a mantra.

"You are who YOU choose to become."

She committed to that choice, and her strength, resilience, and grace have inspired me to commit to that choice too.

We spend so much time believing our past defines us, that our wounds determine our worth. But the truth is our power lies in our choices. She is proof that we are not the sum of our traumas, losses, or failures. We are the sum of our decisions—the decision to get up, to try again, to rewrite the narrative we have been given.

Her story is a lesson for every woman who has ever felt defeated.

No matter what happened to you, you are still the author of your story. You are who YOU choose to become.

And with that in mind, Melissa and I invite you to step boldly into your higHERself™— to choose not just who you've been but who you are becoming.

Building Unshakeable Emotional Resilience

Life will always bring unexpected challenges. The difference between those who thrive and those who spiral is emotional resilience. Resilience is not about avoiding difficult emotions—it's about learning how to move through them with grace, holding the belief that even in the hardest moments, we are not lost.

HOW TO STAY GROUNDED DURING UNCERTAINTY AND CHANGE

Embrace the flow. Ayurveda teaches that life moves in cycles, like the seasons. Struggle is not permanent; it is a phase. Just as winter eventually gives way to spring, your hardships will pass, making way for renewal.

+ **Regulate your nervous system:** When emotions feel overwhelming, place one hand on your heart and breathe deeply for thirty seconds. This simple act signals safety to the brain. Your breath is your anchor; it reminds you that no matter what is happening outside you, you can always return to yourself.

+ **Reframe negative thoughts:** Instead of asking, "Why is this happening to me?" shift to "How is this happening for me?" This one shift in perspective turns obstacles into opportunities and pain into wisdom.

+ **The power of self-compassion:** Speak to yourself like you would a best friend. Research shows that self-compassion increases resilience and decreases stress. Instead of thinking, "I'm failing," reframe it as "I'm learning something valuable." The words you speak to yourself shape the way you experience your challenges.

Resilience is a choice—a choice to keep going, to trust in your strength, and to believe that your story is far from over. And the most powerful thing about resilience? It is contagious. When you rise, you show others they can rise too.

Emotional Regulation Techniques from Ayurveda and Modern Psychology

1. BREATHWORK FOR EMOTIONAL STABILITY

Deep, controlled breathing activates the parasympathetic nervous system, reducing stress.

Try box breathing (inhale for four, hold for four, exhale for four, hold for four) whenever you feel overwhelmed.

2. GROUNDING PRACTICES FOR ANXIETY

When the mind spirals into fear, ground yourself with the five senses.

✦ Name 5 things you can see.

✦ Name 4 things you can hear.

✦ Name 3 things you can touch.

✦ Name 2 things you can smell.

✦ Name 1 thing you can taste.

This immediately brings you back to the present moment.

3. THE POWER OF GRATITUDE AND SURRENDER

Science has proven that gratitude rewires the brain for resilience. At the end of each day, write down

✦ one thing that challenged you

✦ one thing you learned

✦ one thing you are grateful for

And lastly, surrender. You don't need to control everything. Trust that the universe is working in your favor.

Awaken the Healer Within Through the Breath

If you're drawn to these practices and feel called to go deeper, we offer a Vedic Breathwork Practitioner Training through the Ayurveda Alchemist Academy. This training blends ancient pranayama techniques, nervous system science, and spiritual embodiment to support emotional regulation and inner healing.

Whether you're seeking tools for personal transformation or looking to guide others through their own healing journey, Vedic breathwork is a powerful and sacred practice that reconnects you to your highest self. You can learn more about our training at the end of this book or visit **https://www.harmonyinspiredhealth.com.au/breathwork/**.

The Rituals That Shape Your Future

Your mindset is not shaped by one big breakthrough—it is built in the small daily rituals that anchor you into your higHERself™. You don't have to do everything at once. Choose one practice from this chapter and integrate it into your routine. What daily ritual will you start today?

Harnessing Feminine Wisdom and Intuition: The Bridge to Dharmic Impact

As we move from the Empowered Mind Paradigm into the final pillar of the higHERself™ Method—Dharmic Impact—there is one last, essential piece to integrate: the wisdom of your intuition.

You've done the work of reframing limiting beliefs, rewiring your thought patterns, and learning how your unique mind-body constitution influences your perspective. But stepping into your dharma—your true purpose—is not purely an intellectual process. It requires something deeper: trusting your inner guidance, your sacred knowing, your feminine wisdom.

Science has begun to validate what ancient traditions have always known—intuition is real. Research in neuroscience suggests that the subconscious mind processes vast amounts of information before the conscious mind can register it. This is why we sometimes get a feeling about something before we have words to explain it.

Ayurveda, too, recognizes intuition as a higher form of intelligence. It is linked to *Vijnanamaya Kosha*, the wisdom body, which allows us to access truth beyond what the rational mind can comprehend. When we are in tune with this layer of awareness, decisions come easily, and life flows effortlessly.

However, when we ignore our intuition, we often experience doubt, misalignment, and emotional distress. How many times have you looked back and thought, *I knew I shouldn't have done that, or I felt something was off, but I ignored it?* The more we silence our intuition, the quieter it becomes. The more we trust it, the stronger and clearer it grows.

Reflection on Resilience

Remember: "You are who YOU choose to become."

1. When in my life have I felt broken, and how did I begin to rebuild myself?

_____

_____

_____

_____

_____

_____

2. What stories or beliefs am I still holding from past pain, and am I ready to choose a new story?

_____

_____

_____

_____

_____

3. What does resilience mean to me—not as a concept but as a lived experience?

_____

_____

_____

_____

_____

4. What daily rituals or practices help me stay grounded when life feels uncertain or overwhelming?

_____

_____

_____

_____

_____

5. When have I surprised myself with my own strength?

_____

_____

_____

_____

_____

_____

_____

6. If I were mentoring another woman going through a difficult time, what would I tell her?

_____

_____

_____

_____

_____

_____

_____

_____

_____

CHAPTER 23

The Missing Piece: Intuition as Your Guide

We live in a world that teaches us to rely on logic, data, and external validation. We are taught to second-guess ourselves, to weigh every decision against societal expectations, and to trust experts over our own inner knowing. But the truth is, your intuition has been speaking to you all along.

You've felt it—that deep knowing in your gut that told you to walk away from something that didn't serve you. The inexplicable pull toward a new path, even when it didn't seem logical. The whisper that told you this is the way, even when no one else could see it.

This is the bridge between mindset and dharma—learning to listen to that voice, trust it, and act on it. Because without this step, all the mindset work in the world won't move you forward. If you are still looking outside yourself for the answers, you will remain stuck.

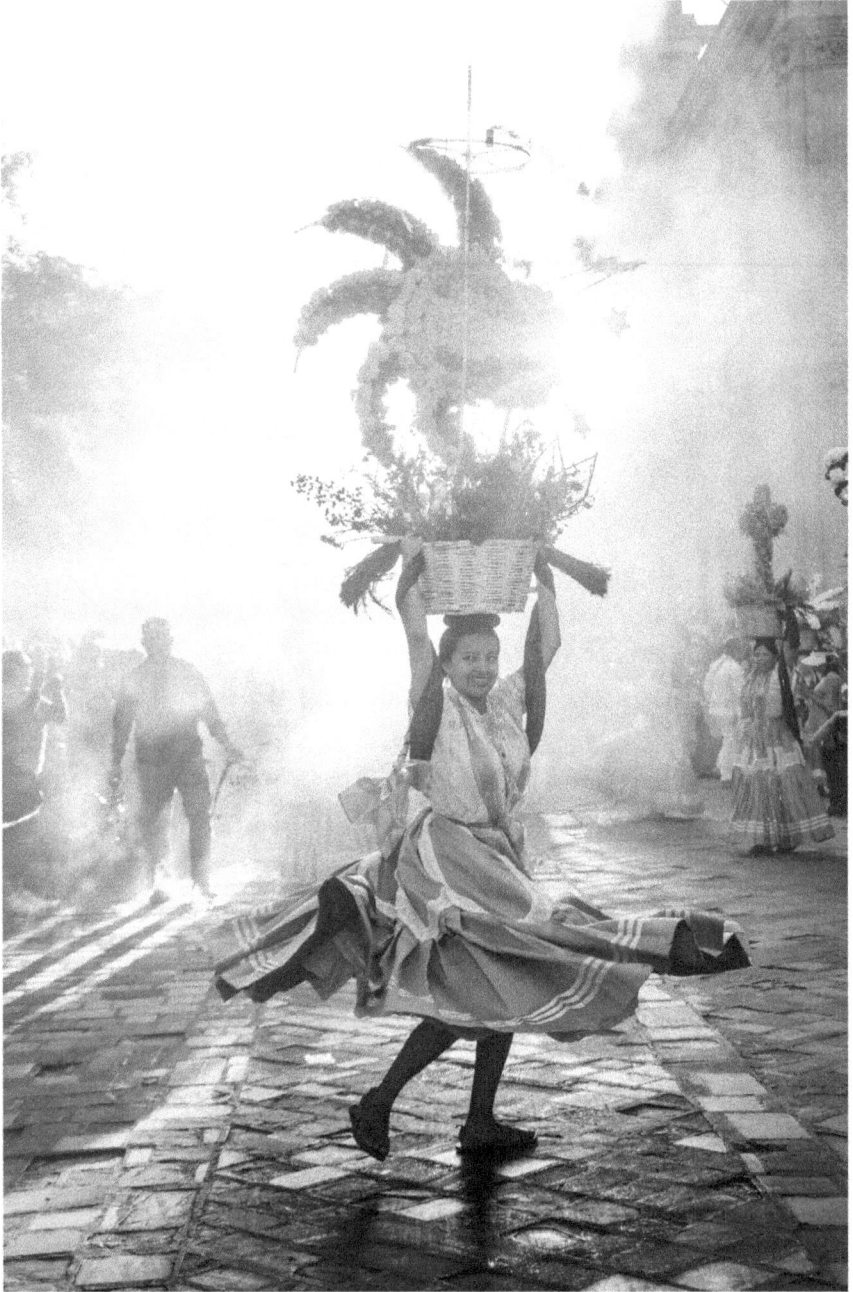

"THEY TRIED TO BURY HER, BUT THEY DIDN'T KNOW SHE WAS A SEED." – MEXICAN PROVERB

Tuning into Your Intuition: The Feminine Way of Knowing

In Vedic and yogic philosophy, intuition is not seen as abstract or mystical—it is understood as a higher faculty of intelligence, arising from the subtle layers of the mind and body. This inner knowing, often called prajñā or viveka (discerning wisdom), allows us to make decisions in alignment with our true nature, even when the logical mind offers no clear path.

Contrary to modern views that place intuition solely in the brain or gut, ancient teachings describe three energetic centers in the body that give rise to intuitive awareness. Each of these centers reflects a different aspect of knowing—mental, emotional, and embodied— and when in balance, they allow us to access deep guidance from within.

AJNA CHAKRA—THE THIRD EYE: INNER VISION AND SPIRITUAL DISCERNMENT

Traditionally regarded as the primary seat of intuition, the Ajna Chakra is located between the eyebrows. It governs perception, insight, and the ability to see clearly—both outwardly and inwardly. When this center is activated and balanced, we feel mentally clear, spiritually connected, and able to access an inner vision that transcends fear or confusion. In the classical texts such as the Yoga Kundalini Upanishad, the Ajna Chakra is described as the gateway to higher consciousness.

ANAHATA CHAKRA—THE HEART: EMOTIONAL TRUTH AND SOUL ALIGNMENT

The Anahata Chakra, or heart center, bridges the physical and spiritual realms. While the third eye provides intuitive vision, the heart allows us to feel what is true. This is where emotional intelligence resides—a kind of intuition that speaks in sensations, connection, and resonance. When the heart chakra is open, we feel more in tune with ourselves and others, more capable of sensing what aligns with our deeper values.

SWADHISTHANA CHAKRA—THE WOMB SPACE: FEMININE KNOWING AND CREATIVE POWER

While not always explicitly called an intuitive center in the classical texts, the Swadhisthana Chakra—located in the sacral area—is the seat of feminine creation and embodied wisdom. In many contemporary feminine-centered Ayurvedic and yogic traditions, this space is honored as the womb center. It holds ancestral memory, cyclical intelligence, and the deep instincts that arise from the body itself. For women especially, this center often becomes a wellspring of guidance when mental clarity is unavailable.

Together, these three centers—mind, heart, and womb—form a trinity of intuitive power. You might receive guidance through a clear thought, a subtle feeling, or a physical sensation. The more we learn to tune in to each layer, the more naturally we align with our inner truth.

Tia's Story: The Barefoot Gypsy and the Art of Flowing with Intuition

Some women move through life like architects, carefully constructing each step with plans and blueprints. Others, like Tia, move like the ocean—pulled by unseen force, trusting the rhythm beneath them.

I first met Tia in Bali, on the cliffs of Uluwatu. She had a quiet confidence. The kind that comes from knowing yourself, trusting your path, and letting life unfold without forcing it. You can see that same alignment in her photography—her content draws you in, capturing moments with a beauty and depth that reflect the way she moves through life. She has trusted her intuition not only in the way she lives but in the art she creates, building a career as a photographer by following what feels right.

While many hesitate, overthink, and second-guess, Tia listens, moves, and flows. She follows her instincts across continents, through seasons of change, and into the unknown, never needing certainty—only trust.

She has traveled the world, couch surfed at random people's places, lived in ways most wouldn't dare, and gathered wisdom far beyond her years. When we spoke about happiness, purpose, and intuition, her answer was beautifully simple: "Happiness to me is living a life that feels deeply fulfilling—one where I can express myself creatively, stay active, surround myself with inspiring people, and take small, intentional steps toward my goals every day."

Unlike many who seek security first and purpose later, Tia embodies feminine flow in motion. She doesn't force clarity—she surrenders to it, allowing it to unfold like the shifting tides.

"It's not about a single calling. It's a way of living that aligns with who we truly are."

I have always felt drawn to the idea of unbound freedom—to roam barefoot without an itinerary, to surrender to wherever life takes me. But my path has taken a different form. My dharma has led me to build roots—with family, business, and a community I deeply cherish. Tia's dharma is different, yet just as true.

The beauty of feminine intuition is it does not demand one path; it whispers a thousand possibilities and asks only that we trust.

As Tia reflected, "Purpose gives life direction, and with that, happiness becomes more than a fleeting emotion but instead it becomes a state of being." She reminds me that intuition is not about chasing clarity—it is about having the courage to flow without always needing to see the shore. Whether we seek freedom in movement or in stillness, our highest self is always guiding us.

The question is: Can we quiet the noise long enough to hear her?

How to Strengthen Your Feminine Intuition

If you're struggling to hear your intuition, it's not because you don't have it—it's because you've been conditioned to doubt it. Reconnecting with this sacred wisdom is not about acquiring something new; it's about remembering what has always been there.

SLOW DOWN AND LISTEN

Your intuition speaks in whispers, not shouts. If your mind is constantly racing, you won't hear it. Create quiet moments in your day—whether through meditation, journaling, or simply sitting in stillness.

FEEL IT IN YOUR BODY

Your intuition doesn't come as thoughts—it comes as sensations. Pay attention:

+ Does something feel light and expansive? That's often a yes.
+ Does it feel heavy or constricting? That's often a no.

Your body is always speaking. Your job is to listen.

TRUST THE FIRST WHISPER

Intuition is quick and subtle. The first feeling you get is usually the most accurate. The longer you analyze or doubt, the more the logical mind takes over.

ALIGN WITH NATURAL CYCLES

Women are cyclical beings. If you still have a menstrual cycle, track when your intuition feels strongest—it's often during menstruation, when the veil between the conscious and subconscious is thin. If you are postmenopausal, align with the moon's phases—the new moon for introspection, the full moon for action.

USE INTUITIVE WRITING

Write a question at the top of a page, then let yourself write freely without judgment. Your intuition will start flowing onto the page.

CONNECT WITH NATURE

Spending time outdoors, walking barefoot on the earth, or simply observing natural rhythms can help you reconnect with your own instincts.

CREATE A RITUAL FOR SELF-TRUST

Every morning, set an intention to trust yourself that day. Repeat affirmations like:

"I trust my inner wisdom."

"My intuition is strong and clear."

"I am always guided toward my highest path."

The Final Shift: Owning Your Mental Power

As we close this section on the Empowered Mind Paradigm, take a moment to reflect on how far you've come—not only in reading these pages but in your own self-awareness. You've explored the power of mindset, the depth of Ayurvedic psychology, and the unique way your dosha shapes your thoughts and emotions. You've uncovered how past conditioning has influenced your beliefs, and most importantly, you've gained the tools to rewrite your narrative.

A shift in mindset isn't just a mental exercise; it's a catalyst for transformation in every area of your life.

When you choose empowering thoughts, you create a ripple effect—your relationships become more fulfilling, your health improves, and your sense of purpose becomes clearer. This is the essence of stepping into your higHERself™— the version of you that leads with wisdom, clarity, and confidence.

From Empowered Mind to Dharmic Impact

Now that you've laid the foundation of a resilient and expansive mindset, you are ready for the final pillar: Dharmic Impact. This is where you take everything you've cultivated—your health, your mental clarity, your emotional resilience—and channel it into your greater purpose.

This next section will guide you through aligning your actions with your truth, stepping into the work you're meant to do, and creating an impact that resonates beyond yourself. Because when you show up as your highest self, you don't just transform your own life—you inspire and uplift those around you.

Your mindset is your greatest tool. Your purpose is waiting. Let's step forward into your dharma.

Reflection on Intuition

If you haven't been already, this is an excellent time to practice your intuitive writing. Write the question at the top of a page, then let yourself write freely without judgment for a set amount of time (say, ten minutes). Your intuition will start flowing onto the page.

1. When was the last time I had a strong intuitive feeling—and did I listen to it?

_____

_____

_____

_____

_____

_____

_____

2. What does my intuition feel like in my body?

_____

_____

_____

_____

_____

_____

_____

3. What past experiences have taught me to doubt or disconnect from my intuition?

_____

_____

_____

_____

_____

_____

_____

4. In what areas of my life do I trust myself most? Where do I still seek outside validation?

_____

_____

_____

_____

_____

_____

_____

_____

_____

5. How can I create more space in my life to hear my intuition clearly?

_____

_____

_____

_____

_____

_____

_____

_____

6. What does my intuition want me to know right now about the next step on my path?

_____

_____

_____

_____

_____

_____

_____

_____

_____

_____

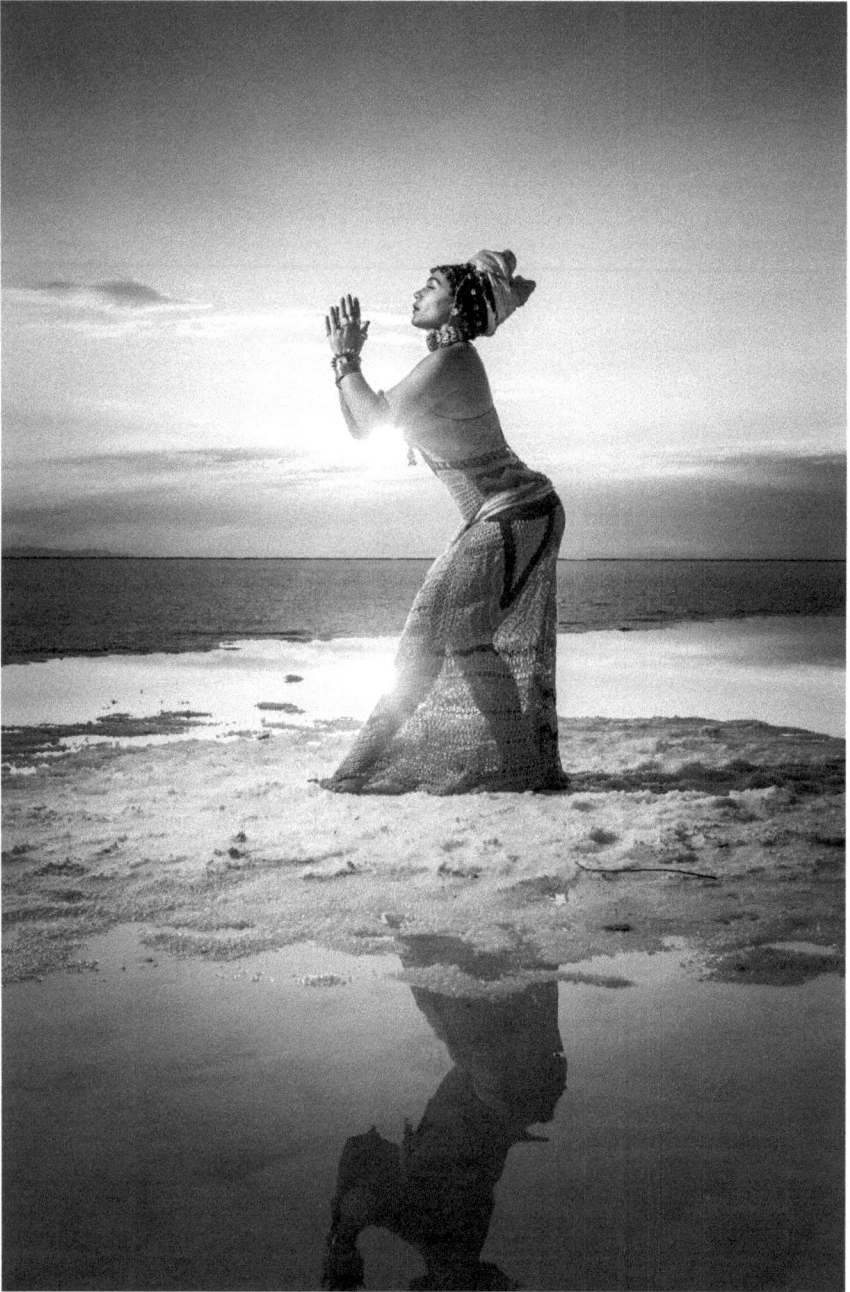

"YOUR PURPOSE IS NOT SOMETHING YOU FIND—IT IS SOMETHING
YOU REMEMBER."

PART 4

Dharmic Impact

Living on Purpose, Leading with Soul

There comes a point in every woman's journey where the inner work must meet the outer world— where healing becomes service, and self-discovery ripens into legacy. This is the essence of dharma: living in alignment with your soul's highest calling, and allowing your presence, purpose, and power to ripple out in meaningful ways.

Part 4 is about remembering why you're here—not in the roles you play but in the deeper truth of who you are and what you are here to give. It is not about chasing productivity or performance. It is about *impact that feels sacred*, sustainable, and soul-led.

In this section, we explore how to embody your dharma in a world that often asks women to shrink, conform, or overextend. We look at how your unique gifts, voice, and vision come together to form a path that no one else can walk but you. Through the lens of Vedic philosophy, Ayurvedic psychology, and feminine leadership, we redefine success as living from your highest integrity—not just achieving but aligning.

Your dharma is not a job title or a role. It's the frequency you hold, the medicine you carry, and the difference only *you* can make— whether that's in your home, your community, your business, or the quiet influence you offer simply by being your most authentic self.

This is the chapter where you stop asking for permission and start leading from embodiment. Where your life becomes a transmission of your truth. Where you stop striving and start serving—from a place of fullness.

You've done the inner work. Now, we rise—not alone but together. Let us walk this final path home: the path of dharmic impact.

CHAPTER 24

Awakening Your Dharma: The Path to Purpose and Fulfillment

What Does It Truly Mean to Live on Purpose?

In the modern wellness world, dharma is often equated with career passion or a sense of life direction—something we're here to "find." But in the ancient Vedic tradition, dharma is not about what you do—it is who you are when you are in right relationship with life itself.

The word dharma comes from the Sanskrit root "dhr," meaning to uphold, to sustain, to support. It's the internal alignment between what you believe, how you show up, and the impact you have. It's the steady framework that helps you make decisions with integrity and move through life with purpose.

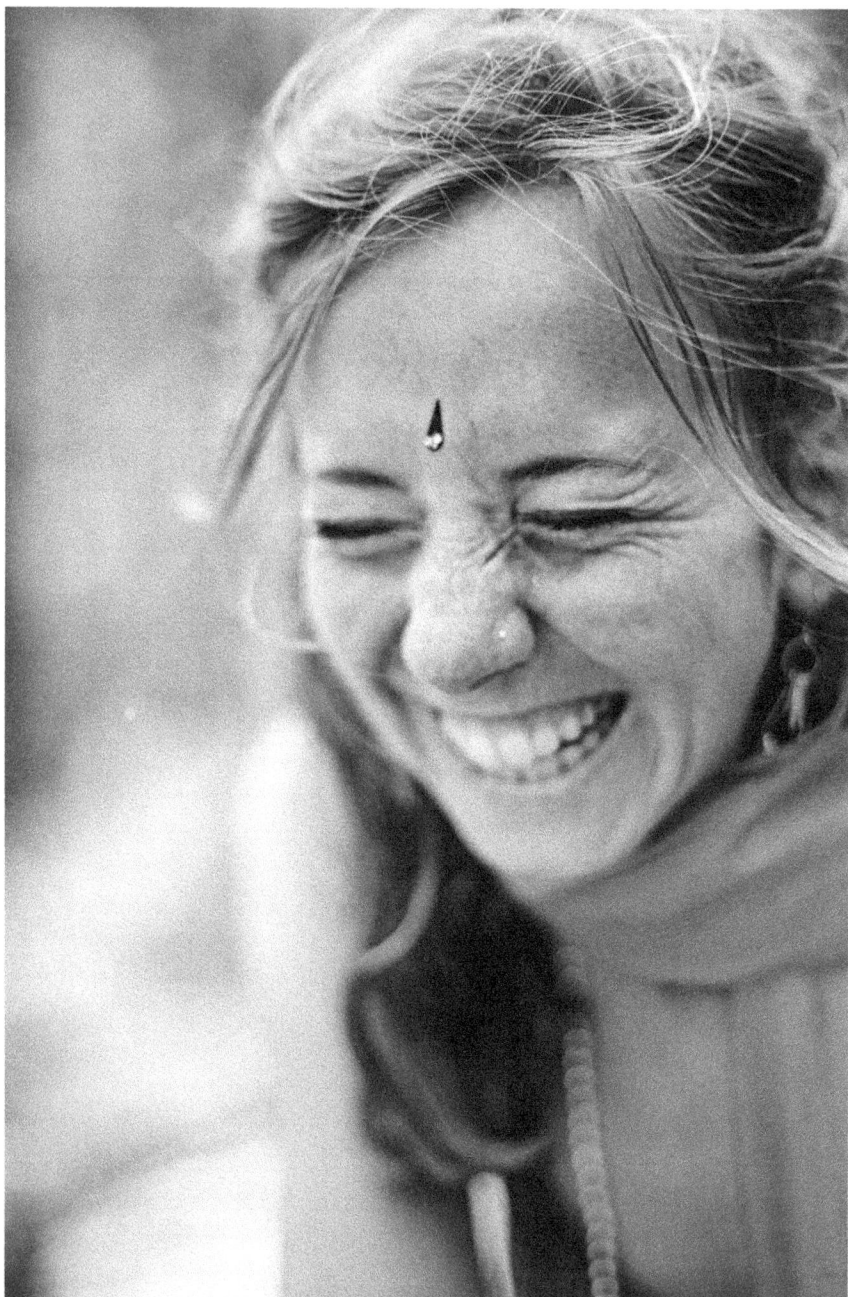

"THE INTUITIVE MIND IS A SACRED GIFT AND THE RATIONAL MIND IS A FAITHFUL SERVANT." – ALBERT EINSTEIN

When you live in alignment with your dharma, life feels more connected—not only to your goals, but to the people and world around you.

You don't need to be a spiritual teacher or healer to live your dharma. A mother raising children with presence, patience, and intention is living her dharma. A nurse who brings empathy into every shift—even under pressure—is in alignment. A creative who uses her art to inspire change, or even simply express truth, is walking her path. A woman who decides to change careers in her forties, not because it's easy, but because she knows she's meant for something more—that's dharma in action.

It's not about the title or the platform. It's about the energy and intention behind how you live. When your actions reflect your values, you begin to feel a deeper sense of fulfilment—even when the work is hard. That's the difference between burnout and purpose-driven momentum.

It is your contribution—not just for our own fulfilment but for the collective good.

In the Bhagavad Gita, Lord Krishna reminds Arjuna that one's dharma is not about chasing personal ambition but about fulfilling one's sacred role in the cosmic order (Rta), even when that role feels uncertain, complex, or inconvenient. Your dharma is not something you chase—it's something you live, moment by moment.

The Four Aims of Life: The Purusharthas

According to Vedic philosophy, dharma is one of the four foundational aims of human life, known as the Purusharthas.

✦ **Dharma (Right Living):** Acting in alignment with universal truth, ethics, and soul integrity.

✦ **Artha (Material Prosperity):** Creating financial and material stability that supports your purpose—not consumes it.

✦ **Kama (Pleasure and Joy):** Enjoying love, sensuality, creativity, and beauty without attachment.

✦ **Moksha (Liberation):** The journey toward self-realization and spiritual freedom.

These four aims are not separate paths but interconnected forces. Dharma comes first because when we abandon our values in pursuit of money and material possessions (Artha) or pleasure (Kama), we disconnect from deeper meaning. Likewise, we cannot authentically seek spiritual freedom (Moksha) if we haven't first honored the responsibilities of the human experience. In this way, dharma is the stabilising force. It keeps us anchored in purpose, even as we engage in the material and emotional realms of life. It invites us to ask: Am I living in a way that reflects who I truly am?

Why Dharmic Health Is the Missing Piece

We live in a world that glorifies productivity, comparison, and performance. Many women strive to "find their purpose," yet feel burned out, disconnected, and confused about where to begin. But what if dharma isn't a destination? What if it's a devotion?

Your dharma isn't limited to your job title or business goals. It's how you show up in the world:

✦ the way you speak to your child when you're tired

✦ the care you put into preparing a meal

✦ the presence you bring to a friend in need

✦ the decisions you make when no one is watching

You don't need to have a perfect five-year plan to live your dharma. You need to choose truthful action over reaction. Clarity over convenience. Integrity over performance.

A woman may be called to become a healer, a teacher, or an entrepreneur, but if she builds her dream through burnout, self-betrayal, or constant comparison, she is out of alignment with her dharma. Right action matters as much as the path itself.

Dharma Is Not Just About Purpose —It's About Presence

This chapter is an invitation to redefine what purpose really means. Not as something far away, waiting to be discovered—but as something alive in you right now.

Dharma lives in the micromoments. It grows each time you choose courage over comfort, honesty over illusion, and contribution over self-doubt. When you learn to honor the sacred responsibilities of your life, even the ordinary ones, you awaken the extraordinary within.

This is the path to dharmic health—a life where your purpose is not a performance but a practice.

The Ayurvedic View of Dharmic Health

In Ayurveda, living in alignment with your dharma directly affects your health. When you resist your natural path—whether through fear, societal expectations, or self-doubt—you create Vikriti (imbalance) in the body and mind.

✦ A Vata imbalance may manifest as restlessness, anxiety, or feeling lost.

✦ A Pitta imbalance may show up as frustration, burnout, or obsession with achievement.

✦ A Kapha imbalance may lead to stagnation, feeling stuck, or resisting change.

When we honor our dharma, we cultivate Ojas (vitality), Tejas (inner radiance), and Prana (life force). Our digestion improves, our nervous system regulates, and we experience inner peace, no matter what stage of life we are in.

Dharmic Impact in Wise Womanhood: A Time of Transformation

For many women entering the phase of wise womanhood in their thirties, forties, and fifties, they are presented with a dharmic crossroads—a time when roles shift; children are getting older, and for some, they have come to the conclusion that having children is not for them in this lifetime; careers reach a plateau, expand, or pivot; relationships evolve or end; and the identity the midlife woman once held so firmly begins to feel uncertain. These women come to me seeking support for a myriad of distresses, such as irregular or painful periods, hot flashes, weight gain, anxiety, and fatigue—valid and real symptoms of perimenopause and menopause. But as we dive deeper into conversation, a different root cause emerges: they feel disconnected from their purpose.

Nicole, a fifty-six-year-old mother, initially booked a consultation with me for menopausal symptoms—low energy, low libido, and brain fog. She spent decades raising her children, and now, with her youngest leaving for university, she found herself completely untethered.

"I don't even know who I am outside of being a mother. I feel like I don't have a purpose anymore."

Nicole's physical symptoms were real, but they were also a reflection of something deeper—a loss of connection to herself. When we explored her past, she spoke about her love of writing, something she abandoned years ago in the busyness of motherhood. Through our sessions, we worked on balancing her hormones with nourishing foods, herbal support, and lifestyle shifts. But we also worked on rekindling her inner fire. I encouraged her to start writing again—not for anyone else but for herself. She begun each morning putting pen to paper, writing poetry, then started a blog about embracing midlife transitions.

Nicole's dharma wasn't lost—it had simply evolved. She had moved from nurturing children to nurturing women through her words. As she stepped into this new chapter, her energy improved, her mood lifted, and her symptoms softened. Her body had been trying to get her attention all along—guiding her back to herself.

Midlife, or any transitional time in a women's lives, is not a loss of identity; it is an invitation to rediscover who she is now. The woman you were at twenty-five is not the woman you are at fifty. Your wisdom, desires, and purpose expand with you.

Many women suffer not just from hormonal imbalance, but from dharmic imbalance—a disconnection from their soul's calling. When we begin to nourish both the body and the spirit, we don't just reclaim our health—we step into the most powerful chapter of our lives. Your purpose is not behind you; it is calling you forward.

Practical Exercises: Discovering Your Dharmic Path

If you feel disconnected from your dharma, start by reflecting on these questions:

1. What activities make you feel fully alive?

2. What have you always been naturally good at? (Skills, talents, things others come to you for help with)

3. What challenges have you overcome that you can now help others navigate?

4. If you had no fear, what would you do with your life?

5. What kind of energy do you want to bring into the world?

6. Once you have reflected, begin small steps toward alignment.

   ✧ Say yes to what excites you.

   ✧ Say no to what drains you.

   ✧ Make choices from your truth, not fear.

Dharma is not something you find—it is something you live.

As we move forward in this section, we will explore how to embody your dharma in real, tangible ways—through the way you show up in relationships, your career, your creativity, and your service to others. Your dharma is not a destination—it is the way you move through life.

It is not about waiting for the perfect moment.

It is about living in truth, right now.

Let's step into it together.

Dharma's Relationship to Happiness and Impact

Happiness. It's a word that carries different meanings for everyone. Some associate it with freedom, love, stability, adventure, or success, while others describe it as a state of contentment, inner peace, or alignment with purpose.

But what truly brings happiness? Is it a fleeting emotion, or a deeper, more sustainable way of living? I interviewed some people who I thought would have an insightful take of these questions as I didn't just want to give my opinion and thoughts, but rather a collective answer from people all over the world.

Lessons from the Road: Gusti's Perspective on Happiness and Dharma

Over the past decade, my travels have connected me with incredible people—each with their own story, wisdom, and understanding of happiness and purpose. One of those people is Gusti, a Balinese driver and tour guide whom I met on a trip to Bali with my husband and twin boys when they were just two years old. His warmth, wisdom, and kind-hearted nature immediately stood out, and over the years, he has become more than just a guide—he has become a trusted friend.

From bustling markets to serene temples, from hidden waterfalls to sacred water purifications, Gusti has guided me through the depths of Bali's spiritual and cultural landscape. One of my fondest memories with him was the time he took me to the holy water temples for a traditional Balinese spiritual cleansing. It was a moment of deep reflection and renewal, a reminder that purification isn't solely for the body—it's for the mind and soul as well.

Through the years, I've come to deeply respect his outlook on life. When I decided to include the voices of others in this book—

real people from different walks of life who have discovered their own meaning of happiness and dharma, Gusti was one of the first people I thought of.

When I asked him the three questions about happiness, dharma, and fulfillment, his answers were profound in their simplicity.

What does happiness mean to you,
and do you consider yourself truly happy?

"Happiness is being grateful for all the gifts we have received—whether that's wealth, a harmonious family, or mental and physical health."

Gusti's words reflect a core teaching of Ayurveda and Vedic philosophy: happiness isn't something we chase; it is something we cultivate within. It is a state of gratitude, an acceptance of what is, rather than a longing for what is not.

How do you personally understand
the concept of dharma and/or purpose?

"Dharma comes from good thoughts, speaking good, and doing good. The goal of life is to achieve the perfection of dharma itself."

This response mirrors the Vedic view that dharma is not just about personal fulfillment—it is about how we show up in the world. Dharma is integrity in thought, word, and action. It is living in alignment with our highest truth, no matter how big or small our role may seem.

How does living in alignment with your dharma influence your sense of fulfillment and happiness?

"Happiness is something we create for ourselves, not something others can define for us. Just like a journey—someone might tell us that a destination is beautiful, but when we arrive, it may not feel the same for us. This is because happiness is not found outside of us; it is found within."

Gusti's analogy is a powerful reminder that no one else can dictate our happiness. Just as one person may find joy in a busy city while another finds peace in the quiet countryside, our dharma—and the happiness it brings—is unique to us. We must stop looking for it outside and instead turn inward to discover what truly lights us up.

A Lesson in Presence and Gratitude

Gusti's perspective highlights something we often forget in our modern, fast-paced lives: happiness is not found in the next goal, achievement, or external validation—it is found in the simple act of being grateful for what we have right now.

When we focus on aligning with our dharma—our truth—rather than chasing someone else's version of success, we unlock a deeper sense of peace.

Gusti has shown me this time and time again through his humble, contented way of life. His joy is not derived from material possessions or achievements, but from living in alignment with his values, his family, and his service to others.

If you ever find yourself in Bali and need a kind-hearted, knowledgeable guide to show you the island's beauty, I highly recommend connecting with Gusti. You can message me, and I'll put you in touch.

Eslana's Story:
Strength Through Unimaginable Loss

I met Eslana over twenty years ago when we studied nursing together in college. Though we were never particularly close, our paths seemed destined to cross—working in the same emergency departments over the years, bumping into each other at the gym, or reconnecting through business events. Recently, our connection deepened as she bravely shared her story—one of profound loss, resilience, and the redefinition of self.

Eslana lost her eldest daughter to suicide, witnessing the tragedy only moments later. The depth of pain and suffering she has endured is something few comprehend. And yet, in the wake of unimaginable grief, Eslana remains one of the strongest, most self-aware women I know. When I asked her about happiness and purpose, she shared insights that can only come from someone who walked through the fire and emerged with wisdom.

HAPPINESS: A PERSPECTIVE SHIFT

For Eslana, happiness is not about constant joy but rather the ability to embrace both the simplicities and complexities of life— the inevitable mix of love, loss, sadness, and beauty. She believes that happiness is not found in striving but in presence, in fully experiencing the moment rather than always reaching for something else.

She explained that many people mistake happiness for something to be attained—some destination they must reach. But true contentment comes from realizing that some things in life can be changed, and others simply are. Learning to differentiate the two, and shifting perspective accordingly, is key.

She illustrates this with a powerful metaphor: imagine a group of people sitting in a circle with a child in the center. Although they all look at the same child, their views differ depending on where they sit. Some see the child's face, others only the back of their head. The only way to truly see another perspective is to stand up, move, and shift your position.

This is how happiness works—it is a conscious choice, a shift in perception. And yet, most people remain stuck, unwilling to move, unaware that they can choose to see things differently.

DHARMA AND THE REDEFINITION OF SELF

For years, Eslana's identity was deeply tied to her roles as a nurse, midwife, and mother. Losing her daughter shattered her world, forcing her into a painful reckoning—not only with grief, but with who she was beyond these roles.

Her career in nursing and midwifery, once something she imagined doing until retirement, became unbearable. Trauma and PTSD made it nearly impossible to return to the profession. At first, she grieved this as another loss, but then she realized something profound:

"I held onto my identity as a nurse too tightly. But nursing is not who I am—it's simply a hat I wore. And now, that hat no longer fits. Instead of mourning its loss, I choose to celebrate the opportunity to redefine myself."

This realization echoes what so many women experience in their wise womanhood years when roles shift—whether it's children leaving home, changing careers, or unexpected life changes. We become so attached to our identities that we forget we are not the roles we play; we are something much greater.

FINDING PURPOSE THROUGH PAIN

Eslana's greatest lesson came through grief: that happiness and fulfillment are found in embracing all of life's experiences, not only the ones we deem positive. She learned that perspective is a choice, that purpose can evolve, and that healing is not about erasing pain but learning to live with it in a way that still allows joy.

She now channels her energy into work that aligns with her new reality—helping others in a way that nurtures her own peace rather than retraumatizing her. She is living proof that purpose is not static. It shifts, as we do, and it's our willingness to adapt that determines whether we remain stuck in suffering or move forward into a new expression of self.

A LESSON IN PERSPECTIVE

If there's one thing Eslana's story teaches us, it's this: You are not your job, your role, or your past. You are not even your pain. You are the force that moves through all of it—the one who can shift perspectives, rewrite narratives, and embrace life even when it doesn't look the way you expected.

Her words remind us that grief and joy coexist. That purpose is not something we cling to but something that evolves with us. And most importantly, that happiness is not something to chase—it is something to choose.

Suman's Story: The Evolution of Dharma and the Power of Self-Identity

Suman came into my life in a way that I would have ordinarily ignored. As a business owner, I receive countless messages from people pitching their services, and usually, my responses are limited. But when Suman reached out about social media management, something told me to reply.

That simple decision led to a powerful working relationship—and an even deeper understanding of her as a person.

Suman lives in Mumbai, India, and over time, I've come to see a lot of myself in her. She is ambitious, spiritual, and deeply reflective. When I asked her about happiness and dharma, her responses struck a chord, as they mirrored many of the realizations I had in my own journey.

HAPPINESS: THE ART OF RECOGNIZING, NOT SEARCHING

For Suman, happiness is not something to be chased—it is something to be recognized. She believes that too many people wait for happiness to come to them, expecting it to arrive with external achievements or perfect circumstances. But true happiness, she says, is about creating joy from whatever situation life presents.

"Happiness for me is seeing my loved ones healthy and safe, but personally, I find joy in the smallest moments—watching a sunset at the beach, tending to my garden, painting, or simply being surrounded by nature."

She considers herself happy, but not completely. "There's more to achieve," she says, a reminder that happiness and fulfillment can coexist with ambition and the desire for growth.

DHARMA: A SHIFTING PURPOSE AT EVERY STAGE OF LIFE

Suman's understanding of dharma is deeply influenced by her Hindu upbringing and spiritual studies. She sees dharma as an ever-evolving force—one that changes at each stage of life. In Hindu philosophy, life is divided into four main stages:

1. **Brahmacharya (student life):** The phase of learning and self-discipline.

2. **Grihastha (householder life):** The phase of family, work, and responsibility.

3. **Vanaprastha (retirement):** A gradual detachment from material life.

4. **Sannyasa (renunciation):** The pursuit of spiritual liberation (Moksha).

Right now, as a young married woman, her dharma is centered around building a life of independence, success, and self-identity. She is driven to create her own wealth, not out of greed, but out of a deep desire to stand on her own feet, to be able to support herself and her dreams without reliance on anyone else.

"I want to earn more than my husband," she laughs, half-joking, but then adds seriously, "I want to create something that makes me proud, that allows me to serve others. But most importantly, I want to be independent—to have my own financial security and freedom."

Yet, she is also aware that dharma will not remain the same forever. She envisions that in her later years, her purpose will shift toward letting go of material attachments and surrendering fully to spirituality.

"My biggest realization is that at its highest level, dharma is about love, kindness, compassion, and service. Before we are daughters, mothers, or employees, we are humans first. And our first dharma is to contribute positively to the world."

LIVING IN ALIGNMENT WITH PURPOSE: THE EMOTIONAL IMPACT

Suman spoke about something many of us experience but don't always recognize—the emotional toll of living out of alignment with our purpose.

"When I go to bed at night, I need to feel at peace, knowing that I did my best. Even if I failed, that's okay, as long as I tried. But when I stray too far from my dharma—when I ignore my purpose for too long—I feel restless, frustrated, and even angry at myself. That energy spills into my interactions with others. It's as if my soul knows I'm not doing what I'm meant to do."

Her words are a reminder that purpose is not just about career success or spiritual enlightenment—it is about inner peace. When we are aligned with our dharma, we move through life with a sense of calm and clarity. When we are out of alignment, we feel unsettled, disconnected, and irritable, even if everything externally seems fine.

A LESSON IN SELF-IDENTITY AND GROWTH

Suman's story beautifully illustrates the dynamic nature of dharma. Purpose is not something we find once and cling to forever—it is something that evolves as we do. Right now, her dharma is about independence, financial empowerment, and personal growth. In the future, it may be about surrender and spiritual liberation. And that's okay.

Her words remind us that our desires, ambitions, and even our struggles are not separate from our dharma—they are dharma in motion. Each phase of life presents a different calling, and when we listen, adapt, and evolve with it, we live with a sense of fulfillment, no matter what stage we're in.

Her journey is proof that dharma is a living, breathing path. And the most important thing we can do is keep walking it.

Helena's Story: The Connection Between Happiness, Dharma, and Presence

Helena is an Ayurvedic practitioner from Brazil who recently moved to Australia, where she now works at my clinic, Harmony Inspired Health. Our shared passion for Ayurveda brought us together, and over time, we've developed not only a professional collaboration but a deep friendship.

She has taught in my Ayurveda Alchemist Academy, sharing her wisdom with students eager to learn this ancient healing science.

When I asked Helena about happiness and dharma, her answers reflected the profound depth of her spiritual practice and understanding. Her perspective reminds us that true happiness isn't about fleeting pleasure or external success—it's about connection, presence, and alignment with something greater than ourselves.

HAPPINESS: A STATE OF CONNECTION AND FREEDOM

For Helena, happiness is not an isolated or self-centered experience; rather, it is the feeling of connection.

"It is the alignment between attitude and thought—the connection with yourself, with nature, with all other beings, with God, and with the universe."

She describes happiness as a state of presence—the ability to fully immerse oneself in the moment without being caught up in worries about the past or future. Yet, paradoxically, happiness is also the feeling of freedom—the ability to move through life with ease, unburdened by the expectations and constraints that weigh us down.

Although she finds moments of happiness in her life, she acknowledges that suffering still arises, as it does for all humanity. "Perhaps, like all people on the path of wisdom, I am still learning."

Her words serve as a powerful reminder that happiness is not an end point—it is a practice. A practice of deep connection, alignment, and being fully present *now*.

DHARMA: THE EFFORTLESS PATH OF SERVICE

Helena's understanding of dharma is simple yet profound: "Dharma is the right, effortless, and natural path of serving the community with your innate skills, no matter the occupation, wage, certificates, or awards."

In other words, dharma is not about prestige or external validation—it is about finding the work that feels natural and aligned. It is about contributing to the world in a way that flows effortlessly from who you already are, rather than forcing yourself into a role that doesn't fit.

This perspective is liberating because it removes the pressure of needing to be a certain kind of person or achieve a particular level of success. Your dharma is not something you have to chase—it is already within you, waiting to be expressed in the way that feels most true to you.

LIVING IN ALIGNMENT WITH PURPOSE: THE KEY TO FULFILLMENT

When asked if living in alignment with dharma affects her sense of happiness and fulfillment, Helena didn't hesitate: "Totally!"

That single word carries immense weight. It is a confirmation that when we follow the path that is meant for us—the path that feels natural and effortless—fulfillment and happiness become inevitable.

When we resist our true calling, we feel stuck, disconnected, and unfulfilled. But when we align with it, life flows with ease. The struggles may still come, but they no longer feel like obstacles—they feel like lessons guiding us further into alignment.

THE TAKEAWAY: FINDING HAPPINESS
IN PRESENCE AND SERVICE

Helena's story teaches us two invaluable lessons:

1. Happiness is found in presence and connection. True joy is not about having more—it's about being more present, more aligned, and more connected to yourself, others, and the universe.

2. Dharma is effortless. Your purpose is not something you need to earn, prove, or force—it is already within you. When you embrace the work that flows naturally from your being, fulfillment follows.

Helena's wisdom reminds us that happiness is not about accumulating more, nor is dharma about striving—it is about allowing. Allowing yourself to be fully present. Allowing yourself to serve in a way that feels true. And allowing life to unfold as it is meant to, with grace and ease.

Hannah's Story: Adventure, Alignment, and the Layers of Dharma

I met Hannah through our kids when they started school, and from the moment we connected, we could have deep, open conversations with ease. She has a rare energy—both adventurous and laid back, a beautiful balance of flow and intention. I've always admired her openness to life, her willingness to embrace new experiences, and her deep understanding of what truly matters.

When I asked Hannah about happiness and dharma, her answers reflected a grounded wisdom that comes from truly knowing oneself.

HAPPINESS: A FEELING, NOT A DESTINATION

For Hannah, happiness is simple: "Happiness to me is when I feel good in my heart." It's not about chasing external success or accumulating more—it's about feeling right within. For her, this feeling comes from

+ spending quality time with family and friends

+ eating good food

+ feeling healthy—physically and mentally

+ practicing yoga, getting massages, walking on the beach, or even just chilling out with her dog

Hannah disclosed "I used to rely on outside influences to bring me joy, but as I've gotten older, I know myself better, and I know what I need."

Happiness comes from understanding yourself deeply and honoring what nourishes your soul.

DHARMA: THE MANY LAYERS OF PURPOSE

Unlike the idea that dharma is a singular, grand life mission, Hannah sees dharma as having many layers—and this perspective is beautifully practical.

"Dharma for me has many layers. It can look like career goals, my spiritual path, being a good wife or mum, or even paying bills on time. These are all duties I have, and I try to do them well. It's not always linear though."

She reminds us that dharma is more than what you do for a living—it's about how you show up in every aspect of your life.

+ Your career can be an expression of your dharma.

+ Your relationships can be an expression of your dharma.

+ Even the simple, everyday responsibilities—like paying bills or keeping your home in order—can be done with a sense of dharma.

This understanding removes the pressure of having to find one singular "purpose." Instead, it allows us to embrace the fullness of our lives and see every role we play as part of a greater alignment.

ALIGNMENT: THE KEY TO FLOW AND FULFILLMENT

Hannah is deeply attuned to what it feels like to be in alignment and what it feels like to be out of it.

"I feel very agitated and 'out of whack' if I'm not living in alignment. I've learnt to quickly pivot back to my path when I've fallen off the wagon."

This is such a valuable skill—knowing when you are off course and having the awareness to realign quickly. Too often, people drift away from what feels right, and instead of pausing to course-correct, they stay stuck in discomfort, fear, or avoidance.

Hannah teaches us that dharma is not rigid—it's fluid. It's okay to veer off the path sometimes. What matters is how quickly you notice and how willing you are to return.

THE TAKEAWAY: DHARMA IS A WAY OF LIVING

Hannah's story reminds us that:

+ **Happiness is an inside job.** The more you know yourself, the more you can create happiness from within—without relying on external circumstances.

+ **Dharma is layered.** Your purpose is not just one big thing; it is woven into all areas of life—your work, your relationships, your daily responsibilities.

+ **Alignment is key.** When you're out of alignment, you feel it. The quicker you recognize this and make adjustments, the more ease and fulfillment you'll experience.

When you stay connected to what feels true, happiness becomes a natural byproduct of an aligned life.

Anna's Story: From Chasing Happiness to Embracing Contentment

Anna was an initial graduates of the Ayurveda Alchemist Academy, but over the years, she has become a dear friend. Originally from the UK, she now calls New Zealand home, and like so many of us, she has spent her life searching for something elusive: happiness.

For years, Anna was driven by an insatiable need to achieve more, earn more, be more. No matter what milestone she reached, there was always another goal in the distance, always another level of success she thought would bring her lasting fulfillment. But it never did.

One day, she asked her father a simple but profound question: "Why am I always like this? Why am I never fully satisfied?"

His answer stopped her in her tracks: "Because you're always chasing happiness, rather than contentment."

THE ILLUSION OF HAPPINESS

Anna realized she spent years tying her happiness to external achievements—especially how much money she was earning. But the more she chased it, the more happiness felt out of reach. She came to understand something powerful: Happiness is an emotion, and like all emotions, it is fleeting. It rises, it falls, it shifts with circumstances. Expecting to feel happy all the time is not only unrealistic—it sets us up for constant disappointment.

Through years of personal development, inner work, and deep reflection, Anna stopped chasing happiness. Instead, she discovered contentment.

Contentment is different from happiness. Contentment is a state of being—a deep sense of peace and acceptance, even when life isn't perfect. It's the ability to feel at home within yourself, regardless of external circumstances.

DHARMA: THE SECRET CODE WITHIN US

When our conversation shifted to dharma, Anna's voice shifted, and I could hear the passion in her tone. She described dharma as our secret code—something we are born with, a unique set of strengths and gifts that position us in the world.

"When we're in dharma, we're in flow. Time feels like it stands still. I feel completely present and like my true self, as opposed to when I'm critically thinking."

Her words perfectly capture what it means to live in alignment with dharma. It's not overanalyzing, planning, or trying to force things—it's allowing yourself to step into the flow of life and serve in a way that feels natural and expansive.

Anna also made an important distinction: "Dharma is not about our job. It's about being of service with the right attitude."

Many people believe they have to turn their passion into their career to live their dharma. But Anna has found that this is not always the case. Dharma is how we show up, not just what we do.

"We can bring our passion into our work, but we don't necessarily have to make our passion our work."

This perspective is so freeing. It removes the pressure to turn every personal joy into a career and instead encourages us to find fulfillment in how we contribute to the world—whether that's through our job, relationships, or the energy we bring into daily interactions.

THE TAKEAWAY: LET GO OF THE CHASE AND TRUST THE FLOW

Anna's story teaches us:

✦ Happiness is fleeting, but contentment is lasting. When we stop chasing temporary highs and instead cultivate inner peace, we free ourselves from the cycle of constant striving.

✦ You don't have to turn your passion into your profession to live your purpose.

✦ Dharma is about how you serve, not just what you do.

For Anna, the shift from chasing happiness to embracing contentment has been life-changing. She now moves through life with a deep ease, knowing she doesn't have to force or control everything—she simply has to trust the flow and live in alignment with what feels true.

The Role of Impact in Happiness

After speaking with people from vastly different backgrounds—entrepreneurs, tour guides, healers, and mothers—one truth stood out: true fulfillment is deeply intertwined with impact.

When I asked, "How does making a positive impact on others influence your happiness?" their answers were strikingly similar:

"Helping others makes life meaningful."

"If I keep my gifts to myself, what is the point? Happiness comes when you share."

"When you give, you receive."

This wisdom isn't new. In Ayurveda, the concept of Seva—selfless service—teaches that when we act in a way that uplifts others, we align with our highest self. Living in dharma is both about what we do and how we serve.

And the irony? The more we focus on creating a positive impact for others, the more we experience deep, lasting happiness ourselves.

Happiness Is Not Something You Chase —It's Something You Dharmically Align With

This realization shifts the entire way we think about happiness. Many of us have been conditioned to chase happiness as if it's a destination we will one day arrive at—when we make more money, when we achieve a goal, when we find the perfect relationship.

But what if happiness isn't something to pursue?

What if happiness is a byproduct of living in alignment with your dharma?

The people I spoke with weren't necessarily the richest, most famous, or most conventionally "successful," but they all shared a common thread—they found purpose and that was intricately connected with how they showed up in life. How they showed up in their struggles, how they showed up at family gatherings, how they showed up to their weekly Pilates class, how they showed up to their child's soccer game, how they showed up to their best days, and how they showed up in the mundane activities that make up life.

It wasn't what they did, but the energy and intention with which they lived—even in the most ordinary moments.

This is why dharma is so essential to happiness. It provides meaning, direction, and a deep sense of fulfillment that no external achievement can replace.

Tash, my best friend since high school, lives a simple yet deeply fulfilling life in rural countryside, raising her three boys. For her, happiness isn't found in grand achievements or extravagant experiences—it's in the everyday moments that often go unnoticed.

It's in the way her child learns a new word and playfully uses it in every sentence. It's sitting on her balcony, watching the mountains, feeling the wind on her face, and recognizing the beauty in both the calm and the chaos of motherhood. She considers herself truly happy—not because life is perfect, but because she chooses to embrace it as it is.

When it comes to dharma, Tash believes that life has a way of guiding us where we need to be. Go with your gut. If something doesn't feel right, change it. Life's too short to stay misaligned.

She found when you live in alignment with your own truth, it becomes easier to tune out external noise and trust your instincts. And in doing so, happiness follows naturally.

Your Dharma Is Bigger Than You

Many of us think of purpose as something deeply personal—a path we must discover for our own fulfillment. And while it's true that aligning with dharma brings profound inner transformation, it's also much bigger than just you.

In Vedic philosophy, dharma isn't simply an individual calling— it's a universal force. It's a way of moving in harmony with the greater whole, of contributing to something beyond yourself. When you align with your dharma, you naturally uplift others—your family, your community, even the world.

When you step into your higHERself™, you don't only transform your own life—you become a catalyst for transformation in others.

The Ripple Effect of Dharma

Time and time again, I've seen women reclaim their sense of purpose and, in doing so, positively impact everyone around them:

✦ A mother who prioritizes her own growth models self-worth and resilience for her children.

✦ A businesswoman who steps into her higher calling creates jobs, mentorship, and inspiration for those around her.

✦ A healer who follows her true path offers relief to those in need.

✦ A teacher who infuses her work with purpose shapes the lives of countless students.

Your dharma is not a selfish pursuit—it is an act of service.

This brings us to the "butterfly effect," the idea that even the smallest action—when done with intention—create ripples of change far beyond what can be seen. In physics, it's the theory that a butterfly flapping its wings on one side of the world could set off a chain of atmospheric events leading to a storm elsewhere.

In the realm of dharma, this means no action taken from a place of purpose is ever insignificant. A kind word. A shared story. A shift in your own energy. These things may seem small in the moment, but they have the power to create waves of transformation in ways you may never fully understand.

The Dharma Effect: Women Creating Ripples of Change

THE NURSE WHO BECAME A HOLISTIC HEALER

Becca had been a nurse for eight years, dedicating her life to caring for others. But after years of working in a high-pressure hospital, she felt burned out, emotionally drained, and unfulfilled. She loved helping people, but something felt off.

During one of our sessions, she admitted, "I know I'm meant to help people heal...but not like this. The system feels broken. I feel like I'm putting Band-Aids on people instead of truly helping them heal."

Becca's dharma was shifting. The skills and compassion that

made her a great nurse weren't meant to be abandoned—they were meant to be redirected.

Through Ayurvedic psychology and deep self-inquiry, Becca discovered her passion for Ayurveda holistic healing and nervous system regulation. She studied Ayurveda Vedic breathwork through our Ayurveda Academy and transitioned from traditional nursing to integrative wellness coaching and breathwork, where she could help patients heal physically, emotionally, and spiritually.

Her impact didn't decrease when she left the hospital—it expanded. Her patients didn't lose her—she found a way to serve them more deeply.

Alana: The Corporate Accountant Who Built a Yoga and Ayurveda Community

Alana had been an accountant for decades. She was successful, respected, and secure. But deep down, she felt something missing.

"I want to do something more meaningful," she told me. "I've spent my life helping people build financial wealth, but what about emotional wealth? What about community?"

She had always been the person who women came to for support—for career advice, for life guidance, for encouragement when they felt lost. Yet she had never seen this as a calling—just something she happened to be good at.

Through our work together, Alana realized her gift was holding space for other women—creating environments where they felt seen, heard, and empowered. She took a leap and studied Ayurveda and yoga training. In a quick timeframe, she shifted gears and opened her own yoga studio teaching yoga, breathwork, and running Ayurvedic cleanses and international retreats, which all combined her financial knowledge with emotional and spiritual mentorship.

At first, she doubted herself.

"Who am I to do this?" she asked.

But the question reframed is "who are you to *not* do this?" Why withhold your dharmic gifts from the world when we need them more than ever.

Dharma doesn't care about your titles or credentials.
It cares about the wisdom you are meant to share.

Her dharma wasn't about choosing between finance and wellness—it was about integrating them in a way that felt aligned. Her accounting background was the backbone to running a financially successful business in such a short timeframe.

How to Align Your Purpose with the Collective Good

So, how do you ensure your dharma isn't solely personal fulfillment but is focused on making an impact on the world?

1. IDENTIFY YOUR UNIQUE GIFTS

Every single person has gifts—something they do naturally, something that lights them up and serves others effortlessly. Maybe it's teaching, writing, healing, organizing, leading, creating, or nurturing.

Reflection Prompt: What do people naturally come to you for? What do you love doing, even when no one is watching?

---

2. FIND THE INTERSECTION OF PASSION AND SERVICE

Your dharma isn't only what you love—it's what the world needs from you. The sweet spot lies at the intersection of

+ what you love

+ what you're naturally good at

+ what people need

Reflection Prompt: How can your unique skills, knowledge, and experiences serve others?

---

3. ALIGN WITH SEVA (SELFLESS SERVICE)

In Ayurveda, Seva means selfless service—contributing to others without attachment to outcomes or rewards. When we serve from a place of love and alignment, we naturally receive abundance in return—whether it's fulfillment, connection, or success.

Reflection Prompt: How can I use my gifts in service to others, without expectation?

_____

_____

_____

_____

_____

_____

If we are aligning our business with our dharma, financial abundance is a natural and necessary outcome—but it should not be the driving force. When we lead with service, purpose, and integrity, success follows organically. By prioritizing impact over income, we create a business rooted in authenticity, one that naturally attracts opportunities, prosperity, and fulfillment. Money becomes the byproduct of living in alignment, rather than the sole motivation.

4. TRUST THE PATH UNFOLDING BEFORE YOU

Dharma is rarely a straight line—it's a series of doors opening, small nudges from the universe, unexpected invitations. Many women hesitate to step into their true calling because they expect a clear roadmap. But dharma doesn't always work that way. It requires trust. Surrender. Courage. Follow what feels right—even if you don't have all the answers yet.

Reflection Prompt: Where am I hesitating because I don't have all the details? What if I simply took the first step?

_____

_____

_____

_____

_____

You Are Here to Make an Impact

You are not here only to exist. You are here to impact, inspire, and uplift. Your dharma is more than a personal journey—it is a collective responsibility.

The world needs more women stepping into their power, more voices speaking their truth, more leaders leading with wisdom and love. So as we move into the final chapters of this book, ask yourself:

1. How am I meant to serve?

2. What impact do I want to leave?

3. Who do I become when I fully step into my higHERself™?

This is where we take everything we've built—our health, our mindset, our self-awareness—and use it to create change, within ourselves and beyond. This is where we stop only thinking about dharma—and start living it.

As we move into the next chapter, we will explore how to practically align with your dharma, break through fears, and step into your highest expression. Because when you are living in alignment, happiness is no longer something you seek—it is something you embody.

CHAPTER 25

Manifesting and Living in Your Highest Expression

You have come so far.

Through this book, you have uncovered hidden layers of yourself, reclaimed your health, transformed your mindset, and awakened your dharma. You have begun to see that you are not bound by past limitations, old beliefs, or external expectations.

Now, the real work begins—not in learning,
but in embodying.

This final chapter is about living fully as your higHERself™—not restricted to moments of inspiration, but in daily actions, thoughts, and choices. Let's weave together Ayurvedic wisdom, modern science, and deep spiritual alignment into a life that feels abundant, expansive, and truly your own.

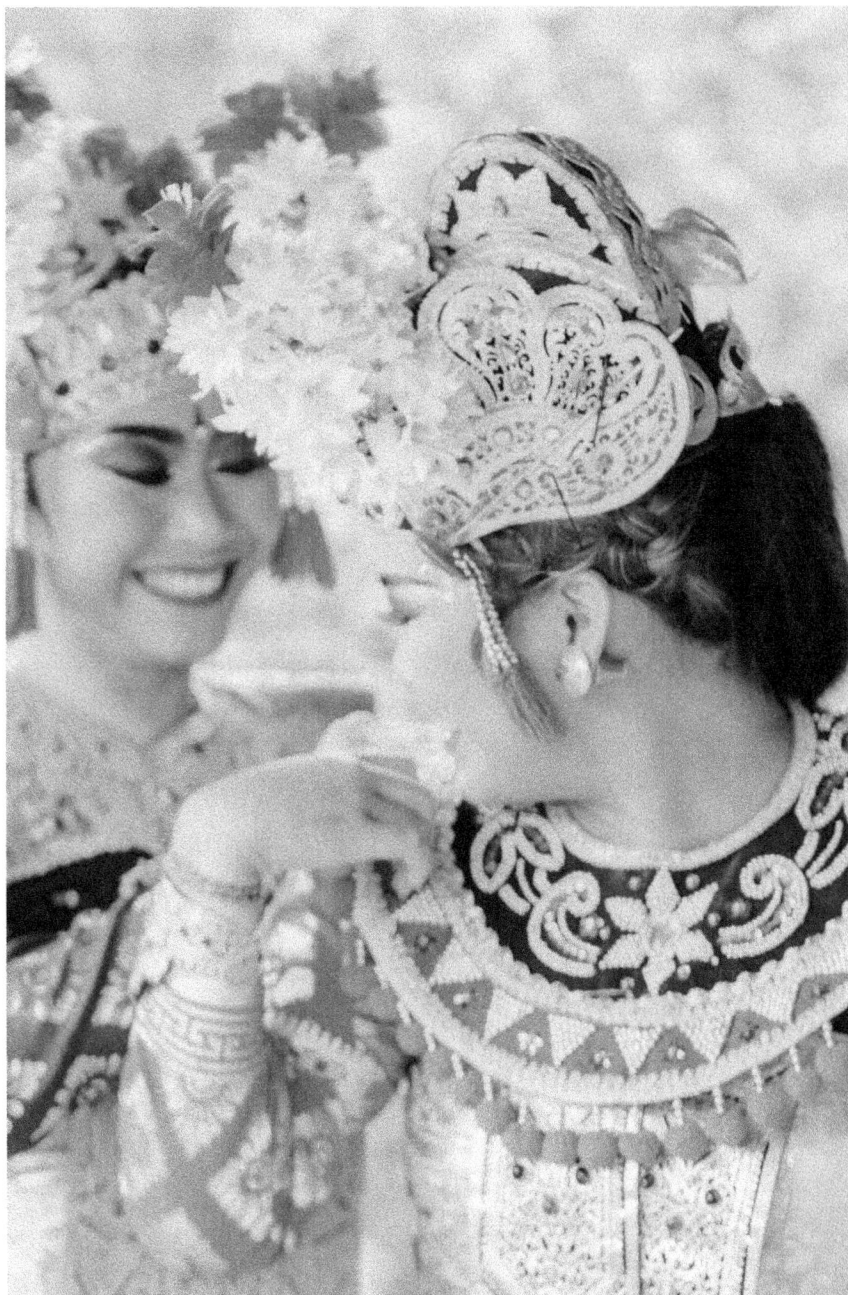

"WHEN YOU DO THINGS FROM YOUR SOUL, YOU FEEL A RIVER MOVING IN YOU, A JOY." – RUMI

Your Highest Expression: What Does It Look Like?

There is no singular definition of living in your highest expression. For one woman, it might be building a thriving business; for another, it might be finding peace in motherhood or traveling the world solo. It could mean stepping into leadership, creating art, serving others, or simply experiencing each day with presence, joy, and gratitude.

Living as your higHERself™ is not about achieving a specific outcome—it's about showing up fully, powerfully, and unapologetically in every aspect of your life.

+ Your body feels strong, balanced, and nourished.

+ Your mind is clear, resilient, and focused.

+ Your emotions are honored, processed, and understood.

+ Your spirit is aligned with your purpose.

+ Your actions reflect your truth.

This is the culmination of Health Alchemy, the Empowered Mind Paradigm, and Dharmic Impact—the integration of everything you've learned into your daily existence.

The Roadmap to Embodiment: Bringing It All Together

To fully embody your higHERself™, you must cultivate rituals, habits, and mindset shifts that support continued growth. Integrate each pillar of this book into your daily life.

1. HEALTH ALCHEMY: HONORING YOUR BODY AS A SACRED VESSEL

You cannot live in your highest expression if your body is depleted. Your physical health is the foundation for everything else—your energy, clarity, and emotional balance. When you treat your body with respect, you create a strong, vibrant vessel to support your dharma.

Daily Ayurvedic Rituals for Health Alchemy

+ Wake up early and align with the Ayurvedic clock.
+ Hydrate daily with clean water.
+ Eat nourishing, seasonal foods that support your dosha.
+ Move your body daily—yoga, walking, strength training, or any way that supports your movement goals.
+ Prioritize rest and deep, restorative sleep.
+ Mantra: "My body is sacred, strong, and filled with vitality."

2. THE EMPOWERED MIND PARADIGM: STRENGTHENING YOUR INNER WORLD

Your mind is your greatest tool or your greatest limitation—the choice is yours. To stay in alignment, you must continuously cultivate clarity, resilience, and self-awareness. This means recognizing negative thought patterns, dismantling limiting beliefs, and actively choosing an empowered perspective.

Daily Mindset Practices

+ Morning intention setting—what energy do you want to bring into your day?
+ Replacing negative thoughts with affirmations.

✦ Journaling to reflect on limiting beliefs and reframe them.

✦ Breathwork or meditation to cultivate mental stillness.

✦ Gratitude practice—write three things you are grateful for each morning and night.

✦ Mantra: "I choose thoughts that empower, uplift, and expand me."

Emotional Mastery: Feeling Fully Without Fear

Your emotions are not your enemy—they are your guide.

To embody your higHERself™, you must allow emotions to flow without suppression or resistance. This means honoring grief, anger, sadness, and joy—seeing them as teachers rather than obstacles.

Daily Emotional Resilience Practices

✦ Ask yourself, "What am I feeling right now? What does it need?"

✦ Allow emotions to move—through journaling, movement, or expression. Use cooling practices for Pitta anger, grounding for Vata anxiety, and energizing for Kapha stagnation.

✦ Set boundaries—protect your energy from what drains you.

✦ Cultivate self-compassion—speak to yourself like you would a loved one.

✦ Mantra: "I honor my emotions as sacred messengers of my truth."

3. DHARMIC IMPACT: LIVING YOUR PURPOSE EVERY DAY

Dharma is not a career—it's the way you show up in the world. Living as your higHERself™ means acting in alignment with your values, making choices that feel true, and showing up in a way that uplifts both yourself and others.

Daily Practices for Living Your Dharma

+ Align your actions with your core values—ask, "Does this choice reflect who I want to be?"

+ Serve others in small, meaningful ways.

+ Follow the path that lights you up, even if it's unconventional.

+ Trust that the universe supports you when you walk your true path.

+ Celebrate your growth, no matter how small.

+ Mantra: "I am walking my true path, and every step is divinely guided."

If you feel called to the dharmic path of diving deeper into the wisdom of Ayurveda, I would love to invite you to become an Ayurveda Alchemist and study with us at our Ayurveda Academy: **www.harmonyinspiredhealth.com.au/ayurveda-alchemist**.

A Mother's Wisdom: A Life of Growth, Purpose, and Presence

Throughout this book, my mother's story has been woven into these pages—her journey of resilience, loss, healing, and transformation. When I asked her to reflect on the higHERself™ pillars, she offered words that reflect a lifetime of searching, evolving, and ultimately, embracing the beauty in life's simplest moments.

She speaks of mindset and growth as a continuous unfolding—sometimes light and graceful, other times turbulent and uncertain. She has walked through storms, felt lost, and at times, disconnected from herself. But she never stopped seeking. Through personal transformation and deep introspection, she learned that the greatest shift comes from within. As she beautifully put it, "It's as if I'm wearing a new set of glasses."

Sobriety gifted her clarity, and with that clarity came a deep reverence for life. Today, she walks through her days with gratitude, curiosity, and playfulness, embracing the unexpected gifts of existence. She has discovered that joy isn't found in grand achievements but in the trees' whisper, the birdsong, the laughter of grandchildren, and the privilege of simply waking up to see the beauty in the world.

When it comes to purpose, she believes it was always there, waiting to be recognized. Her purpose is not focused on accolades or external validation. It is as simple and profound as existing in kindness—showing up as a present and loving partner, mother, grandmother, and friend.

She finds fulfillment not in the pursuit of more but in the deep connection she shares with nature, in caring for orphaned koalas and wallabies, in listening to the creek dance over boulders, in feeling the earth beneath her feet. This, to her, is what it means to be alive.

Health to her is to keep an active mind, body, and soul. To nurture, to play, to rest, to learn, to laugh and to cry. To keep her body moving...walking barefoot on grass...to keep her senses stimulated... smelling the summer rains...to keep her mind delighted...watching fireflies dancing in the dark.

Her words are a reminder that life doesn't need to be constantly fixed or figured out—it simply needs to be lived. That happiness is found in presence, that purpose is found in love, and that true health is about experiencing life fully, with all its textures, seasons, and emotions.

CHAPTER 26

The Final Ritual: A Sacred Commitment to Your higHERself™

Transformation doesn't happen in an instant—it happens in daily choices.

To close this chapter, I invite you to make a commitment to yourself. Not to perfection, not to achieving everything overnight— but to continuously choose growth, alignment, and authenticity.

Take a deep breath. Place your hands over your heart. And say:

"I commit to honoring my body, my mind, my emotions, my soul and my purpose. I commit to stepping into my highest expression, every single day, with love, trust, and courage. I am ready to live as my higHERself™."

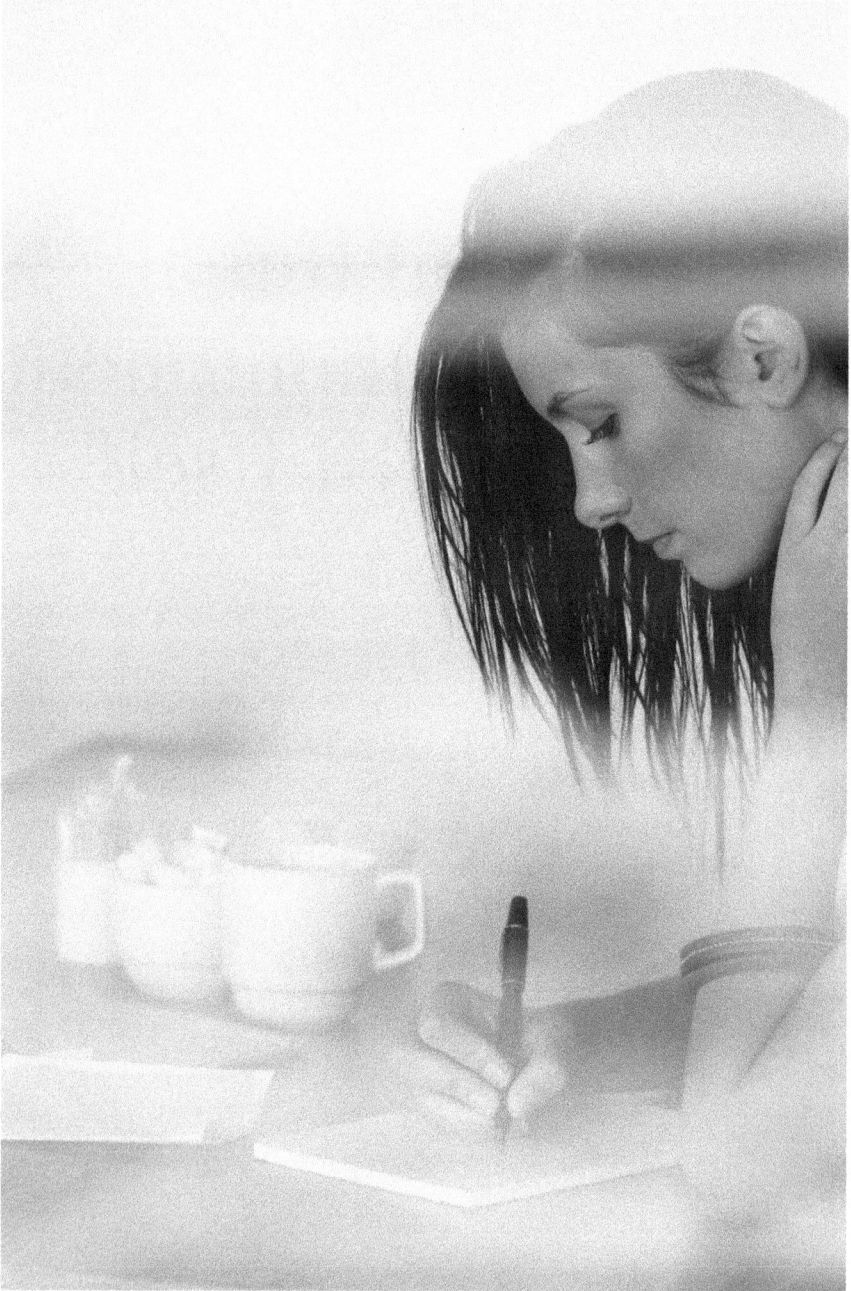

"YOUR LIFE IS YOUR MESSAGE TO THE WORLD. MAKE IT INSPIRING."

Your Next Step: Walking Forward as Your higHERself™

You have everything you need. The wisdom. The tools. The power. The final pages of this book guide you through sustaining this transformation—how to stay aligned, navigate setbacks, and continue evolving. Because this is not the end of your journey—it is the beginning. Let's step forward together.

The Continuous Journey to Your higHERself™

You have arrived at the final pages of this book, but this is not the end. It is a beginning. Becoming your higHERself™ is not a destination; it is a lifelong unfolding.

Like the cycles of nature, you will evolve, shift, and expand. Some seasons bring clarity and momentum; others ask you to slow down and reflect.

Both are necessary. Both are beautiful.

You are not meant to stay the same. The woman you were at the beginning of this book is not the woman reading these words now. You have changed. You have shed old beliefs, embraced new wisdom, and stepped into a deeper understanding of who you are meant to be.

But growth does not stop here. This work is continuous.

The wisdom of Ayurveda, the power of your mindset, and the depth of your dharma are always available to you. This book was never meant to be read once and set aside—it is a guide to return to, again and again, as you navigate the ever-changing seasons of your life.

Revisiting Your Path, Again and Again

As you evolve, so will your needs. The practices that serve you today may not be the ones that serve you a year from now.

✦ When you feel disconnected from your body, return to Health Alchemy—reignite your Agni, realign your hormones, nourish your vitality.

✦ When self-doubt creeps in, revisit the Empowered Mind Paradigm—shift your perspective, rewrite your story, reclaim your truth.

✦ When you question your path, seek clarity in Dharmic Impact— ask yourself how you can serve, how you can create, how you can step further into alignment.

This book is your compass, but you are the one walking the path. Trust yourself. Keep going.

The Power of Women Rising Together

Your transformation is not only for you. When you step into your higHERself™, you become a spark—a living, breathing invitation for other women to rise. Your presence, courage, and alignment ripple outward, touching your daughters, sisters, friends, and community. Empowered women *empower* women.

We've been conditioned to believe that success is an individual journey. But in truth, feminine power has always been collective. Women have gathered in circles for generations—to share stories, pass down wisdom, cry, laugh, and remind one another of their innate strength. This is not new—it is ancient. And it is time we remembered.

We rise stronger when we rise together. When one woman reclaims her voice, it echoes in the hearts of many. When you heal your body, you heal your lineage. When you live your truth out loud, you become a permission slip for others to do the same.

So gather your women. Form circles, book clubs, rituals, or simple coffee dates. Share what you've learned. Reflect together. Celebrate together. Hold space for one another without judgment. This is sacred.

Let your voice be heard—not because it is perfect, but because it is real. Let your story be known—not because it's resolved but because it's brave. When you support another woman's rise, you raise the frequency of us all.

Let us choose collaboration over comparison. Let us become the generation that healed together.

A Final Invitation: Stay Open, Stay Committed, Stay Expansive

This is my invitation to you:

+ Stay open to growth. Keep learning. Keep questioning. Keep expanding.

+ Stay committed to yourself. Choose your well-being, your joy, and your purpose every single day.

+ Stay expansive in your vision. Dream boldly. Trust that you are capable of more than you ever imagined.

+ The world needs women who are awake, aligned, and unapologetically themselves. The world needs *you*.

Take a breath. Place your hand on your heart. And know that you are exactly where you are meant to be. Step forward, not as the woman you were yesterday, but as your higHERself™.

The Daily Practice of Living as Your higHERself™

There is no perfect way to do this. Some days, you will feel deeply aligned. Other days, you may struggle. This is all part of the process.

The key is consistency. Small, intentional rituals practiced daily will create profound shifts over time.

You are your greatest healer. You are your greatest teacher. And you hold the power to live every single day as your higHERself™.

This is only the beginning.

Go forward. Live fully. Shine brightly.

Trust that everything you need is already within you.

You are ready.

With love and gratitude,

Dr. Harmony x x x x

Top 10 Takeaways from
Ayurveda and the Alchemy of HER

1. YOU ARE NOT BROKEN; YOU ARE BECOMING.

Healing is not about fixing yourself—it's about returning to wholeness and remembering who you truly are beneath the layers of conditioning, self-doubt, and societal expectations.

2. YOUR HEALTH IS MORE THAN PHYSICAL—IT IS MENTAL, EMOTIONAL, SPIRITUAL, AND DHARMIC.

True wellness is not just the absence of disease; it's the presence of vitality, clarity, and alignment in every aspect of your being.

3. YOU DON'T NEED TO FIND YOUR IDENTITY—YOU NEED TO FREE YOURSELF FROM IT.

You are not defined by labels, roles, or expectations. You are infinite, evolving, and capable of stepping into any version of yourself that aligns with your truth.

4. YOUR THOUGHTS SHAPE YOUR REALITY.

The stories you tell yourself—about your worth, your abilities, your limitations—become your lived experience. If you change your mind, you change your life.

5. HORMONES DO NOT CONTROL YOU; YOU CAN WORK WITH THEM.

Ayurveda teaches that by balancing your dosha, nourishing your Agni, and living in harmony with nature, you can transition through every stage of womanhood with grace and ease.

6. DHARMA IS NOT JUST PURPOSE—IT IS RIGHT LIVING.

Your dharma is not just a job or a passion; it is the way you show up in the world every single day, in every action, with integrity and alignment.

7. MIDLIFE IS NOT A CRISIS—IT IS AN AWAKENING.

The shift you feel in your late thirties, forties, and beyond is not an ending; it is a powerful initiation into your next evolution, an invitation to step into your wisdom and power.

8. ABUNDANCE IS NOT ABOUT HOW MUCH YOU HAVE—IT'S ABOUT HOW MUCH YOU ALLOW YOURSELF TO RECEIVE.

Scarcity is a mindset, not a circumstance. You are worthy of more—more joy, more success, more love, more fulfillment.

9. HEALING IS NOT A SOLO JOURNEY.

Your growth, your expansion, and your dharmic impact are amplified when you surround yourself with a community of like-minded, high-vibrational women who uplift and inspire you.

10. YOU ARE YOUR OWN HEALER, YOUR OWN GURU, YOUR OWN GUIDE.

Ayurveda, mindset work, and dharmic living are tools—but the power has always been within you. Your higHERself™ is not something outside of you; it has been waiting for you all along.

Let these truths sink in. Let them become part of your inner knowing. And most importantly—let them guide you as you rise into the woman you were always meant to be.

Bonus Section: Practical Ayurveda for Everyday Life

Ayurveda is not just about knowledge; it's about embodiment. True transformation happens through consistent daily rituals that nourish the body, calm the mind, and awaken the soul. These practices are designed to reconnect you with nature's rhythms, balance your doshas, and align you with your higHERself™.

Whether you're starting your morning, winding down in the evening, or syncing with your menstrual cycle, these Ayurveda-inspired recipes and rituals will support your health, energy, and intuition.

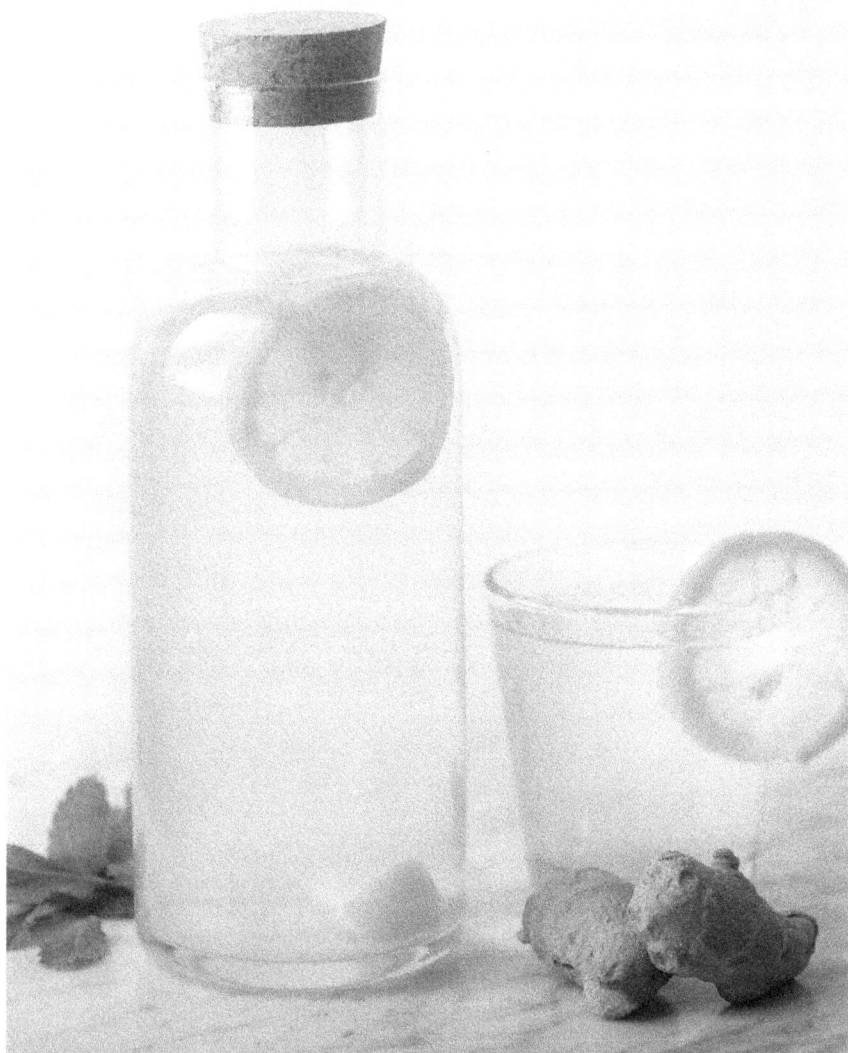

DAWN WATER

Ayurvedic Dawn Water:
A Ritual for Detox & Digestion

Purpose: Supports digestion, flushes toxins (Ama), and awakens Agni (digestive fire)

Best for: All doshas (adjust for season and personal constitution)

RECIPE

1 cup warm water (filtered)

1/2 tsp freshly squeezed lemon juice (omit if Pitta is high)

1/4 tsp raw honey (optional, but do not heat)

1 slice fresh ginger (omit if feeling too hot or inflamed)

a pinch of Himalayan pink salt (for electrolyte balance)

How to Use: Drink first thing in the morning before food or caffeine. This hydrates the body, gently detoxifies the liver, and stimulates digestion.

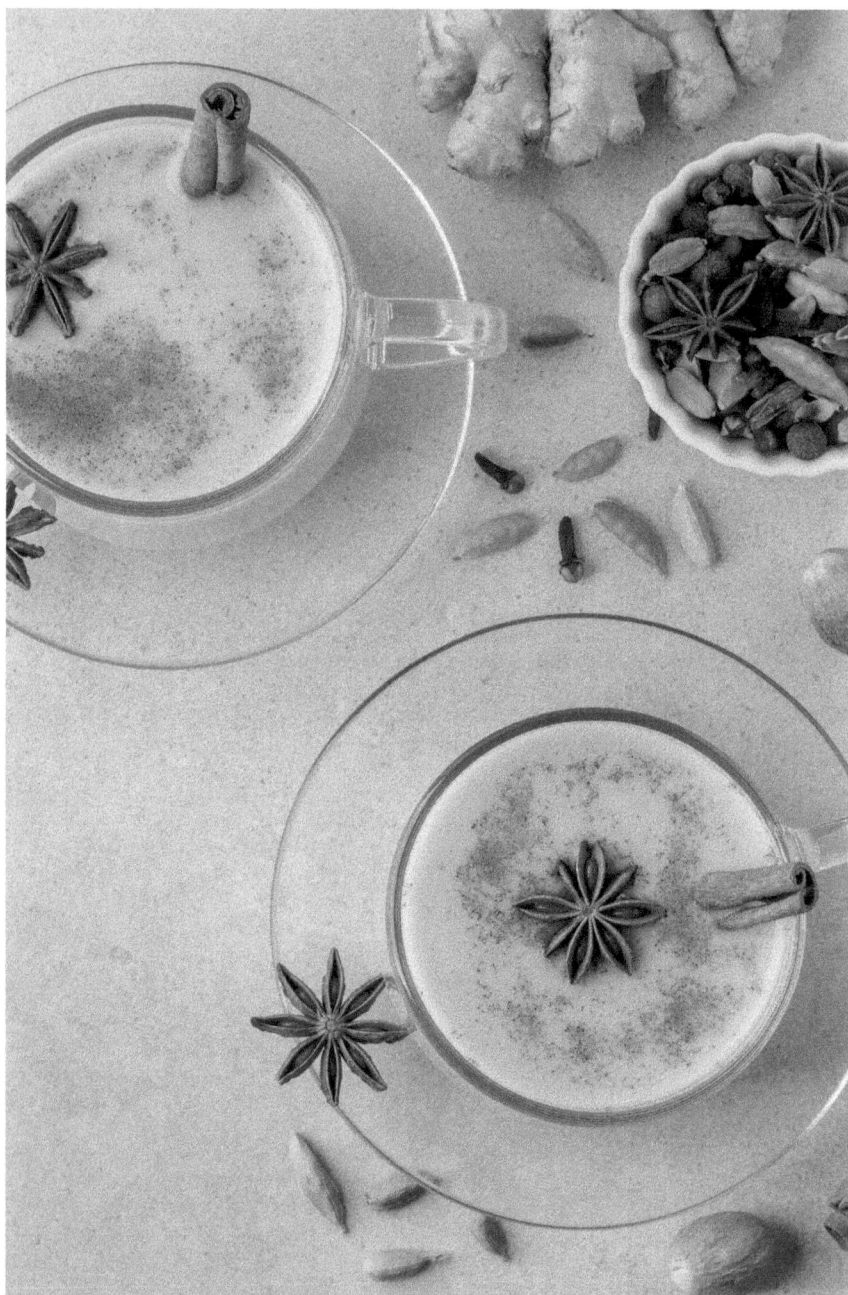

OJAS ELIXIR

Ojas Drink: The Ayurvedic Elixir for Radiance and Vitality

Purpose: Replenishes Ojas (vital essence), boosts immunity, and enhances feminine glow

Best for: Vata & Pitta (Kapha should drink in moderation)

RECIPE

1 cup warm almond or oat milk

1/2 tsp ashwagandha powder (adaptogen for stress and vitality)

1/2 tsp cinnamon (balances blood sugar and improves digestion)

1/4 tsp nutmeg (calms the nervous system and supports sleep)

1 tsp ghee (builds Ojas and nourishes the tissues)

1 tsp raw honey (only add once drink is warm, not hot)

Option: Superpower the elixir by blending 3 dates with the ingredients above.

How to Use: Enjoy before bed or during the luteal phase (PMS support) to calm the nervous system and restore feminine energy.

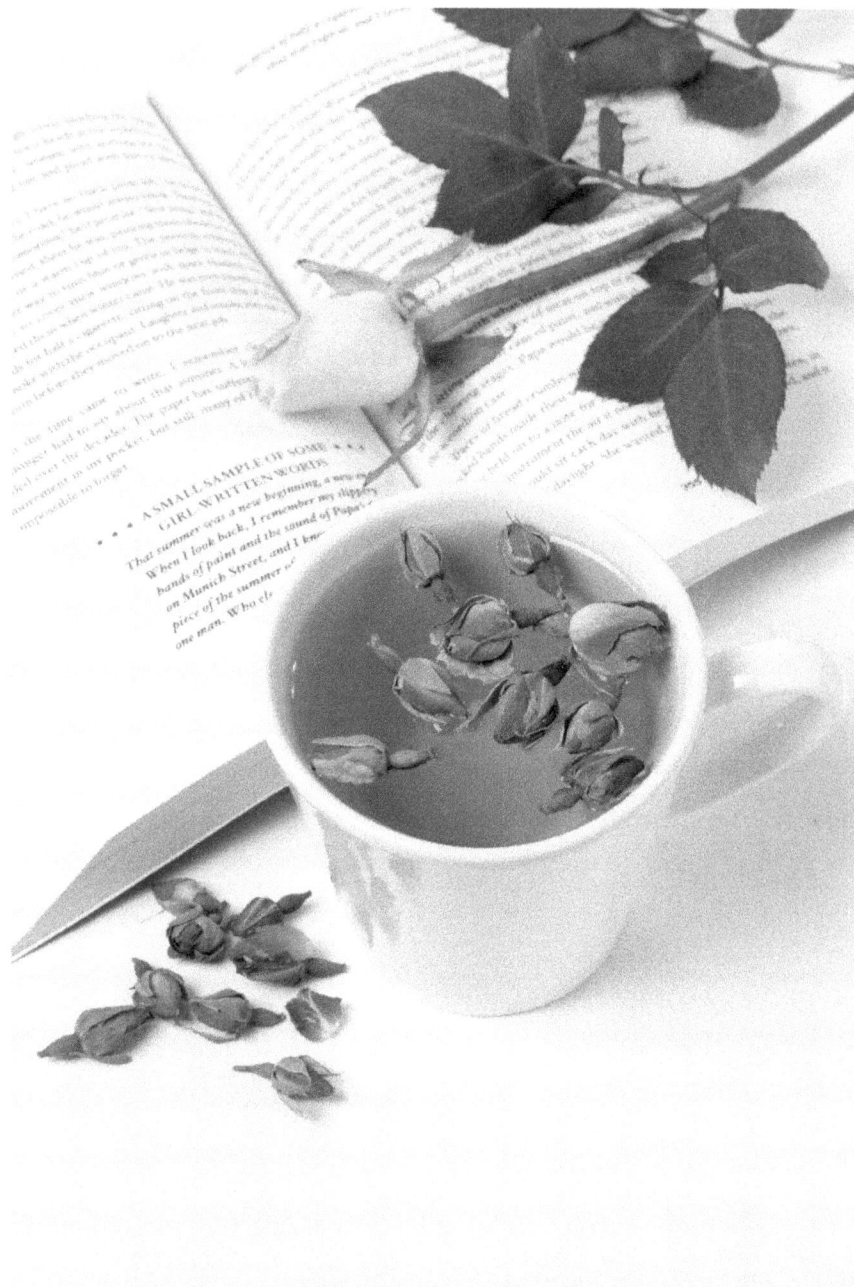

HERBAL DOSHA TEA

Ayurvedic Herbal Teas for Every Dosha

Purpose: Nourishes the body and mind, balances doshas, and supports digestion

VATA-PACIFYING TEA (CALM AND GROUNDING)

1 tsp dried chamomile

1 tsp fennel seeds

1/2 tsp fresh-grated ginger

1 cup hot water

Steep for 5 minutes and drink before bed to calm the nervous system.

PITTA-PACIFYING TEA (COOLING AND SOOTHING)

1 tsp dried rose petals

1 tsp licorice root

1/2 tsp coriander seeds

1 cup hot water

Best for hot flashes, stress, or irritability.

KAPHA-PACIFYING TEA (ENERGIZING AND CLEANSING)

1 tsp tulsi (holy basil)

1/2 tsp cinnamon

1/2 tsp dried orange peel

1 cup hot water

Perfect for sluggish digestion or morning sluggishness.

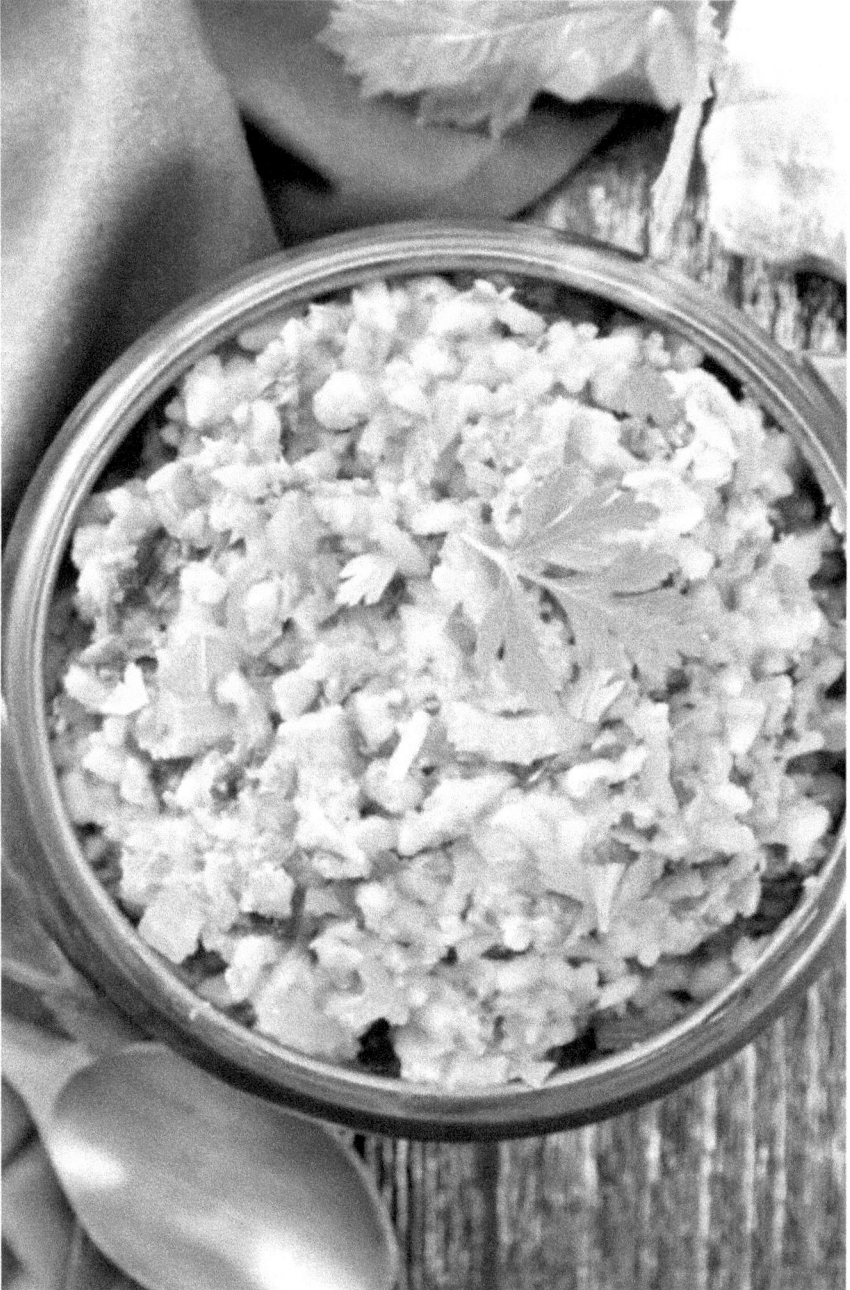

KITCHARI

Kitchari: Ayurveda's Ultimate Healing Meal

Kitchari is one of the most revered dishes in Ayurveda—a simple yet deeply nourishing meal that supports digestion, detoxification, and overall well-being. This traditional one-pot dish combines basmati rice, split mung dal, and warming spices to create a balanced meal that is easy to digest and packed with essential nutrients. Often used in Ayurvedic cleansing, kitchari provides the body with nourishment while allowing the digestive system to rest and reset. It is tridoshic, meaning it can be adapted to balance Vata, Pitta, and Kapha doshas, making it an ideal meal for everyone.

THE BENEFITS OF KITCHARI

✦ **Easy to Digest:** The combination of rice and mung dal is light on the stomach, making it perfect for those with weak digestion or recovering from illness.

✦ **Balances Agni (digestive fire):** The spices help stimulate digestion without overwhelming the system.

✦ **Detoxifying:** Kitchari helps eliminate Ama (toxins) while providing deep nourishment.

✦ **Sattvic and Grounding:** It calms the mind and body, making it ideal during times of stress, transition, or cleansing.

TRADITIONAL AYURVEDIC KITCHARI RECIPE

1/2 cup basmati rice

1/2 cup split yellow mung dal (soaked for 1–2 hours and rinsed)

4–5 cups water (adjust for desired consistency)

1 tbsp ghee or coconut oil

1 tsp cumin seeds

1 tsp mustard seeds

1 tsp coriander powder

1 tsp turmeric powder

1/2 tsp fennel seeds

1/2 tsp ground ginger (or 1 tsp fresh grated ginger)

1/4 tsp hing (asafoetida, optional for digestion)

1 small carrot, chopped (optional)

1 handful of leafy greens (like spinach or kale)

Pink Himalayan salt to taste

Fresh cilantro and lemon juice for garnish

Instructions

1. **Prepare the ingredients:** Rinse the rice and soaked mung dal well until the water runs clear. This removes excess starch and improves digestibility.

2. **Heat the spices:** In a large pot, heat the ghee or coconut oil over medium heat. Add the cumin and mustard seeds and let them pop. Then, add the coriander powder, turmeric, fennel, ginger, and hing. Stir for a few seconds to release their aroma.

3. **Cook the dal and rice:** Add the mung dal and rice to the pot, stirring to coat them with the spices. Pour in the water and bring to a gentle boil.

4. **Simmer gently:** Reduce the heat, cover, and let it cook for about 30–40 minutes, stirring occasionally. If adding vegetables, add them halfway through cooking.

5. **Final touches:** Once everything is soft and creamy, add salt to taste.

6. **Remove from heat:** Garnish with fresh cilantro, and squeeze a little lemon juice on top.

7. **Serve and enjoy:** Eat warm and mindfully, savoring each bite. For enhanced nourishment, serve with extra ghee on top.

HOW TO CUSTOMISE KITCHARI FOR YOUR DOSHA

Vata-Balancing Kitchari

+ Add extra ghee for grounding.

+ Use more warming spices like cinnamon and cloves.

+ Cook to a soft, soupy consistency to soothe digestion.

Pitta-Balancing Kitchari

+ Use coconut oil instead of ghee.

+ Reduce mustard seeds and add fennel for cooling.

+ Include cooling veggies like zucchini or cilantro.

Kapha-Balancing Kitchari

+ Reduce oil and keep it on the drier side.

+ Add extra black pepper, ginger, or chili for stimulation.

+ Avoid excess salt and make it lighter with more leafy greens.

WHEN TO EAT KITCHARI

+ **During cleansing periods:** Kitchari is the staple meal of Ayurvedic detoxes (Panchakarma).

+ **When feeling run-down:** It provides deep nourishment while being easy on digestion.

+ **After travel or stressful periods:** Helps reset the gut and bring grounding energy.

+ **Seasonal transitions:** A great meal to ease into the change of seasons, keeping Agni strong.

Kitchari is not just food; it is a healing ritual, a way to honor your body and digestion. Whether eaten for a gentle cleanse or as a nourishing meal, it is a beautiful example of Ayurveda's wisdom—balancing, grounding, and deeply restoring.

Enjoy this sacred dish as a way to connect with your body, reset your digestion, and realign with your highest self.

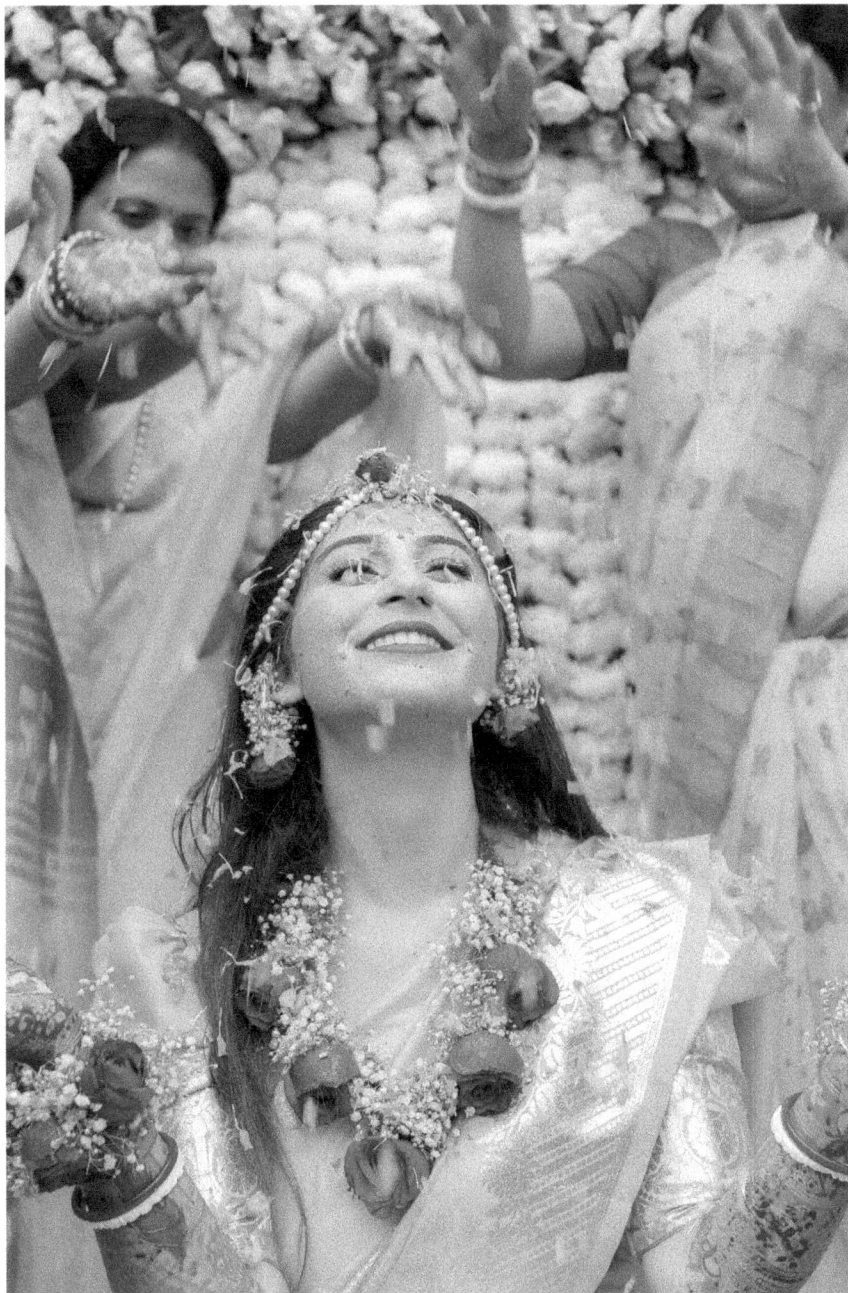

IN AYURVEDA, DAILY RITUALS ARE MEDICINE FOR THE SOUL AS MUCH AS FOR THE BODY.

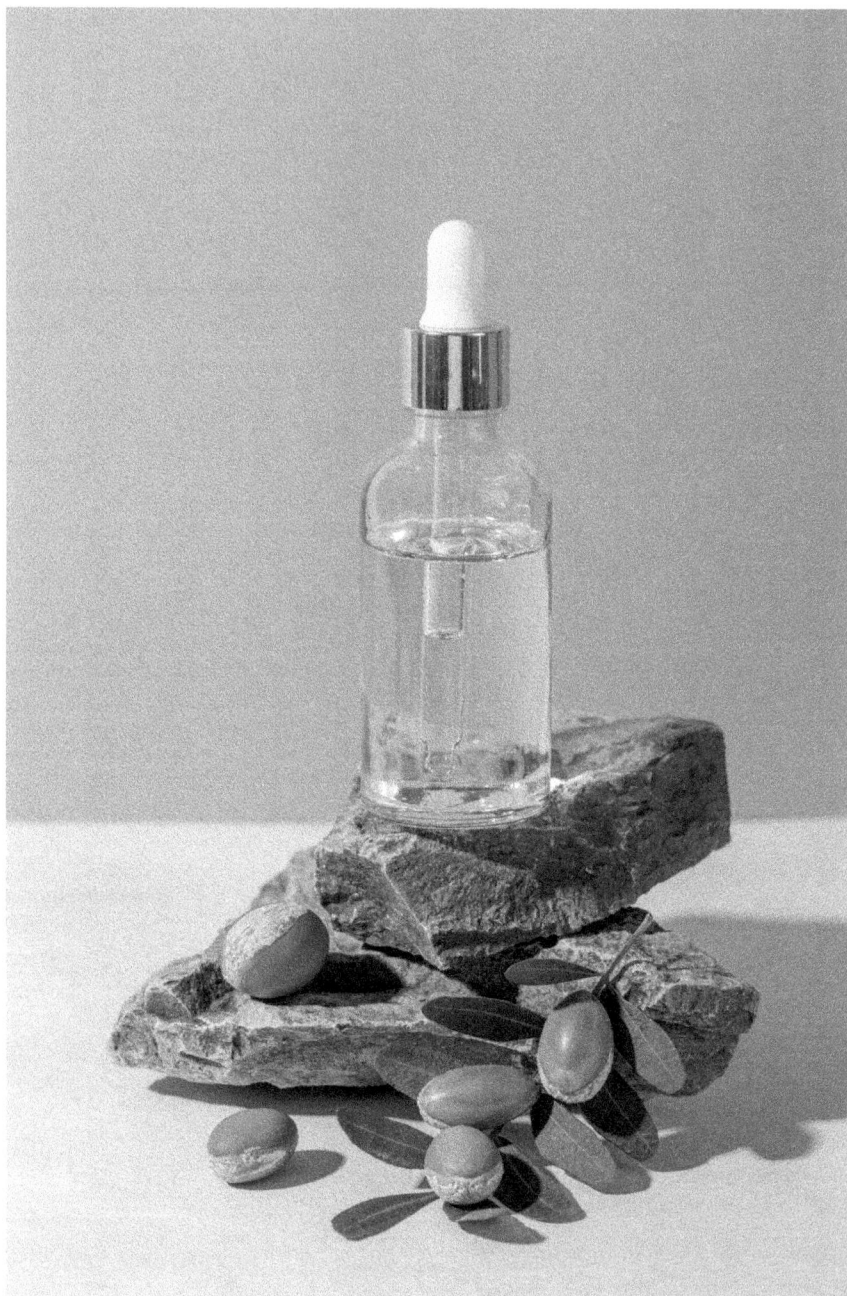

GLOW SKIN OIL

Glow Skin Oil: A Rejuvenating Face and Body Serum

Purpose: Enhances skin radiance, prevents premature aging, and nourishes all doshas

Best for: Vata (hydration), Pitta (cooling), Kapha (circulation)

RECIPE

2 tbsp organic sesame oil (Vata) *or* coconut oil (Pitta) *or* mustard oil (Kapha)

3 drops rose essential oil (Pitta) *or* sandalwood essential oil (Vata) *or* eucalyptus (Kapha)

1 tsp turmeric-infused oil (anti-inflammatory and brightening)

How to Use: Massage onto damp skin after showering for deep hydration and lymphatic support.

MOON GAZING MEDITATION

Moon Gazing Meditation: Balancing Feminine Energy

Purpose: Aligns your energy with the moon, enhances intuition, and supports hormone balance

Best for: Women wanting to reconnect with their cycles, regulate emotions, and access deeper wisdom

HOW TO PRACTICE

1. Go outside at night and find a quiet place under the moonlight.

2. Sit comfortably, placing one hand over your womb space.

3. Take seven deep breaths, inhaling through the nose and exhaling through the mouth.

4. Soften your gaze and look at the moon, allowing its light to wash over you.

5. Whisper an intention for the cycle ahead: "I allow myself to surrender and receive."

6. Stay for 5–10 minutes, absorbing the energy and feeling the stillness.

Bonus: Track how you feel before and after. Over time, this meditation helps sync your energy with the moon phases, deepening your connection to your inner cycles.

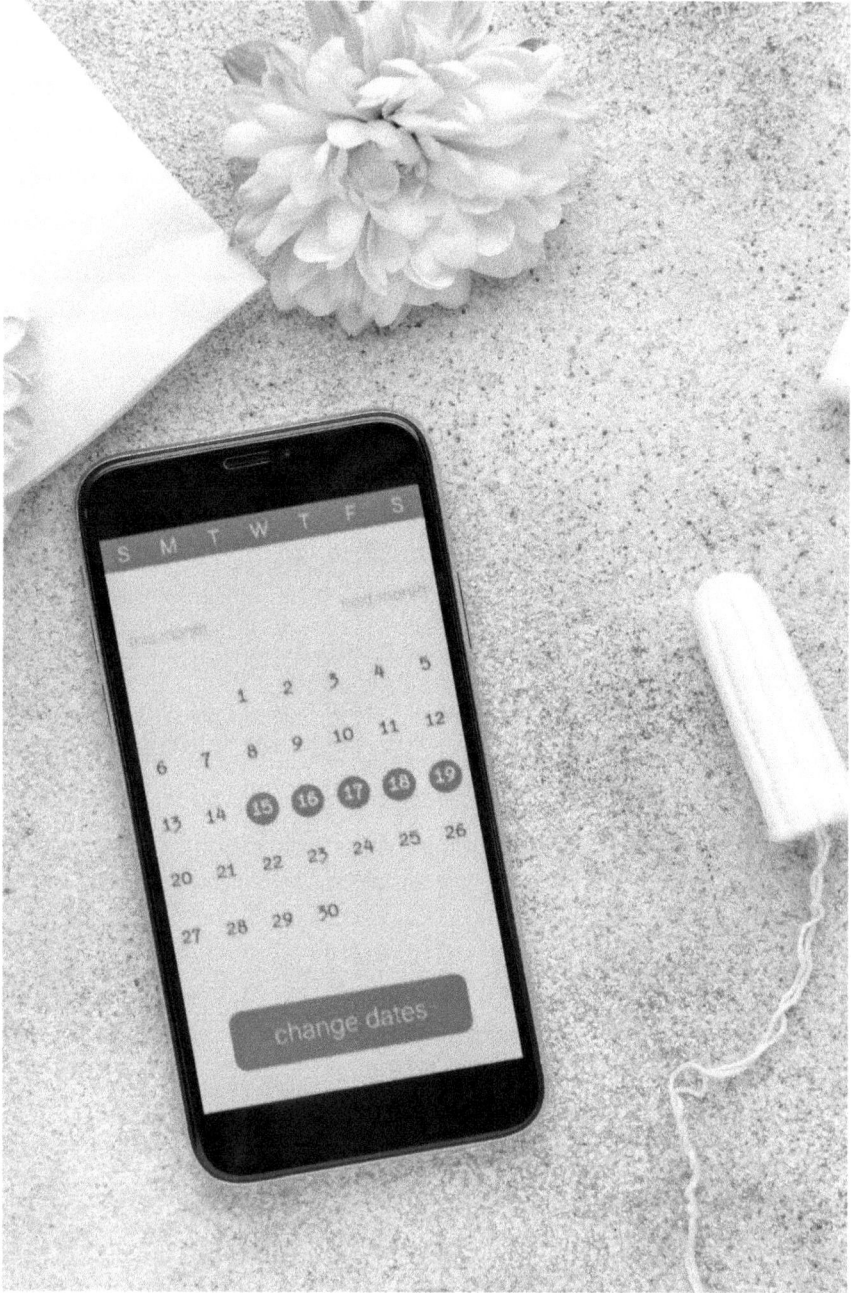

MENSTRUAL CYCLE TRACKER

Cycle Tracker:
Aligning with Your Feminine Rhythms

Purpose: Helps you track hormonal shifts, emotions, and energy levels throughout your cycle

Best for: Women who want to understand their menstrual phases (aligning with the moon), even postmenopause.

TRACKING YOUR CYCLE

1. **Menstrual Phase (Days 1–5): The New Moon**
   - ✧ Energy: Low, inward-focused
   - ✧ Ayurvedic dosha: Vata
   - ✧ Self-care: Rest, hydrate, warm foods

2. **Follicular Phase (Days 6–14): The Waxing Moon**
   - ✧ Energy: Rising, creative, social
   - ✧ Ayurvedic dosha: Kapha, Pitta
   - ✧ Self-care: Light movement, creative projects

3. **Ovulation Phase (Days 15–17): The Full Moon**
   - ✧ Energy: Peak vitality, magnetic, radiant
   - ✧ Ayurvedic dosha: Pitta
   - ✧ Self-care: Socializing, manifestation rituals

4. **Luteal Phase (Days 18–28): The Waning Moon**
   - ✧ Energy: Slowing down, reflective
   - ✧ Ayurvedic dosha: Pitta, Vata
   - ✧ Self-Care: Journaling, yin yoga, early bedtime

How to Use: Start journaling your symptoms, mood, and energy levels. Over time, you'll notice patterns that help you plan your schedule, workouts, and self-care accordingly.

Bibliography

American Thyroid Association. 2024. "Targeting Thyroid Receptor Antibodies to Treat Graves' Hyperthyroidism and Eye Disease." *Clinical Thyroidology for the Public* 17 (5): 5–6.

Armour, M., Dahlen, H. G., Zhu, X., Farquhar, C., and Smith, C. A. 2018. "The Role of Treatment Timing and Acupuncture Type in the Management of Primary Dysmenorrhea: An Exploratory Randomized Controlled Trial." *PLoS One* 13 (3): e0193037.

Bajalan, Z., Alimoradi, Z., and Moafi, F. 2019. "Nutrition as a Potential Factor of Primary Dysmenorrhea: A Systematic Review of Observational Studies." *Gynecologic and Obstetric Investigation* 84 (3): 209–224.

Black Dog Institute. 2025. " Suicide Prevention: Building the Evidence-base for Effective Suicide Prevention." Accessed May 22. https://www.blackdoginstitute.org.au/research-areas/suicide-prevention/.

Bernstein, Gabrielle. 2016. *The Universe Has Your Back: Transform Fear to Faith*. Hay House Inc.

Chen, Zhangling, Qian, Frank, Hu, Yang, Li, Yanping, Rimm, Eric B., Sun, Qi, et al. January 2023. "Dietary Phytoestrogens and Total and Cause-specific Mortality: Results from 2 Prospective Cohort Studies." *The American Journal of Clinical Nutrition* 117 (1): 130–140. https://ajcn.nutrition.org/article/S0002-9165(22)10533-2/fulltext .

Chou, S. H., Chamberland, J. P., Liu, X., et al. 2011. "Leptin Is an Effective Treatment for Hypothalamic Amenorrhea." *Proceedings of the National Academy of Sciences* 108 (16): 6585–6590. doi:10.1073/pnas.1019874108.

Creswell, J. David, Dutcher, Janine M., Klein, William M., Harris, Peter R., Levine, and John M. 2013. "Self-affirmation Improves Problem-solving Under Stress." *PLoS One* 8 (5): e62593.

Desmawati, Desmawati, and Sulastri, Delmi. February 14, 2019. "Phytoestrogens and Their Health Effects." *Open Access Macedonian Journal of Medical Sciences* 7 (3): 495–499. https://doi.org/10.3889/oamjms.2019.044.

The Endocrine Society. 2022. "Endocrine Library." https://www.endocrine.org/patient-engagement/endocrine-library.

Gua, C., and Zhang, C. 2024. "The Role of Gut Microbiota in the Pathogenesis of Endometriosis: A Review." *Frontiers in Microbiology* 15. doi:10.3389/fmicb.2024.1363455.

Han, Q., Wang, J., Li, W., Chen, Z. J., and Du, Y. 2021. "Androgen-induced Gut Dysbiosis Disrupts Glucolipid Metabolism and Endocrinal Functions in Polycystic Ovary Syndrome." *Microbiome* 9 (1): 101.

Harvard Medical School. "How Does Exercise Reduce Stress? Surprising Answers to This Question and More." Harvard Health Publishing. July 7, 2021. https://www.health.harvard.edu/mind-and-mood/exercising-to-relax.

Karayiannis, Dimitrios, Kontogianni, Meropi D., Mendorou, Chrisina, Mastrominas, Minas, and Yiannakouris, Nikos. 2018. "Adherence to the Mediterranean Diet and IVF Success Rate Among Non-obese Women Attempting Fertility." *Human Reproduction (Oxford, England)* 33 (3): 494–502. doi:10.1093/humrep/dey003.

Lally, P., van Jaarsveld, C. H., Potts, H. W., and Wardle, J. 2010. "How Are Habits Formed: Modelling Habit Formation in the Real World." *European Journal of Social Psychology* 40 (6): 998–1009.

McLean, Carmen P., Asnaani, Anu, Litz, Brett T., and Hofmann, Stefan G. 2011. "Gender Differences in Anxiety Disorders: Prevalence, Course of Illness, Comorbidity, and Burden of Illness." *Journal of Psychiatric Research* 45 (8): 1027–1035. doi:10.1016/j.jpsychires.2011.03.006.

Muffone, Ann R. M. C., de Oliveira, Paola D. P., and Rabito, Labito I. 2023. "Mediterranean Diet and Infertility: A Systematic Review with Meta-analysis of Cohort Studies." *Nutrition Reviews* 81 (7): 775–789. doi:10.1093/nutrit/nuac087.

National Sleep Foundation. "How Can Menopause Affect Sleep?" January 18, 2024. https://www.sleepfoundation.org/women-sleep/menopause-and-sleep.

Osborn, E., Brooks, J., O'Brien, P. M. S., and Wittkowski, A. September 16, 2020. "Suicidality in Women with Premenstrual Dysphoric Disorder: A Systematic Literature Review." *Archives of Women's Health* 24 (2): 173–184. https://doi.org/10.1007/s00737-020-01054-8.

Prasad, Divya, Wollenhaupt-Aguiar, Bianca, Kidd, Katrina, de Azevedo Cardoso, Taiane, and Frey, Benico N. December 16, 2021. "Suicidal Risk in Women with Premenstrual Syndrome and Premenstrual Dysphoric Disorder: A Systematic Review and Meta-analysis." *Journal of Women's Health* 30 (12): 1693–1707. https://doi.org/10.1089/jwh.2021.0185.

Rahbar, N., Asgharzadeh, N., and Ghorbani, R. 2012. "Effect of Omega-3 Fatty Acids on Intensity of Primary Dysmenorrhea." *International Journal Gynaecology and Obstetrics* 117 (1): 45–47.

Reebs, B. 2018. "Cortisol and Thyroid: How Stress Affects Your Health." Dr. Ben Reebs Blog. July 9, 2018. https://www.drreebs.com/cortisol-thyroid-stress/.

Sacher, J., Zsido, R. G., Barth, C., et al. 2023. "Increase in Serotonin Transporter Binding in Patients with Premenstrual Dysphoric Disorder across the Menstrual Cycle: A Case-control Longitudinal Neuroreceptor Ligand PET Imaging Study." *Biological Psychiatry* 93 (12): 1081–1088.

Sharma, P. V. 1998. *Sushruta Samhita* vol 1. Chaukhambha Visvabharati.

Smith, Rhianna-Lily. "How Do Minerals Affect the Menstrual Cycle?" *Technology*

Networks. April 18, 2024. https://www.technologynetworks.com/ proteomics/news/how-do-minerals-affect-the-menstrual-cycle-385891.

Takahashi, J. S., Hong, H. K., Ko, C. H., and McDearmon, E. L. 2008. "The Genetics of Mammalian Circadian Order and Disorder: Implications for Physiology and Disease." *Nature Reviews Genetics* 9 (10): 764–775. doi:10.1038/nrg2430.

US Department of Veterans Affairs. March 19, 2025. "Whole Health Library: Estrogen Dominance." https://www.va.gov/WHOLEHEALTHLIBRARY/ tools/estrogen-dominance.asp.

Vaillant, George Eman. 2012. *Triumphs of Experience: The Men of the Harvard Grant Study*. Harvard University Press.

Wentz, I. 2025. "The Benefits of Vitamin D for Your Thyroid." *Thyroid Pharmacist*. February 14. https://thyroidpharmacist.com/articles/vitamin-d-benefits-thyroid/.

Glossary

AYURVEDIC TERMS

Agni (Digestive Fire)	The body's metabolic energy responsible for digestion, absorption, and transformation of food and experiences. Balanced Agni leads to good health, while weak or excessive Agni results in disease.
Ama (Toxins)	Undigested waste and metabolic toxins that accumulate in the body due to poor digestion, leading to disease and imbalance.
Abhyanga	Ayurvedic self-massage using warm herbal oils to nourish the body, calm the nervous system, and balance the doshas.
Ayurveda	A 5,000-year-old system of natural medicine from India that promotes health through diet, lifestyle, herbs, and mind-body balance.
Chakras	Energy centers in the body that correspond to different aspects of physical, mental, and spiritual health. There are seven main chakras aligned along the spine, each associated with specific functions and elements:

1. Root Chakra (Muladhara)—Located at the base of the spine. Governs safety, stability, and survival. Element: Earth. Color: Red.

2. Sacral Chakra (Svadhisthana)—Located below the navel. Governs creativity, sensuality, and emotional flow. Element: Water. Color: Orange.

3. Solar Plexus Chakra (Manipura)—Located in the upper abdomen. Governs personal power, confidence, and willpower. Element: Fire. Color: Yellow.

4. Heart Chakra (Anahata)—Located at the center of the chest. Governs love, compassion, and relationships. Element: Air. Color: Green.

5. Throat Chakra (Vishuddha)—Located at the throat. Governs communication, self-expression, and truth. Element: Ether. Color: Blue.

6. Third Eye Chakra (Ajna)—Located between the eyebrows. Governs intuition, insight, and inner wisdom. Element: Light. Color: Indigo.

7. Crown Chakra (Sahasrara)—Located at the top of the head. Governs spiritual connection, consciousness, and enlightenment. Element: Cosmic Energy. Color: Violet or White.

Dinacharya (Daily Routine)	Ayurvedic self-care practices that align with nature's rhythms to promote balance and well-being.
Doshas	The three primary energies governing the body and mind:
	Vata (Air & Ether)—Governs movement, creativity, and nervous system regulation. Imbalance causes anxiety, dry skin, and bloating.
	Pitta (Fire & Water)—Governs digestion, metabolism, and transformation. Imbalance leads to inflammation, anger, and digestive issues.
	Kapha (Earth & Water)—Governs structure, stability, and lubrication. Imbalance results in sluggishness, weight gain, and congestion.
Gunas (Mental States)	The three qualities influencing the mind:
	Sattva—Purity, clarity, balance.
	Rajas—Activity, restlessness, passion.
	Tamas—Inertia, heaviness, ignorance.
Jatharagni	The main digestive fire responsible for breaking down food and nutrients.
Manas (Mind)	The mind, which processes thoughts, emotions, and experiences.
Marma Points	Vital energy points in the body similar to acupuncture points in TCM.
Nadi Shodhana (Alternate Nostril Breathing)	A pranayama (breathwork) technique to balance the nervous system.
Ojas (Vital Energy)	The essence of immunity, vitality, and longevity. It is nourished by healthy food, rest, and positive emotions.
Prakriti (Constitution)	A person's unique Ayurvedic blueprint determined at birth, consisting of a combination of doshas.
Prana (Life Force Energy)	The vital energy flowing through the body, responsible for sustaining life and consciousness.
Samskaras (Mental Impressions)	Deep-seated patterns, beliefs, and past experiences that shape one's perception and behavior.
Shatavari	A revered Ayurvedic herb known as "Queen of Herbs," used for female reproductive health and hormonal balance.
Srotas (Channels)	The body's energetic pathways responsible for circulation, digestion, and detoxification.

Trigunas (Three Mental States)	Sattva, Rajas, and Tamas-qualities that shape thoughts, emotions, and personality.
Vikruti (Current State of Imbalance)	The present doshic imbalance influenced by lifestyle, diet, stress, and environment.

TRADITIONAL CHINESE MEDICINE (TCM) TERMS

Qi (Life Force Energy)	The vital energy that flows through the body's meridians and is essential for health.
Jing (Essence)	The foundational energy inherited from parents, governing growth, reproduction, and aging.
Meridians	Pathways through which Qi flows in the body, used in acupuncture and energy healing.
Shen (Mind/ Spirit)	The spirit housed in the heart, associated with consciousness, emotions, and mental clarity.
Yin & Yang	The dual forces in nature that must be in balance for optimal health.
	Yin—Cooling, nourishing, feminine energy
	Yang—Heating, active, masculine energy

WOMEN'S HEALTH TERMS

Amenorrhea	The absence of menstrual periods, which can be caused by hormonal imbalances, stress, or low body weight.
Cortisol	The primary stress hormone, which, when chronically elevated, can disrupt menstrual cycles and overall hormonal health.
Cycle Syncing	Aligning diet, movement, and self-care practices with the four phases of the menstrual cycle.
DHEA (Dehydroepian- drosterone)	A hormone precursor to estrogen and testosterone, influencing energy, libido, and aging.
Dysmenorrhea	Painful menstruation, often caused by hormonal imbalances or conditions like endometriosis.

Estrogen Dominance	A hormonal imbalance where estrogen levels are too high relative to progesterone, leading to PMS, fibroids, and mood swings.
Follicular Phase	The first half of the menstrual cycle, when estrogen levels rise, promoting ovulation and energy.
Insulin	A hormone that regulates blood sugar levels. Insulin resistance, common in PCOS, can lead to weight gain, irregular cycles, and metabolic disorders.
Luteal Phase	The second half of the cycle, marked by increased progesterone to support a potential pregnancy.
Menorrhagia	Heavy or prolonged menstrual bleeding, often caused by hormonal imbalances, fibroids, or underlying health conditions.
Menopause	The permanent cessation of menstruation, typically occurring between ages forty-five and fifty-five, signaling the end of reproductive years.
PCOS (Polycystic Ovary Syndrome)	A common hormonal disorder affecting 1 in 10 women, characterized by irregular periods, ovarian cysts, excess androgens (male hormones), insulin resistance, and difficulty with fertility.
Perimenopause	The transitional phase before menopause, characterized by hormonal fluctuations, irregular cycles, and symptoms like hot flashes.
PMDD (Premenstrual Dysphoric Disorder)	A severe form of PMS that impacts mood, mental health, and daily functioning.
Progesterone	A hormone essential for menstrual cycle regulation, pregnancy, and calming the nervous system.
Second Spring	A term used in Eastern medicine to describe the postmenopausal years as a period of renewal, wisdom, and transformation.
Testosterone in Women	An important hormone for libido, bone density, and muscle strength, often declining with age.
Thyroid Dysfunction	Imbalances in thyroid hormones (hypothyroidism or hyperthyroidism) that impact metabolism, mood, and menstrual cycles.
Xenoestrogens	Synthetic compounds that mimic estrogen in the body, found in plastics, pesticides, and cosmetics, contributing to hormonal imbalances.

Work with Harmony

Dr. Harmony Robinson-Stagg (acupuncture) integrates the ancient wisdom of Ayurveda and Traditional Chinese Medicine with modern science to help women reconnect with their health, vitality, and purpose. Whether you're here for personal healing or seeking professional training in holistic wellness, there's a pathway that meets you where you are and supports where you're meant to go.

The Ayurveda Alchemist Academy

This is the heart of my work and my highest calling.

A leading Ayurvedic education and coaching academy for women ready to transform their lives and the lives of others through ancient wisdom and modern mentorship. Whether you dream of becoming a certified Ayurvedic coach or simply want to study Ayurveda to deepen your personal journey, the Academy offers two powerful learning tracks.

+ **Pathway One: Personal Transformation:** For the woman who wants to study Ayurveda to heal herself, deepen self-awareness, and live in alignment—without the business component.

+ **Pathway Two: Professional Certification:** For aspiring coaches and wellness professionals who want to become certified Ayurveda Holistic Health Coaches and guide others toward balance and vitality.

Both pathways offer mentorship, community, and a soul-aligned curriculum.

Learn more or enroll:
https://www. harmonyinspiredhealth.com.au/ayurveda-alchemist

Other Certifications and Educational Courses

AYURSOUL VEDIC BREATHWORK PRACTITIONER TRAINING

A powerful program teaching ancient Vedic breathwork techniques for emotional healing, nervous system regulation, and deep spiritual connection.

https://www.harmonyinspiredhealth.com.au/breathwork/

AYURVEDA MASSAGE AND BODYWORK THERAPIST CERTIFICATION

Learn the sacred art of Ayurvedic massage and body therapies, integrating healing touch with traditional Ayurvedic principles.

https://www.harmonyinspiredhealth.com.au/ayurveda-massage-bodyworks-therapist-certification/

INTRO TO AYURVEDA—SELF-PACED COURSE

Perfect for beginners, this course provides a foundational understanding of Ayurveda, including doshas, digestion, and daily self-care practices.

https://www.harmonyinspiredhealth.com.au/academy/

WOMEN'S HEALTH, KNOW THY SELF—SELF-PACED COURSE

A powerful short course exploring women's health, hormones, and nutrition through the lens of Ayurveda.

https://www.harmonyinspiredhealth.com.au/academy/

Interested in integrating Ayurveda into your existing health or wellness practice? This free masterclass will introduce you to the fundamentals of Ayurveda and how you can incorporate this ancient wisdom into modern health coaching and holistic healing.

https://www.harmonyinspiredhealth.com.au/masterclass-ayurveda-for-wellness-professionals/

1:1 Ayurveda and Women's Health Consultations
(Servicing Clients World Wide)

Personalized guidance using Ayurvedic principles, functional medicine, and holistic health strategies to support:

- ✦ hormonal imbalances (PMDD, PCOS, perimenopause and menopause)

- ✦ digestive health and metabolism

- ✦ stress, anxiety, and emotional well-being

- ✦ fertility, pregnancy, and postpartum support

- ✦ chronic fatigue, burnout, and adrenal health

https://www.harmonyinspiredhealth.com.au/womens-health-clinic-services/

Acupuncture and Women's Health Treatments

Harness the power of Traditional Chinese Medicine to regulate hormones, reduce stress, and promote overall well-being. Acupuncture sessions are tailored to support women's health and balance the mind-body connection.

https://www.harmonyinspiredhealth.com.au/acupuncture-burleigh-heads-gold-coast/

Business Mentorship for Wellness Practitioners

Turn your passion for Ayurveda and holistic health into a thriving business with mentorship and guidance from Harmony. This mentorship is designed to help new and established practitioners confidently step into their dharma and make a meaningful impact.

https://www.harmonyinspiredhealth.com.au/business-mentorship-coaching/

Listen to the Harmony Inspired Health Podcast

On my podcast, I share empowering conversations, ancient wisdom, and modern insights on Ayurveda, women's health, hormones, mindset, and purpose. If you loved the themes of this book, you'll feel right at home here—real talk, practical tools, and soulful guidance to help you embody your higHERself™.

https://www.harmonyinspiredhealth.com.au/podcasts/

Ready to Begin?

Explore how you can work with Harmony by visiting
https://www.harmonyinspiredhealth.com.au
or connecting on Instagram:
@harmony.inspired.ayurveda

Acknowledgments

Writing this book has been a journey of deep reflection, learning, and growth, and I could not have done it alone. I am filled with immense gratitude for the incredible people who have supported, guided, and inspired me along the way.

To my husband Phil, thank you for your unwavering support, patience, and belief in me. Your encouragement has been the foundation upon which I've built this dream.

To my beautiful children, Xavier and Cruiz—you are my greatest teachers. Your unconditional love and the privilege of being your mother have shaped me in ways I could never have imagined. Thank you for reminding me daily of what truly matters.

To Melissa, my business cheerleader—your support, encouragement, and faith in my mission have meant the world to me. Thank you for always being there to remind me of my power.

To my late grandmother, whose love, wisdom, and spirit continue to guide me: You are forever in my heart.

To my mum, for courageously sharing your story, allowing your experiences to be woven into these pages with such honesty and wisdom. Your journey has not only shaped my own but will inspire so many others.

To my dad, for your quiet strength and presence. Thank you for your support and the values you instilled in me.

To my brother, for being a part of the foundation that made me who I am today.

To Julie Postance, my brilliant book coach—your guidance, wisdom, and unwavering belief in my voice helped shape this book into what it is today. Thank you for keeping me focused, pushing me when I needed it, and reminding me of the impact these words could have.

To Cortni Merritt, my editor—your keen eye, attention to detail, and ability to bring clarity and flow to my words have been invaluable. Thank you for refining my message while honoring my voice and vision.

To Neat Designs—your artistry and ability to capture the essence of this book in a single image is truly a gift. Thank you for creating a cover that feels as powerful as the message inside.

To Sophie White, for your expertise in typesetting and layout—thank you for bringing this book to life in a way that is beautiful, cohesive, and a joy to read.

To everyone who contributed their stories and wisdom, thank you for your vulnerability, insight, and willingness to share your experiences. Your words add richness and depth to this book.

And finally, to you, the reader—thank you for choosing to embark on this journey with me. May this book serve as a guide, a source of inspiration, and a reminder that you are capable of stepping into your most empowered, radiant, and authentic self.

With love and gratitude,

Dr. Harmony

Testimonials

I first met Harmony in person at a Panchakarma retreat in Bali. It was my introduction to Ayurveda and holistic healing, and while I was intrigued, I initially turned down her invitation to join the Ayurveda Alchemist course, as I was focused on other ideas at the time. After completing the Panchakarma and returning from another contract onboard the yacht (my day job as a seafarer), I felt a deep desire to explore Ayurveda further, especially to address my own health challenges.

Enrolling in Harmony's course was one of the best decisions I've ever made. The course offers an in-depth exploration of Vedic wisdom, beautifully broken down into twelve easy-to-follow modules. Each module dives into different aspects of Ayurveda, from understanding the doshas to creating personalized healing protocols. Harmony's ability to blend the ancient wisdom of Ayurveda with modern Western medicine is truly remarkable and provides a holistic understanding of both worlds.

Her teaching style is engaging and practical, making the content accessible even for beginners like myself. She also provides ample support throughout the course, ensuring that each student not only understands the material but feels empowered to apply it in their own life. This course didn't just teach me about Ayurveda— it ignited a passion in me to help other women on their wellness journeys. Whether you're new to Ayurveda or looking to deepen your knowledge, I highly recommend the Ayurveda Alchemist course. You will not be disappointed. —*Samantha Morris*

Harmony is incredible! I felt I was in such capable hands from the moment I met her. She was able to put me at ease and extract everything I needed from exactly where I was at, and give me a practical, simple plan back to better health I could start straight away. I am already feeling more energized. Such an inspirational woman with extensive holistic knowledge of women's health and all things Ayurveda. She genuinely wants to help and lift women to their fullest potential. Highly recommend her business and services. —*Laura Fekete*

The Ayurveda Alchemist program was such a great experience. I was halfway through a Women's Wellness Coaching Course when I decided to pivot and sign up with Harmony. I changed because I felt the course I was doing had not hit the holistic mark I was wanting and the Ayurveda Alchemist was exactly what I needed. Harmony's approach made it easy and joyful to learn—so much support form Harmony and all of the beautiful women associated. —*Julie Manners*

Before enrolling in the Ayurveda Alchemist Program, I had already unknowingly embarked on a self discovery/philosophy of life journey. I had a passion to want to be of service to the emerging generation somehow but couldn't quite put my finger on how to get there or what to do.

I subconsciously knew of Ayurveda, having traveled to India before, but never considered it to be something that I could peruse a path in, until one day I stumbled across Harmony's website and her plethora of knowledge and expertise.

I decided within twenty-four hours that this was the path I was meant to take, and I have never looked back. I pushed through the self-doubt, the worry, the overwhelm, and feeling like I may be in over my head about starting my journey.

With the help of Harmony, the support system, in-depth course material, abundant resources, and the beautiful community she has built, I now have a clear vision and path ahead of me. For anyone seeking direction, purpose, or a deeper understanding of themselves and their place in the world and in nature, I wholeheartedly recommend Harmony's Ayurveda Alchemist program. It has been a profound and transformative journey that has left an indelible mark on my life. —*Lilly Underwood*

Highly recommend! Harmony provides professional service and with such a vast background of professional knowledge in many styles of health specialties, you know you are in great hands.

Harmony is dedicated to ensuring optimal health is reached in comfortable, compassionate environment with your choice of online or in person consultations. —*Simone Kelly*

I've suffered from IBS for most of my adult life, and Harmony has truly provided me with the knowledge and skills to help combat the symptoms. An Ayurvedic approach has been a true blessing. I cannot recommend Harmony more highly. —*Bianca*

I will use Harmony time and time again for the moments in my life when I need some clarity or guidance. Her ability to use her knowledge and wisdom in both Western and Eastern medicine, philosophy, and psychology to help with physical and emotional situations is a skill not many people have. *Highly* recommend, any day of the week! —*Anna Veale*

I came to study Ayurveda through my interest in alternative methods of healing. The Ayurveda Alchemist course with Harmony provided the tools to discover our unique body types and mindset (Prakriti), and with the framework provided by Harmony, I am now on my way to becoming a lifestyle and wellness coach, fully equipped with the skills to provide Ayurvedic coaching services for people ready to embark on a journey of self-discovery and health using Ayurvedic principles. If you are contemplating studies in holistic health, reach out to Harmony. You will not regret it! —*Wendy Augutis*

The Ayurveda Alchemist program will change your life! Harmony delivers the most amazing program, providing easy to digest, in-depth knowledge on all aspects of Ayurveda, inspiring guest speakers, and a life-changing cleanse. It is a fantastic program for beginners and people looking to continue their study. The business coaching has inspired me to open a yoga studio and now run Ayurveda cleanses confidently. Something I wouldn't be doing if I didn't complete the Ayurveda Alchemist. I couldn't recommend this program enough. Thank you, Harmony! —*Emma Windle*

It was coincidence (or perhaps divine intelligence) that caused me to sign up for Harmony's three month Thrive program. When I signed up for the program, I knew I wasn't firing on all burners. I have worked with natural healers in the past who decried medical intervention, and I ended up spending a fortune on herbal medications that gave me an allergic reaction. I have also worked with doctors whose specialized skills don't factor in metaphysical conditions so to say that I was a skeptic of the healing world at large is probably an understatement.

I was particularly drawn to Harmony's position at the intersection of East and West medicine and felt satisfied that with her connection to Ayurveda and her medical background things wouldn't get too woo-woo. What I didn't realize the day I signed up was that I had an extensive blood clot in my calf. The clot was discovered on the morning of my first meeting with Harmony—which I had to cancel.

Because everything is linked, a list of health issues simultaneously appeared the moment I started working with Harmony. It was almost as if my body was waiting for some attention before going into a complete meltdown. During the three-month Thrive program, I have been able to eliminate all the pain I was in without the use of medications whereas before, I had been on daily anti-inflammatories. The clot has reduced by 95 percent, and my body is in a much better place.

Harmony's medical background has been invaluable in helping me decode both my body and the medical messages I was receiving from doctors, who mean well but don't always appreciate that you don't speak their language. Her metaphysical knowledge has helped me interrogate the underlying issues that could lead to physical symptoms.

In short, Harmony is a great cheerleader whose medical background and metaphysical knowledge perfectly position her in the healing space. —*Keryn Clark*

My experience with Harmony in the three-month Thrive program was way beyond my expectations, but exactly what I was looking for. I had lived with PCOS for over ten years and spent a few years off the pill, trying to heal it naturally. Despite already living and eating quite healthily, I still was unhappy with my weight, wasn't ovulating, had acne, and really needed support. I wanted someone with experience to support me to make the changes I needed to thrive. I got that and so much more with Harmony. She treated me as an individual, not just someone with PCOS, and supported me on every level. Not only did we work on my diet and lifestyle and implement herbs, we did a limiting core belief session that changed my life and my relationship with food. This really helped me to shift the deeper reason I was struggling to lose weight. Although I was a little hesitant to make the financial investment for three months of 1:1 support, it was a commitment that was worth every penny, and the investment even helped me to stay committed and motivated toward my progress. By the end of our program, I lost 7 kilos, my skin is perfectly clear, and my bloods [periods] came back, showing I've ovulated and am in perfect hormone range. Combining my own dedication to my health with the expertise and support of a holistic practitioner was one of the best things I've ever done for myself. Thank you, Harmony. You have changed my life, and I'm forever grateful! —*Camille Sherer*

I've been seeing Harmony for more than a year, and she has helped me in so many different ways, not only with my ongoing digestive issues but also with mindset, motivation, and personal growth. With Harmony's support, my digestion improved, parasites were eliminated, and most *importantly*, my relationship with food enhanced a lot.

Every time I leave her consultation, I feel valued, understood, and motivated. Harmony promulgates wisdom in Eastern and Western medicine and patiently explains and elaborates so you actually understand where your symptoms are coming from and what to do to get better. I love that she gives you the tools to work on your own health and also prescribes and concocts natural medicine to your individual needs.

When you choose to work with Harmony, you'll get the whole package: a holistic health practitioner that goes above and beyond in order to support their clients on their journey to better health and well-being. Thank you for everything, Harmony! Highly recommend!! —*Jordis Wilsdorf*

I was referred to Harmony at Harmony Inspired Health by a work friend. I'm so glad and grateful I was! After several months of skin and digestive issues, Harmony was able, after one consultation, to pinpoint exactly what was going on, but more importantly, help me understand my health issues and guide me through fixing them. —*Vishakha*

Your Next Step:
Keep the Transformation Going

If this book has inspired or empowered you, don't let the journey stop here—let's create a ripple effect together.

+ **Share the wisdom**: Gift this book to the women in your life—friends, family, colleagues—who are ready to reclaim their health, mindset, and purpose.

+ **Leave a review**: Your words matter! A review on Amazon or Goodreads helps this book reach more women who need this knowledge.

+ **Spread the message**: Share your favorite insights or quotes on social media. Tag me @harmony.inspired.ayurveda so I can celebrate with you!

+ **Deepen Your Journey**—If you're ready to integrate these teachings on a deeper level, explore my courses, mentorships, and practitioner certifications at **www.harmonyinspiredhealth. com.au**

Your transformation is only the beginning. Now, let's inspire others to step into their higHERself™.

Author Contact Page

Email: **inspire@harmonyinspired.com.au**

Website: **https://www.harmonyinspiredhealth.com.au**

Instagram: **@harmony.inspired.ayurveda**

LinkedIn: **Dr Harmony Robinson-Stagg**

Podcast: Ayurveda, Women's Health & Holistic Success
by Harmony Inspired Health
https://www.harmonyinspiredhealth.com.au/podcasts/

YouTube: **Harmony Inspired Health**

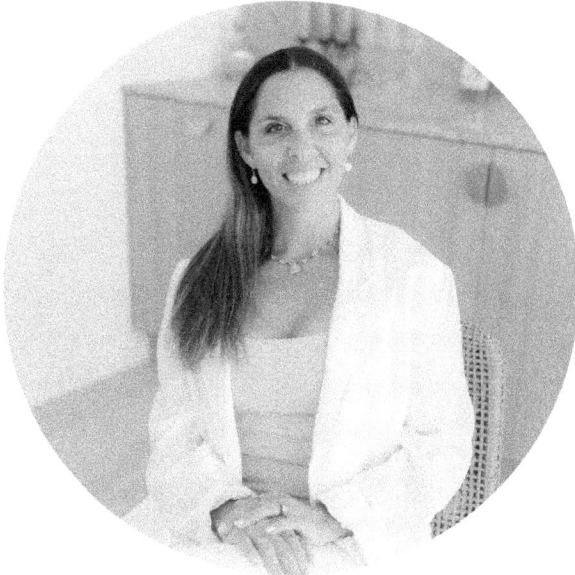

www.ingramcontent.com/pod-product-compliance
Lightning Source LLC
Chambersburg PA
CBHW051242020426

42333CB00025B/3018